Clinical Hepatology

Clinical Hepatology

Editor: Amy McMahon

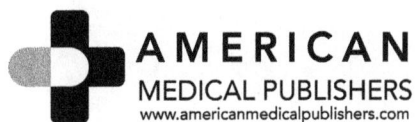

AMERICAN
MEDICAL PUBLISHERS
www.americanmedicalpublishers.com

AMERICAN
MEDICAL PUBLISHERS
www.americanmedicalpublishers.com

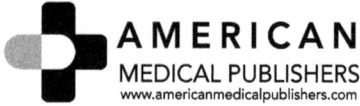

Cataloging-in-Publication Data

Clinical hepatology / edited by Amy McMahon.
    p. cm.
Includes bibliographical references and index.
ISBN 978-1-63927-187-0
1. Hepatology. 2.Gastroenterology--Treatment. 3. Liver--Diseases. I. McMahon, Amy.
RC801 .C55 2022
616.33--dc23

American Medical Publishers,
41 Flatbush Avenue,
1st Floor, New York,
NY 11217, USA

ISBN 978-1-63927-187-0 (Hardback)

Contents

Preface

The field of hepatology is concerned with the study of the liver, biliary tree, gallbladder and pancreas, and their clinical conditions. Some of the diseases affecting the hepatobiliary system include Aagenaes syndrome, Budd-Chiari syndrome, Crigler-Najjar syndrome, Mirizzi's syndrome, HELLP syndrome, Alagille syndrome, etc. The diseases arising due to alcohol consumption and viral hepatitis are the common conditions that are under the scope of this study. There has been a rise in cases of cirrhosis and related complications. Liver function tests detect enzymes in blood which normally are most abundant in liver tissue, such as serum albumin, serum globulin, aspartate transaminase, alanine transaminase, etc. An examination of these levels aids in the diagnosis of liver conditions. The objective of therapy in hepatology is to slow the progression of the disease. This is done with anti-viral medications, steroid-based drugs, medications such as ursodeoxycholic acid, etc. Liver transplantation is an effective treatment for acute or chronic liver conditions with the potential to cause severe and irreversible liver dysfunction. This book explores all the important aspects of clinical hepatology in the modern day. It strives to provide a fair idea about hepatological disorders and to help develop a better understanding of the latest advances in their clinical management. With state-of-the-art inputs by acclaimed experts of hepatology, this book targets students and professionals.

The researches compiled throughout the book are authentic and of high quality, combining several disciplines and from very diverse regions from around the world. Drawing on the contributions of many researchers from diverse countries, the book's objective is to provide the readers with the latest achievements in the area of research. This book will surely be a source of knowledge to all interested and researching the field.

In the end, I would like to express my deep sense of gratitude to all the authors for meeting the set deadlines in completing and submitting their research chapters. I would also like to thank the publisher for the support offered to us throughout the course of the book. Finally, I extend my sincere thanks to my family for being a constant source of inspiration and encouragement.

Editor

Retinoid and carotenoid status in serum and liver among patients at high-risk for liver cancer

Yachana Kataria[1]*, Ryan J. Deaton[2], Erika Enk[2], Ming Jin[2], Milita Petrauskaite[2], Linlin Dong[5], Joseph R. Goldenberg[2], Scott J. Cotler[3], Donald M. Jensen[4], Richard B. van Breemen[5] and Peter H. Gann[2]

Abstract

Background: Approximately 2.7 million Americans are chronically infected with hepatitis C virus (HCV). HCV patients with cirrhosis form the largest group of persons at high risk for hepatocellular carcinoma (HCC). Increased oxidative stress is regarded as a major mechanism of HCV-related liver disease progression. Deficiencies in retinoid and carotenoid antioxidants may represent a major modifiable risk factor for disease progression. This study aims to identify key predictors of serum antioxidant levels in patients with HCV, to examine the relationship between retinoid/carotenoid concentrations in serum and hepatic tissue, to quantify the association between systemic measures of oxidative stress and antioxidant status, and to examine the relationship between retinoids and stellate cell activation.

Methods: Patients undergoing liver biopsy ($n = 69$) provided fasting blood, fresh tissue, urine and completed a diet history questionnaire. Serum and questionnaire data from healthy volunteers ($n = 11$), normal liver tissue from public repositories and patients without liver disease ($n = 11$) were also collected. Urinary isoprostanes, serum and tissue retinoid concentrations were obtained by UHPLC-MS-MS. Immunohistochemistry for αSMA was performed on FFPE sections and subsequently quantified via digital image analysis. Associations between urinary isoprostanes, αSMA levels, and retinoids were assessed using Spearman correlation coefficients and non-parametric tests were utilized to test differences among disease severity groups.

Results: There was a significant inverse association between serum retinol, lycopene, and RBP4 concentrations with fibrosis stage. Serum β-carotene and lycopene were strongly associated with their respective tissue concentrations. There was a weak downward trend of tissue retinyl palmitate with increasing fibrosis stage. Tissue retinyl palmitate was inversely and significantly correlated with hepatic αSMA expression, a marker for hepatic stellate cell activation ($r = -0.31$, $P < 0.02$). Urinary isoprostanes levels were inversely correlated with serum retinol, β-carotene, and RBP4.

Conclusions: A decrease in serum retinol, β-carotene, and RBP4 is associated with early stage HCV. Retinoid and carotenoid levels decline as disease progresses, and our data suggest that this decline occurs early in the disease process, even before fibrosis is apparent. Measures of oxidative stress are associated with fibrosis stage and concurrent antioxidant depletion. Vitamin A loss is accompanied by stellate cell activation in hepatic tissue.

Keywords: Vitamin A, HCV, Diet, Biomarker

* Correspondence: yachana.kataria@childrens.harvard.edu
[1]Department of Laboratory Medicine, Boston Children's Hospital, Boston, MA, USA
Full list of author information is available at the end of the article

Background

The progression of hepatitis C virus (HCV) infection can lead to cirrhosis and in some cases hepatocellular carcinoma (HCC), which has limited treatment options and poor prognosis. Approximately 2.7 million Americans are chronically infected with HCV. HCV patients with cirrhosis form the largest group of persons at high risk for HCC [1–5]. Oxidative stress, resulting from chronic inflammation, is purported to be a major mechanism for hepatic fibrosis and cirrhosis [6]. An imbalance between production of reactive oxygen species and antioxidant defense induces a number of pathophysiological changes in the liver, including activation of hepatic stellate cells (HSCs), oxidative damage to lipids, nucleotides and proteins, and initiation of proliferative processes associated with regeneration. Vitamin A and its carotenoid precursors are an important part of the body's antioxidant defense, due to their ability to scavenge and directly neutralize free radicals in the tissue. In normal liver, quiescent HSCs are responsible for the storage of more than 90 % of the body's vitamin A reserves as retinyl esters. Upon chronic liver injury HSC undergo activation, lose their capacity to store vitamin A while acquiring contractile, proliferative and proinflammatory properties that are believed to play a major role in fibrogenesis [7]. Hepatic αSMA expression in the parenchyma is a marker of activated HSCs due to their myofibroblast phenotype. However, it is uncertain if retinoid loss is required for stellate cell activation and if retinoid loss accelerates activation.

In this context, deficiencies in dietary antioxidants, such as retinoids and carotenoids, could represent a major modifiable risk factor for chronic liver disease (CLD) progression. Two prospective epidemiological studies evaluating the relationship between serum retinoids and liver cancer among subjects with chronic hepatitis B found that higher pre-diagnostic serum retinol was strongly associated with a subsequent reduced risk of liver cancer [8, 9]. More recently, a large cohort study in Finland observed that higher baseline serum retinol and β-carotene were inversely associated, many years later, with the incidence of liver cancer and death from CLD [10]. Additionally, a randomized trial has reported compelling evidence that polyprenoic acid, a synthetic retinoid, reduced the incidence of second primary liver tumors and prolonged survival in HCC patients [11]. A small number of studies to date have found that these serum micronutrients are depleted in cirrhotic patients and only three studies to date have assessed hepatic antioxidant levels in small and generally heterogeneous populations of pre-cirrhotic individuals [12–19].

Despite vast improvements in HCV treatment in recent years, there are potential opportunities for therapeutic or preventive strategies involving antioxidant repletion, particularly in patients who have progressed to cirrhosis even if they achieve virologic cure [20–22]. These limitations highlight a crucial need to develop adjuvant strategies to prevent progression in high-risk individuals [23]. However, supplementation with vitamin A itself must be approached cautiously in individuals with liver disease, as hypervitaminosis A causes accelerated liver fibrosis and may also promote carcinogenesis [24]. Therefore, there is a need for more information on the spectrum and causes of retinoid and carotenoid depletion in the HCV-infected population, so that optimal strategies for clinical trials can be identified.

Among HCV-infected persons, antioxidant depletion could be explained by a combination of dietary, lifestyle, and physiological factors. Apart from processes directly linked to HCV infection, these factors include inadequate dietary antioxidant intake, smoking, alcohol intake or diabetes, all of which have been reported to diminish defense against oxidative stress. The present study aims to: a) determine the prevalence and predictors of retinoid and carotenoid depletion in a well-defined patient population, b) examine the relationships between retinoid and carotenoid concentrations in serum and hepatic tissue, c) quantify the association between systemic measures of oxidative stress and antioxidant status, and d) examine the relationship between antioxidant levels and stellate cell activation. We postulated that lower retinoid and carotenoid concentrations and higher levels of oxidative stress would be associated with fibrosis stage among HCV-infected patients.

Methods
Study population
We conducted a cross-sectional study among patients with HCV at the University of Illinois at Chicago (UIC) and University of Chicago (UC). A total of 91 subjects were included in this study; however not every subject fulfilled every component of the study. We consented and consecutively enrolled patients with confirmed HCV undergoing percutaneous or transvascular liver biopsy ($n = 69$) who provided fasting blood, fresh tissue, urine, and completed a diet history questionnaire. At the time of the biopsy, liver histology was staged into F0-4 according to the Batts-Ludwig scoring system. Subjects with F0 were categorized as having no fibrosis. Subjects with fibrosis stage 1–2 and fibrosis 3–4 were categorized as mild/moderate and severe fibrosis, respectively. The liver histology staging criteria was utilized to define fibrosis stage in our analysis.

All biopsies were performed with 16 or 18-gauge needles; an average of 7.7 mm^3 fresh tissue was taken from the end of each core and snap frozen for research purposes. We collected serum, urine, and questionnaire data from healthy volunteers ($n = 11$). We obtained post-mortem normal liver tissue from the Cooperative Human Tissue Network (CHTN) repository ($n = 8$); there was no corresponding serum, urine and questionnaire data for these individuals. The remaining controls included patients with no chronic liver disease ($n = 3$) who provided serum, tissue, urine, and questionnaire data. The UIC and UC Institutional Review Boards approved the study. An informed consent to participate in the study was obtained from participants.

Dietary assessment

The National Cancer Institute Diet History Questionnaire I (DHQ) was completed by all participants who provided serum. The DHQ was subsequently analyzed by the Diet*Calc Analysis Program (Version 1.4.3. National Cancer Institute, Applied Research Program). This program generated nutrient estimates based on frequency and portion sizes over the past year. Approximate retinoid and carotenoid intake was calculated from the DHQ. Pre-formed vitamin A is primarily found in animal sources such as eggs, dairy produce, fish, and meat. Carotenoids, which are found primarily in plant foods, include α-carotene, β-carotene, β-cryptoxanthin, lutein, and zeaxanthin; of those only α-carotene, and β-carotene are pro-vitamin A carotenoids; i.e., vitamin A precursors. To account for both pre-formed and pro-vitamin A dietary sources, the recommended dietary allowance for vitamin A is expressed in retinol activity equivalents (RAE).

Serological measurements

Serum analyses were performed by the clinical pathology laboratories at UIC. The serum chemistry panel included liver function tests aspartate aminotransferase (AST), alanine aminotransferase (ALT), international normalized ratio (INR), albumin, total bilirubin, total protein, BUN, hemoglobin, creatinine, and platelet count. Fasting serum insulin, glucose, and high sensitivity C-reactive protein, a marker of systemic inflammation (hs-CRP) were measured in single batches on SYNCHRON® Systems from Beckman Coulter (Pasadena, California). Based on blinded duplicates from a quality control pool of serum, intra-batch coefficients of variation (CV) aliquots for fasting serum insulin, glucose, and hs-CRP were 2.4, 0.65, and 0.98 %, respectively. Insulin resistance was measured using the homeostatic model assessment of insulin resistance (HOMA-IR). Predictive markers of fibrosis, aminotransferase to platelet ratio index (APRI) and Fibrosis 4 (FIB4) were calculated using published formulas [25, 26].

Serum retinoid/carotenoid assays

Singlicate measurements of retinoids and carotenoids in fasting serum samples were performed by using atmospheric pressure chemical ionization mass spectrometry as described previously, with the following changes [27]. Ultrahigh pressure liquid chromatography-tandem mass spectrometry (UHPLC-MS/MS) was carried out using a Shimadzu (Kyoto, Japan) LCMS-8040 triple quadrupole mass spectrometer equipped with a Shimadzu Shim-pack XR-ODSIII column (2.0 × 50 mm, 1.6 μm) at 35 °C. After holding at 5:95 (v/v) methyl-*tert*-butyl ether/methanol for 0.3 min, a 0.45-min linear gradient was used from 5 to 30 % methyl-*tert*-butyl ether at a flow rate of 0.6 mL/min. Carotenoids and retinoids were detected by MS/MS during the same analysis using polarity switching and the following selected reaction monitoring transitions: lycopene m/z 536 to 467 (-), $[^{13}C_{10}]$-lycopene (internal standard) m/z 546 to 477 (-), β-carotene m/z 536 to 536 (-), lutein m/z 551 to 135 (+), retinol and retinyl palmitate m/z 269 to 93 (+).

Based on blinded replicates from a quality control pool of serum, mean intra- and inter- batch CVs for retinol in serum samples were 9.3 and 13.9 %, respectively. Average intra- and inter- batch CV for all serum retinoids and carotenoids were 13.9 and 9.7 %, respectively.

The Relative Dose Response (RDR) test has been proposed as a better alternative for determining vitamin A deficiency compared to serum retinol. A retinol increase of greater than 20 % following a challenge dose of retinyl palmitate is considered a positive test indicating deficient liver reserves. Serum delta RDR values were calculated according to the following formula: $100 \times \frac{A_5 - A_0}{A_5}$. A_0 is the serum retinol concentration at baseline, and A_5 is the serum retinol concentration at 5 h post-retinol dose. Test participants provided serum for baseline retinol levels after an overnight fast, and then ingested 1000 RAE of retinyl palmitate dissolved in corn oil on a cracker. Serum retinol levels were measured again five hours later. Of the 24 subjects who completed the RDR, eleven had tissue available.

RBP4 measurement

Serum retinol binding protein 4 (RBP4) was measured in duplicate using an enzyme-linked immunosorbent assay (ELISA) (ALPCO Diagnostics, Salem, NH) according to the manufacturer's instructions. The kit utilized a polyclonal rabbit anti-RBP antibody.

Tissue retinoid/carotenoid assays

Hepatic tissue retinoid and carotenoid measurements were performed using UHPLC-MS/MS as described above, except that the tissue (0.5 to 5 mg) was homogenized in 200 μl water and extracted twice using 600 μl portions of ethanol/hexane (20:80; v/v) containing 0.1 % butylated hydroxytoluene. The same protocol was used for all of the hepatic tissue available. Based on adjacent samples from a random subject within each batch, mean intra-batch CV for hepatic tissue retinyl palmitate, β-carotene, and lycopene were 6.9, 10.0 and 4.1 %, respectively.

Urinary isoprostanes
Urine concentrations of 8-iso-PGF2α, a marker of lipid peroxidation were measured using a rapid UHPLC-MS/MS assay as described previously [28]. Based on anonymous replicates from a quality control pool of urine, mean intra- and inter-batch CV for the urinary isoprostanes measurements were 6.4 and 7.8 %, respectively.

Immunohistochemistry
Tissue sections of 4 μm each were placed on charged slides, dehydrated, and then deparaffinized. Immunostaining was carried out using a BondRX (Lecia Biosystems, Buffalo Grove, IL) autostainer with a mouse monoclonal antibody for αSMA (DAKO, Clone 1A4) in a 1:2000 dilution for 15 min at room temperature to identify HSC. The sections were then incubated in rabbit anti-mouse IgG (Bond Polymer Refine Detection, Leica Biosystems) for 20 min. No antigen retrieval was used for this stain. Color reaction was developed using diaminobenzidine (DAB) as the chromagen, followed by counterstaining with hematoxylin. Positive and negative controls were included in each batch.

Slides were scanned at 20× on an Aperio ScanScope® CS whole-slide digital microscope (Leica Biosystems). A digital draw tool was used to identify hepatic parenchymal areas. Large vessels, inflammation, and artifacts (e.g., folds, debris, etc.) were excluded from analysis. αSMA quantitation was restricted to the hepatic parenchymal region to exclude αSMA positive cells (i.e., portal fibroblasts and bone marrow derived collagen-producing cells) in the portal region [29]. Definiens Tissue Studio® 3.6.1 (Definiens, Munich, Germany), a digital image analysis platform, was used to measure the percent positivity of αSMA stain area within the hepatic parenchyma.

Statistical analysis
Frequency distributions of dietary intake, urinary isoprostanes, retinoid, and carotenoid concentrations were examined for normality. Scatterplots and Spearman rank correlation coefficients were used to examine relationships among the variables of interest. A P-value of < 0.05 was considered statistically significant, and all tests were two-sided. Analyses were performed using SAS Version 9.2 (SAS, Inc., Cary, NC).

Results
Table 1 shows selected demographics and clinical characteristics of the study participants at both institutions by fibrosis stage. Participants in the control group were more likely to be white, overweight, and non-smokers. There were no differences in ethnicity, BMI, smoking status, or diabetes among the disease groups. The no fibrosis group was more likely to be overweight or obese compared to the mild/moderate fibrosis group (94 % vs 59 %). A majority of the HCV-positive subjects had either genotype 1a (52 %) or 1b (38 %) as reported by medical records. The median AST, APRI, and FIB-4 levels in disease subjects were positively associated with the fibrosis stage (Additional file 1: Table S1). However, hs-CRP concentrations were inversely and significantly associated with fibrosis stage ($P < 0.05$) (Additional file 1: Table S1).

Dietary intake of individual retinoids and carotenoids did not differ between controls and HCV subjects. There was evidence of a downward trend for total vitamin A intake (expressed as retinol activity equivalents, RAE) with increasing fibrosis stage, however this trend was weak and not readily distinguishable from chance, as shown in Fig. 1. Total vitamin A, or individual retinoid and carotenoid intake also did not differ by fibrosis stage or predictive markers of fibrosis (APRI and FIB-4). Mean total vitamin A intake was 1182 and 1295 mcg RAE for men and women, respectively; values well above the general population based on data from NHANES III (682 and 606 mcg RAE, for men and women, respectively). Total vitamin A or individual retinoid and carotenoid intake levels were not associated with BMI, smoking status, alcohol consumption, or insulin resistance.

Dietary β-carotene and lutein intake were positively and significantly correlated with their respective serum concentrations (β-carotene: $r = 0.24$, $P = 0.05$; lutein: $r = 0.33$, $P < 0.01$). However, total vitamin A intake did not correlate with serum retinol concentrations ($r = 0.07$, $P = 0.53$). Similarly, no relationships between intake and serum were observed for other dietary carotenoids. Tissue retinoid and carotenoid levels were not associated with dietary intake (data not shown). Figure 2 shows that serum retinol and hepatic retinyl palmitate concentrations, the respective dominant forms of vitamin A in serum and liver, were not correlated ($r < 0.01$, $P = 0.99$). However, serum and tissue concentrations of β-carotene ($r = 0.56$, $P < 0.01$) and lycopene ($r = 0.77$, $P < 0.01$) were moderately correlated in this study population.

Serum retinol and RBP4 concentrations were significantly lower in HCV subjects compared to controls, although no HCV subjects met the standard serum criteria for vitamin A deficiency (<200 ng/mL). Figure 3 shows a significant downward trend of serum retinol and RBP4 concentrations with increasing hepatic fibrosis. Similar relationships were also observed for serum β-carotene, lycopene, and lutein concentrations (Fig. 4). No relationships were observed for serum retinoids and carotenoids with either APRI or FIB-4 scores (data not shown). However,

Table 1 Selected characteristics of the study population by fibrosis stage

Characteristics	Control	No fibrosis	Mild/Moderate fibrosis	Severe fibrosis	Total	P-value*	P-value**
	n = 22	n = 18	n = 34	n = 17	n = 91		
Age - Median (IQR)	45 (42–54)	55 (51–62)	53 (48–58)	56 (53–57)	53 (46–58)	0.17	0.17
Gender							
Male	12	6	18	10	46	0.42	0.27
Female	10	12	16	7	45		
Ethnicity							
Asian	0	0	1	0	1	**<0.01**	0.68
Black	2	12	17	7	38		
White	18	6	15	9	48		
Unknown	2	0	1	1	4		
BMI							
< 25	0	1	13	4	18	**0.02**	0.11
25–30	5	9	12	7	33		
> 30	9	8	8	6	31		
Unknown	8	0	1	1	10		
Smoking Status							
Never	17	7	10	7	41	**0.02**	0.60
Former	2	7	11	7	27		
Current	3	4	13	3	23		
Diabetes							
Yes	3	2	3	4	12	0.56	0.33
No	19	16	31	13	79		
HCV Genotype							
1	–	11	29	13	53	0.15	0.15
2	–	1	0	0	1		
3	–	0	0	1	1		
Unknown	–	6	5	3	14		

*P-values are Fisher exact (2-tailed) for comparison of proportions and Kruskal-Wallis test for comparison of medians amongst all groups
**P-values are Fisher exact (2-tailed) for comparison of proportions and Kruskal-Wallis test for comparison of medians amongst diseased groups
Bold face represents statistically significant values

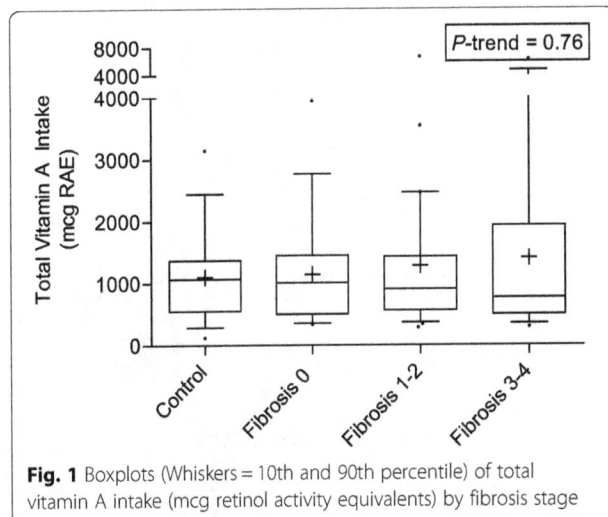

Fig. 1 Boxplots (Whiskers = 10th and 90th percentile) of total vitamin A intake (mcg retinol activity equivalents) by fibrosis stage

RBP4 levels were inversely and significantly correlated with AST and ALT levels ($r = -0.34$, $P < 0.01$; $r = -0.28$, $P = 0.015$, respectively). Individual retinoid and carotenoid concentrations did not vary according to sex, BMI, smoking status, alcohol consumption, or insulin resistance. Of the 24 HCV participants who completed the RDR test, two of them had RDR values >20 %, suggestive of a vitamin A deficiency. There was no apparent relationship between delta RDR retinol concentrations and retinyl palmitate concentrations in hepatic tissue (Spearman $r = -0.03$, $P = 0.92$) or fibrosis stage (data not shown).

Hepatic retinyl palmitate levels were lower in control tissue samples, which were mostly obtained post-mortem, compared to diseased subjects (Wilcoxon $P = 0.04$). In contrast, hepatic lycopene and β-carotene concentrations were higher in controls compared to diseased subjects

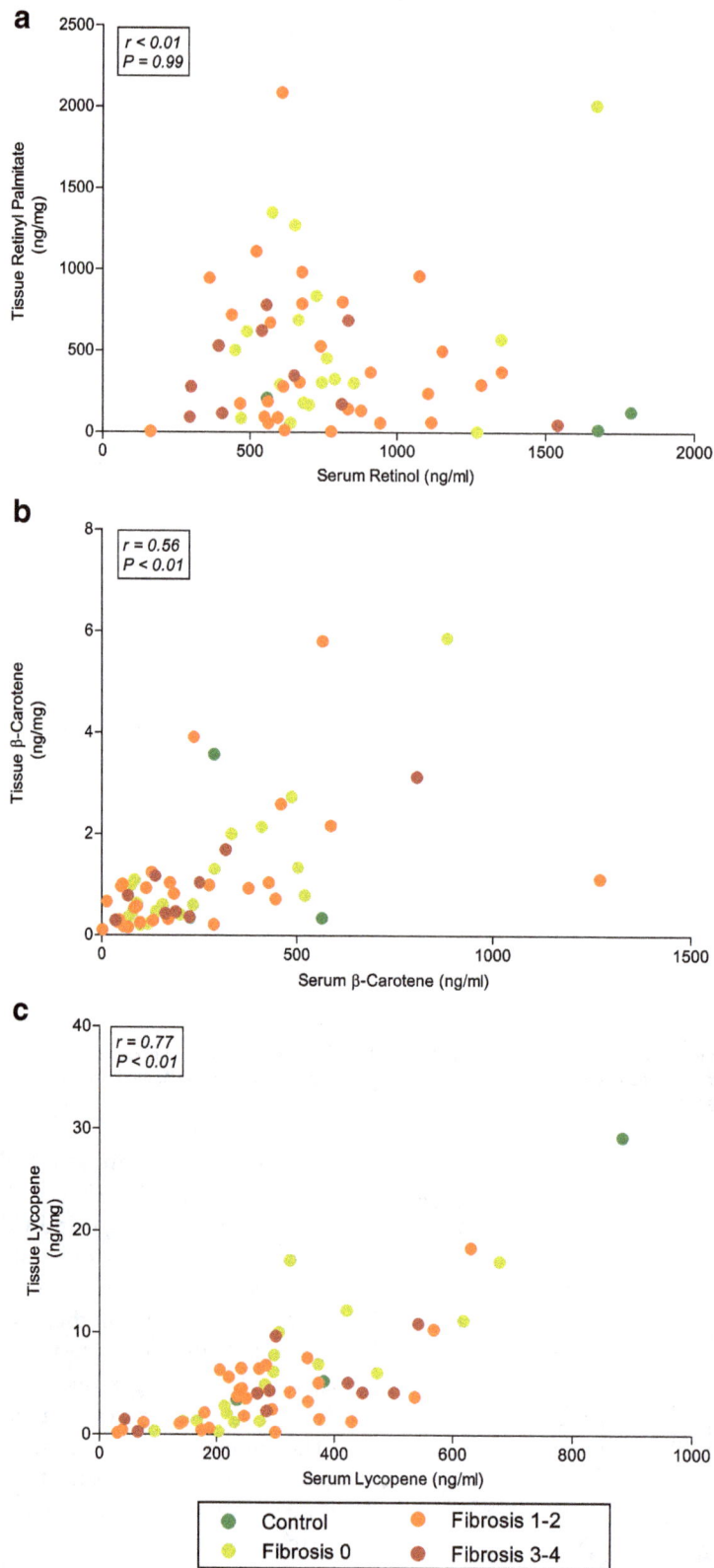

Fig. 2 Scatterplots showing correlations (Spearman r) between **a** Serum retinol and tissue retinyl palmitate (*n* = 60), **b** Serum and tissue β-carotene (*n* = 58), and **c** Serum and tissue lycopene (*n* = 60)

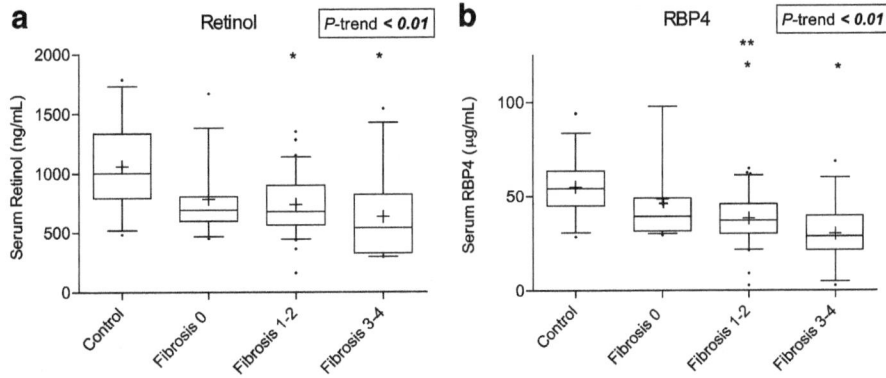

Fig. 3 Boxplots (Whiskers = 10th and 90th percentile) for serum concentrations of **a** retinol and **b** RBP4 by fibrosis stage. *$P < 0.05$ compared to Control **$P < 0.05$ compared to Fibrosis 0 group

(Wilcoxon $P = 0.07$, $P = 0.34$, respectively). There was a weak inverse relationship between hepatic retinyl palmitate concentration and fibrosis stage among all subjects ($P = 0.36$) (Fig. 5). Furthermore, hepatic β-carotene and lycopene concentrations showed a weak downward trend with increasing fibrosis stage. Hepatic retinyl palmitate was positively and significantly correlated with APRI, FIB-4, ALT, and AST ($r = 0.27$, $P = 0.03$; $r = 0.29$ $P = 0.02$; $r = 0.30$, $P = 0.015$; and $r = 0.24$, $P = 0.05$, respectively). These relationships were not observed for tissue carotenoids.

Parenchymal αSMA expression in hepatic tissue appeared to increase only among subjects with fibrosis 3–4 (Additional file 2: Figure S1) (Wilcoxon $P = 0.12$). αSMA expression was not associated with serum retinol concentrations ($r = -0.03$, $P = 0.79$). However, αSMA expression was inversely and significantly correlated with tissue retinyl palmitate concentrations ($r = -0.31$, $P = 0.013$) (Fig. 6). This relationship was not observed for any other tissue carotenoids (data not shown). In particular, hepatic lycopene levels were not correlated with αSMA expression ($r = -0.03$, $P = 0.81$).

Urinary isoprostane levels were positively and significantly associated with fibrosis stage (Additional file 3: Figure S2). Serum retinol, β-carotene, and RBP4 concentrations were all inversely and significantly associated with urinary isoprostane concentrations. Tissue retinoid concentrations were not correlated with urinary isoprostane levels (Table 2). However, both serum and hepatic lycopene were suggestively correlated ($r = -0.18$, $P = 0.12$; $r = -0.22$, $P = 0.09$, respectively).

Discussion

Our results confirm that depletion of vitamin A, lycopene, and β-carotene is widespread among patients with chronic HCV infection. This phenomenon seems to occur early in the disease process, even before fibrosis is apparent, and cannot be explained, based on our results,

by diet, obesity, alcohol intake, smoking, or insulin resistance. Inverse associations with fibrosis progression were more apparent for serum as opposed to hepatic levels of retinoids and carotenoids, and were especially clear for serum retinol and RBP4. While we found relatively strong correlations between serum and liver tissue for lycopene and β-carotene, hepatic retinyl palmitate was poorly correlated with serum retinol, suggesting differential factors modulating these levels [17, 18]. It is also possible that declines in serum retinoids appear earlier in the disease process than declines in hepatic stores. We further observed that depletion of serum antioxidants is linked to increasing levels of urinary isoprostanes, which are reflective of systemic oxidative stress due to lipid peroxidation. An important finding was that hepatic retinyl palmitate levels were significantly and inversely associated with stellate cell activation, as measured by αSMA expression in liver biopsy specimens. Taken together, results from this cross-sectional analysis support the hypotheses that depletion of retinoid and carotenoid antioxidants occurs early in the disease process and that this depletion parallels an increase in oxidative stress and evidence of hepatic stellate cell activation.

In the present study, the reduced serum retinol levels associated with CLD progression were well above the widely accepted WHO cut-off point of 200 ng/mL for vitamin A deficiency. Moreover, only two of the HCV participants had a positive RDR test, indicating inadequate liver vitamin A reserve. Serum retinol and β-carotene levels in our HCV participants were also generally comparable to the NHANES III participants, a nationally representative sample of the US population [30]. Reduced dietary intake of retinoids and carotenoids do not appear to be responsible for the observed associations with fibrosis stage, which could be the result of diminished storage capacity, increased metabolism or defective mobilization

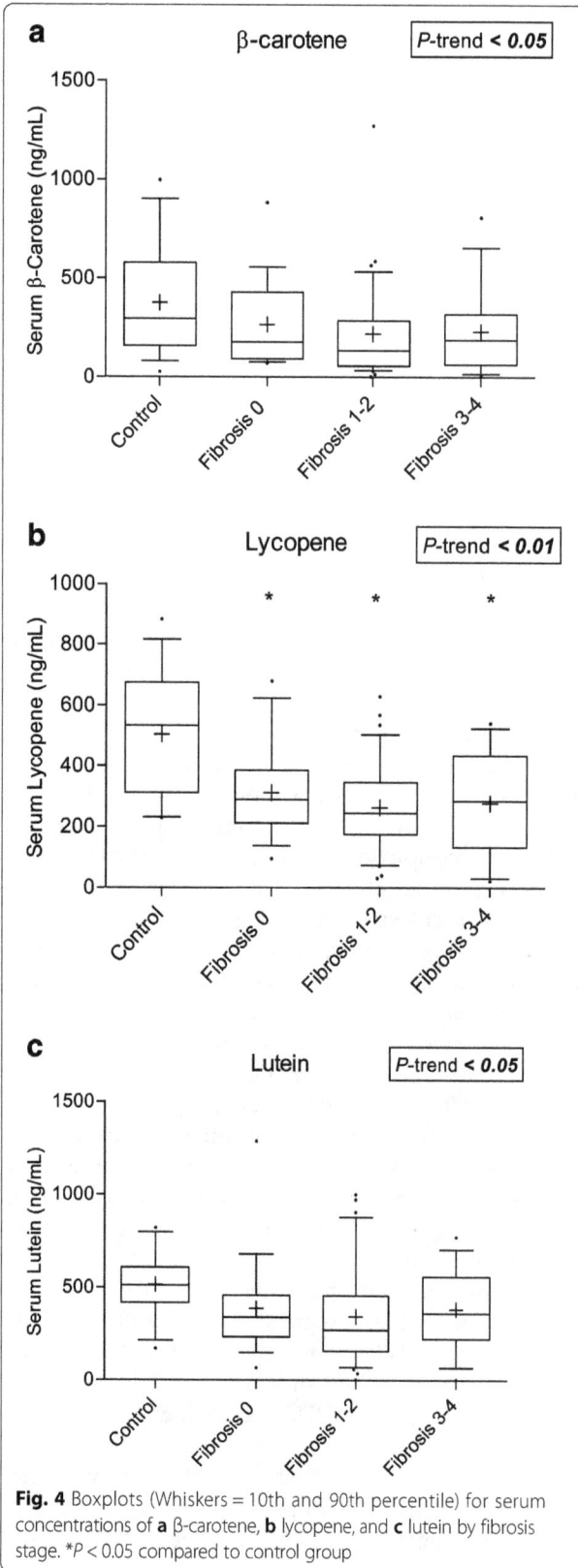

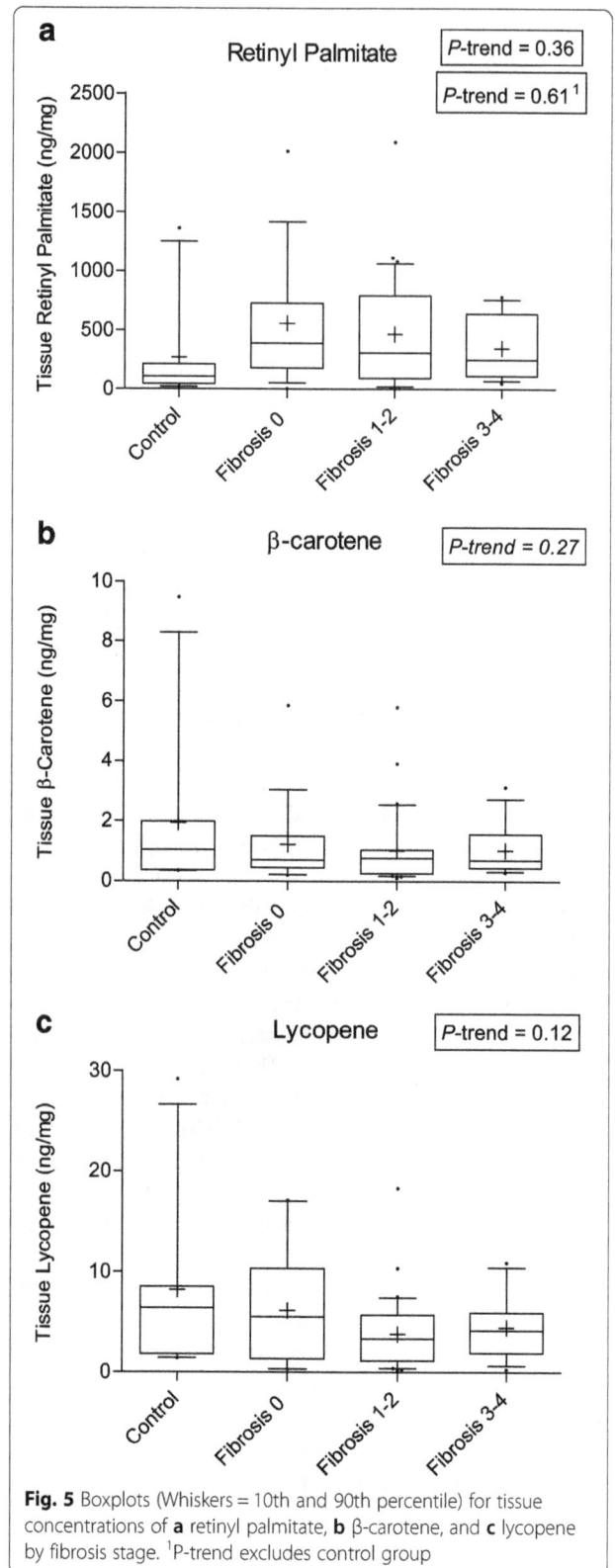

Fig. 4 Boxplots (Whiskers = 10th and 90th percentile) for serum concentrations of **a** β-carotene, **b** lycopene, and **c** lutein by fibrosis stage. *$P < 0.05$ compared to control group

Fig. 5 Boxplots (Whiskers = 10th and 90th percentile) for tissue concentrations of **a** retinyl palmitate, **b** β-carotene, and **c** lycopene by fibrosis stage. [1]P-trend excludes control group

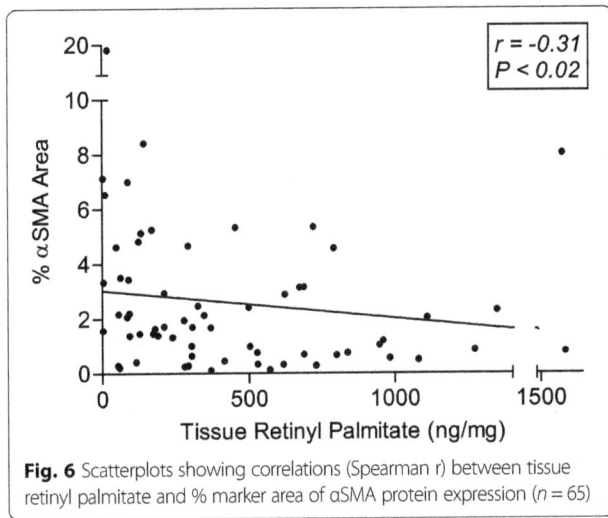

Fig. 6 Scatterplots showing correlations (Spearman r) between tissue retinyl palmitate and % marker area of αSMA protein expression ($n = 65$)

of retinol due to impaired RBP4 synthesis [15, 31, 32]. In any event, a cross-sectional study such as this is unable to determine if antioxidant depletion is a causal factor in fibrosis progression, or simply an epiphenomenon that accompanies progression.

The current study supports prior evidence that serum RBP4 concentrations are inversely related to disease severity in HCV patients [33, 34]. We observed a high correlation between serum RBP4 and retinol ($r = 0.78$, $P < 0.001$). Serum RBP4 measured by an enzyme immunoassay might be a feasible and cost-effective alternative for assessing vitamin A status. No association was detected between RBP4 levels and albumin, suggesting that generally decreased hepatic protein synthesis did not contribute to the reduction in RBP4. However, impaired mobilization of hepatic stores could explain the decrease of RBP4 seen in CLD. Increased serum RBP4 has been reported to

contribute to insulin resistance associated with type 2 diabetes and obesity, which are possible risk factors for CLD progression [35]. We observed no correlation between RBP4 concentrations and BMI, glucose, or insulin levels. The possible effects of reduced RBP4 levels on insulin resistance among CLD patients might warrant further study.

A small number of studies have evaluated serum and tissue concentrations of dietary antioxidants in patients with CLD; although these have focused on more severe, later stage disease. The lack of correlation between serum retinol and tissue retinyl palmitate could be explained by impaired release of retinol from damaged hepatocytes or by the presence of homeostatic mechanisms that maintain hepatic retinol until vitamin A stores are severely depleted. We did not observe a definite decline in hepatic retinyl palmitate concentrations with increasing disease severity in earlier stages of CLD. Yadav et al. reported lower levels of retinyl esters in 20 HCV patients compared to controls [17]. In our study, however, the lower concentration in controls could have been caused by the degradation of retinyl palmitate into retinol in the cadaver tissue by endogenous esterase. Indeed, we observed higher levels of hepatic retinol in the control subjects (data not shown). It has been reported that patatin-like phospholipase domain-containing protein 3 (PNPLA3) regulates retinyl ester release. Specifically, carriers of the I148M mutation in PNPLA3 have intracellular hepatic retention of retinyl palmitate [36]. Subsequently, Mondul et al. found in NAFLD patients that carriers of the PNPLA3 I148M mutation have lower circulating levels of retinyl palmitate and RBP4 but not β-carotene concentrations [37]. PNPLA3 is also a strong determinant for HCC [38]. Taken together, it is possible that the intracellular retention of vitamin A is contributing to fibrosis progression and HCC. The observed reduction in serum Vitamin A levels may reflect a pseudo-deficiency. Future studies investigating the PNPLA3 genotype in this population may provide further insight. The reason for the positive relationship between hepatic retinyl palmitate and liver enzymes is unclear, but this relationship would also be consistent with mechanisms that favor retention of vitamin A in the presence of early but ongoing liver damage.

Lycopene cannot be converted to vitamin A and thus it presents an attractive potential alternative for antioxidant supplementation in CLD. Adverse effects have not been reported with consuming lycopene supplements or high amounts of lycopene-rich foods [39, 40]. We observed an inverse relationship of serum lycopene levels with fibrosis stage. Moreover, unlike vitamin A, there was also a strong correlation between serum and hepatic lycopene levels, thus indicating that dietary supplementation could result in higher hepatic lycopene concentrations. Yuan, et al. demonstrated an inverse association

Table 2 Spearman correlations between urinary isoprostanes, serum and tissue retinoids/carotenoids

Serum Retinoids/Carotenoids (ng/mL) ($n = 77$)	Urinary isoprostanes (ng/mg creatinine)	
	r	P-value
Retinol	**−0.23**	**0.05**
Lycopene	−0.18	0.12
β-Carotene	**−0.22**	**0.05**
Lutein	−0.12	0.31
RBP4 (ug/L)	**−0.25**	**0.03**
Tissue Retinoids/Carotenoids (ng/mg) ($n = 60$)		
Retinol	−0.05	0.72
Lycopene	−0.22	0.09
β-Carotene	−0.08	0.53
Retinyl Palmitate	−0.03	0.79

Bold face represents statistically significant values

between lycopene concentration in baseline serum and risk of developing HCC in China. Lycopene is a potent carotenoid antioxidant that is also thought to affect processes related to mutagenesis, carcinogenesis, cell differentiation, and proliferation [41, 42]. Epidemiological data suggest that lycopene may act as a chemopreventive agent for many cancer types such as prostate, breast, and lung [43]. In vitro studies have observed that lycopene can inhibit mouse and human hepatocytes by inducing cell cycle arrest [44, 45]. However, dietary lycopene did not prevent liver cancer in an in vivo model of spontaneous hepatocarcinogenesis [46]. These discrepant results warrant further investigation.

Serum hs-CRP is synthesized by hepatocytes in response to inflammation and is regulated by pro-inflammatory cytokines such as IL-6. In a recent cohort analysis in China, higher serum CRP levels at baseline were associated with liver cancer incidence and death from CLD [47]. As such, we hypothesized that higher levels of hs-CRP would occur with increasing fibrosis stage. However, in this study, hs-CRP concentrations decreased with increasing fibrosis stage. While these findings are counterintuitive, a few smaller studies have suggested similar results [48–50]. Nasciemento, et al. observed lower hs-CRP to IL-6 ratio compared to controls, suggesting that IL-6 stimulation of CRP production in the liver might be mitigated by HCV [48]. It appears that CRP production is affected early during the natural history of HCV infection, thus negating its utility as a biomarker of inflammation in this population.

F_2-isoprostanes are a sensitive and validated urinary marker of systemic oxidative stress due to lipid peroxidation. In our study, smokers had higher isoprostane levels compared to non-smokers. Our data indicate a positive association between urinary isoprostane concentrations and fibrosis stage. To our knowledge, this extends beyond previous data that have shown patients with CLD and cirrhosis have increased isoprostane levels compared to controls [16]. As hypothesized, we observed a significant inverse association of F_2-isoprostanes with serum retinol, β-carotene, and RBP4 levels. However, tissue retinoid and carotenoid levels were not associated with urinary isoprostane levels with the possible exception of lycopene. Urinary isoprostanes are a measure of total body lipid peroxidation, and therefore do not reliably reflect oxidative stress in the target organ.

As we expected, subjects with moderate to severe fibrosis had higher levels of αSMA expression in hepatic tissue compared to subjects with mild fibrosis or none at all. Thus, it appears that HSC activation might not be apparent, at least by immunohistochemical technique, until substantial fibrosis is present. Our data indicate that vitamin A depletion could occur prior to development of significant fibrosis and evidence of HSC activation. The hepatic

vitamin A depletion might be attributable to either loss of storage capacity or increased consumption via autophagy. Increased metabolism of vitamin A droplets through autophagic mechanism generates substrates needed for energy intensive pathways to meet the metabolic demands of proliferation, fibrogenesis, and contractility [51].

This is the first comprehensive analysis to examine the interrelationships among dietary, serum, and hepatic levels of retinoids and carotenoids with early progression of disease in HCV patients. The present study, to our knowledge, is the largest to date to quantitate hepatic retinoids and carotenoids. In addition, the study benefitted from quantitative image analysis that provided objective and reproducible measures of αSMA expression in liver biopsy specimens. However, certain limitations are acknowledged including, a limited sample size for specific subgroups and a cross sectional design that cannot be used to infer causal direction. Unfortunately, we were unable to administer the RDR to more patients due to the additional blood sample required five hours after the initial retinyl ester dose. Additionally, the postmortem tissue samples of normal liver were not ideal as they could have undergone artifactual changes in retinoid and carotenoid concentrations.

Findings from this study could be applicable to the emerging epidemic of obesity-related non-alcoholic fatty liver disease (NAFLD) and non-alcoholic steatohepatitis (NASH) [52]. Oxidative stress is believed to play a key role in these disease processes, similar to HCV-related liver disease. Currently, there are no specific therapies for NAFLD beyond dietary modifications and exercise. Lower levels of retinoids have been implicated in NAFLD. Transgenic mice with impaired retinoid signaling develop steatohepatits and eventually HCC [23]. It has also been found that NAFLD patients have higher levels of oxidative stress and lower vitamin A intake, independent of metabolic syndrome status, suggesting that adequate vitamin A intake is important in protecting against oxidative stress in NAFLD patients [53].

Conclusions

In conclusion, a decrease in serum retinol, β-carotene, and RBP4 is associated with early stage HCV. Retinoid and carotenoid levels decline as disease progresses, and our data suggest that this decline occurs early in the disease process, even before fibrosis is apparent. Measures of oxidative stress are associated with fibrosis stage and concurrent antioxidant depletion. Vitamin A loss is accompanied by stellate cell activation in hepatic tissue. Our data highlight the potential importance of dietary retinoids and carotenoids as determinants of progression in early chronic liver disease and support the need for mechanistic studies leading to well-designed intervention studies.

Abbreviations
ALT: alanine aminotransferase; APRI: aminotransferase to platelet ratio index; AST: aspartate aminotransferase; CLD: chronic liver disease; FFPE: fresh frozen paraffin embedded; FIB-4: fibrosis-4; HCC: hepatocellular carcinoma; HCV: hepatitis C; hs-CRP: high sensitivity C-reactive protein; HSCs: hepatic stellate cells; NAFLD: non-alcoholic fatty liver disease; NASH: non-alcoholic steatohepatitis; RAE: retinol activity equivalents; RBP4: retinol binding protein 4; UHPLC-MS/MS: ultrahigh pressure liquid chromatography-tandem mass spectrometry; αSMA: α-smooth muscle actin.

Competing interests
The authors declare that they have no competing interests.

Authors' contributions
YK conducted the data analysis and wrote the manuscript. RD contributed with acquisition, analysis, and interpretation of data. Additionally, he critically revised the manuscript for intellectual content. EE participated in design, coordination, and acquisition of data as the sole study coordinator. MJ acquired all of the clinical serum data. MP conducted the digital image analysis. LD completed the serum and tissue retinoid concentrations. JG carried out the RBP4 ELISA assay. SC participated in the design, coordination, and recruitment of the study at UIC as the study hepatologist. SC also made substantial contributions in the interpretation of the data. DJ participated in the design, coordination, and recruitment of the study at UC as the study hepatologist. RB contributed to serum tissue retinoid and carotenoid measurements and assisted in drafting the manuscript. PG conceived the study, participated in its design and coordination and aided in preparation of the manuscript. All authors read and approved the final manuscript.

Acknowledgements
The authors would like to acknowledge Peter Nguyen, Shunyan Mo, Smruti Mohanty, Audrey Silver, Cynthia Bogue, Monique Williams, Soyoun Ahn, Scot Aita, Jamie Berkes, Natasha Walzer and other clinical staff at both participating institutions. This has been supported by R21CA131787 from the National Cancer Institute of the National Institutes of Health.

Author details
[1]Department of Laboratory Medicine, Boston Children's Hospital, Boston, MA, USA. [2]Department of Pathology, University of Illinois at Chicago, Chicago, IL, USA. [3]Department of Hepatology, Loyola University, Chicago, IL, USA. [4]Center for Liver Diseases, University of Chicago, Chicago, IL, USA. [5]Department of Medicinal Chemistry & Pharmacognosy, University of Illinois at Chicago, Chicago, IL, USA.

References
1. Centers for Disease Control and Prevention (CDC). Vital signs: evaluation of hepatitis C virus infection testing and reporting - eight U.S. sites, 2005-2011. MMWR Morb Mortal Wkly Rep. 2013;62(18):357–61.
2. Cardin R, Saccoccio G, Masutti F, Bellentani S, Farinati F, Tiribelli C. DNA oxidative damage in leukocytes correlates with the severity of HCV-related liver disease: validation in an open population study. J Hepatol. 2001;34(4):587–92.
3. Cardin R, D'errico A, Fiorentino M, Cecchetto A, Naccarato R, Farinati F. Hepatocyte proliferation and apoptosis in relation to oxidative damage in alcohol-related liver disease. Alcohol Alcohol. 2002;37(1):43–8.
4. Levent G, Ali A, Ahmet A, Polat EC, Aytac C, Ayse E, et al. Oxidative stress and antioxidant defense in patients with chronic hepatitis C patients before and after pegylated interferon alfa-2b plus ribavirin therapy. J Transl Med. 2006;4:25.
5. Fujita N, Horiike S, Sugimoto R, Tanaka H, Iwasa M, Kobayashi Y, et al. Hepatic oxidative DNA damage correlates with iron overload in chronic hepatitis C patients. Free Radic Biol Med. 2007;42(3):353–62.
6. Ha HL, Shin HJ, Feitelson MA, Yu DY. Oxidative stress and antioxidants in hepatic pathogenesis. World J Gastroenterol. 2010;16(48):6035–43.
7. Friedman SL. Hepatic stellate cells: protean, multifunctional, and enigmatic cells of the liver. Physiol Rev. 2008;88(1):125–72.
8. Yuan JM, Gao YT, Ong CN, Ross RK, Yu MC. Prediagnostic level of serum retinol in relation to reduced risk of hepatocellular carcinoma. J Natl Cancer Inst. 2006;98(7):482–90.
9. Yu MW, Hsieh HH, Pan WH, Yang CS, CHen CJ. Vegetable consumption, serum retinol level, and risk of hepatocellular carcinoma. Cancer Res. 1995;55(6):1301–5.
10. Lai GY, Weinstein SJ, Albanes D, Taylor PR, Virtamo J, McGlynn KA, et al. Association of serum [alpha]-tocopherol, [beta]-carotene, and retinol with liver cancer incidence and chronic liver disease mortality. Br J Cancer. 2014;111(11):2163–71.
11. Muto Y, Moriwaki H, Saito A. Prevention of second primary tumors by an acyclic retinoid in patients with hepatocellular carcinoma. N Engl J Med. 1999;340(13):1046–7.
12. Jinno K, Okada Y, Tanimizu M, Hyodo I, Kurimoto H, Sunahara S, et al. Decreased serum levels of Beta-carotene in patients with hepatocellular-carcinoma. Int Hepatol Commun. 1994;2(1):43–6.
13. Clemente C, Elba S, Buongiorno G, Berloco P, Guerra V, Di Leo A. Serum retinol and risk of hepatocellular carcinoma in patients with child-Pugh class A cirrhosis. Cancer Lett. 2002;178(2):123–9.
14. Peres WAF, Chaves GV, Goncalves JCS, Ramalho A, Coelho HSM. Vitamin A deficiency in patients with hepatitis C virus-related chronic liver disease. Br J Nutr. 2011;106(11):1724–31.
15. Newsome PN, Beldon I, Moussa Y, Delahooke TE, Poulopoulos G, Hayes PC, et al. Low serum retinol levels are associated with hepatocellular carcinoma in patients with chronic liver disease. Aliment Pharmacol Ther. 2000;14(10):1295–301.
16. Jain SK, Pemberton PW, Smith A, McMahon RFT, Burrows PC, Aboutwerat A, et al. Oxidative stress in chronic hepatitis C: not just a feature of late stage disease. J Hepatol. 2002;36(6):805–11.
17. Yadav D, Hertan HI, Schweitzer P, Norkus EP, Pitchumoni CS. Serum and liver micronutrient antioxidants and serum oxidative stress in patients with chronic hepatitis C. Am J Gastroenterol. 2002;97(10):2634–9.
18. Ukleja A, Scolapio JS, McConnell JP, Spivey JR, Dickson RC, Nguyen JH, et al. Nutritional assessment of serum and hepatic vitamin A levels in patients with cirrhosis. Gastroenterology. 2001;120(5):A266-A.
19. Rocchi E, Casalgrandi G, Ronzoni A, Rosa MC, Cioni G, Marazzi A, et al. Antioxidant liposoluble vitamins and carotenoids in chronic hepatitis. Eur J Intern Med. 2001;12(2):116–21.
20. Pearlman BL. Protease inhibitors for the treatment of chronic hepatitis C genotype-1 infection: the new standard of care. Lancet Infect Dis. 2012;12(9):717–28.
21. Scheel TKH, Rice CM. Understanding the hepatitis C virus life cycle paves the way for highly effective therapies. Nat Med. 2013;19(7):837–49.
22. Bruno S, Stroffolini T, Colombo M, Bollani S, Benvegnu L, Mazzella G, et al. Sustained virological response to interferon-alpha is associated with improved outcome in HCV-related cirrhosis: a retrospective study. Hepatology. 2007;45(3):579–87.
23. Yanagitani A, Yamada S, Yasui S, Shimomura T, Murai R, Murawaki Y, et al. Retinoic acid receptor alpha dominant negative form causes steatohepatitis and liver tumors in transgenic mice. Hepatology. 2004;40(2):366–75.
24. Nollevaux MC, Guiot Y, Horsmans Y, Leclercq I, Rahier J, Geubel AP, et al. Hypervitaminosis A-induced liver fibrosis: stellate cell activation and daily dose consumption. Liver Int. 2006;26(2):182–6.
25. Lok AS, Everhart JE, Wright EC, Di Bisceglie AM, Kim HY, Sterling RK, et al. Maintenance peginterferon therapy and other factors associated with hepatocellular carcinoma in patients with advanced hepatitis C. Gastroenterology. 2011;140(3):840–U230.
26. Sterling RK, Lissen E, Clumeck N, Sola R, Correa MC, Montaner J, et al. Development of a simple noninvasive index to predict significant fibrosis in patients with HIV/HCV coinfection. Hepatology. 2006;43(6):1317–25.
27. Zhu D, Wang Y, Pang Y, Liu A, Guo J, Bouwman CA, et al. Quantitative analyses of beta-carotene and retinol in serum and feces in support of

clinical bioavailability studies. Rapid Commun Mass Spectrom. 2006;20(16):2427–32.

28. Yu R, Zhao G, Christman JW, Xiao L, Van Breemen RB. Method development and validation for ultra-high pressure liquid chromatography/tandem mass spectrometry determination of multiple prostanoids in biological samples. J AOAC Int. 2013;96(1):67–76.

29. Knittel T, Kobold D, Piscaglia F, Saile B, Neubauer K, Mehde M, et al. Localization of liver myofibroblasts and hepatic stellate cells in normal and diseased rat livers: distinct roles of (myo-)fibroblast subpopulations in hepatic tissue repair. Histochem Cell Biol. 1999;112(5):387–401.

30. Goyal A, Terry MB, Siegel AB. Serum antioxidant nutrients, vitamin A, and mortality in U.S. adults. Cancer Epidemiol Biomark Prev. 2013;22(12):2202–11.

31. Ross AC, Zolfaghari R. Regulation of hepatic retinol metabolism: perspectives from studies on vitamin A status. J Nutr. 2004;134(1):269S–75.

32. Peres WAF, Chaves GV, Goncalves JCS, Ramalho A, Coelho HSM. Assessment of the relative dose-response test as indicators of hepatic vitamin A stores in various stages of chronic liver disease. Nutr Clin Pract. 2013;28(1):95–100.

33. Huang JF, Dai CY, Yu ML, Shin SJ, Hsieh MY, Huang CF, et al. Serum retinol-binding protein 4 is inversely correlated with disease severity of chronic hepatitis C. J Hepatol. 2009;50(3):471–8.

34. Petta S, Tripodo C, Grimaudo S, Cabibi D, Camma C, Di Cristina A, et al. High liver RBP4 protein content is associated with histological features in patients with genotype 1 chronic hepatitis C and with nonalcoholic steatohepatitis. Dig Liver Dis. 2011;43(5):404–10.

35. Yang Q, Graham TE, Mody N, Preitner F, Peroni OD, Zabolotny JM, et al. Serum retinol binding protein 4 contributes to insulin resistance in obesity and type 2 diabetes. Nature. 2005;436(7049):356–62.

36. Pirazzi C, Valenti L, Motta BM, Pingitore P, Hedfalk K, Mancina RM, et al. PNPLA3 has retinyl-palmitate lipase activity in human hepatic stellate cells. Hum Mol Genet. 2014;23(15):4077–85.

37. Mondul A, Mancina RM, Merlo A, Dongiovanni P, Rametta R, Montalcini T, et al. PNPLA3 I148M variant influences circulating retinol in adults with nonalcoholic fatty liver disease or obesity. J Nutr. 2015;145(8):1687–91.

38. Valenti L, Dongiovanni P, Ginanni Corradini S, Burza MA, Romeo S. PNPLA3 I148M variant and hepatocellular carcinoma: a common genetic variant for a rare disease. Dig Liver Dis. 2013;45(8):619–24.

39. Mayne ST, Graham S, Zheng TZ. Dietary retinol: prevention or promotion of carcinogenesis in humans? Cancer Causes Control. 1991;2(6):443–50.

40. Giovannucci E, Rimm EB, Liu Y, Stampfer MJ, Willett WC. A prospective study of tomato products, lycopene, and prostate cancer risk. J Natl Cancer Inst. 2002;94(5):391–8.

41. Hossain MZ, Wilkens LR, Mehta PP, Loewenstein W, Bertram JS. Enhancement of gap junctional communication by retinoids correlates with their ability to inhibit neoplastic transformation. Carcinogenesis. 1989;10(9):1743–8.

42. Bertram JS, Pung A, Churley M, Kappock TJ, Wilkins LR, Cooney RV. Diverse carotenoids protect against chemically induced neoplastic transformation. Carcinogenesis. 1991;12(4):671–8.

43. Giovannucci E. Tomatoes, tomato-based products, lycopene, and cancer: review of the epidemiologic literature. J Natl Cancer Inst. 1999;91(4):317–31.

44. Park YO, Hwang ES, Moon TW. The effect of lycopene on cell growth and oxidative DNA damage of Hep3B human hepatoma cells. Biofactors. 2005;23(3):129–39.

45. Matsushima-Nishiwaki R, Shidoji Y, Nishiwaki S, Yamada T, Moriwaki H, Muto Y. Suppression by carotenoids of microcystin-induced morphological changes in mouse hepatocytes. Lipids. 1995;30(11):1029–34.

46. Watanabe S, Kitade Y, Masaki T, Nishioka M, Satoh K, Nishino H. Effects of lycopene and Sho-saiko-to on hepatocarcinogenesis in a rat model of spontaneous liver cancer. Nutr Cancer. 2001;39(1):96–101.

47. Chen W, Wang JB, Abnet CC, Dawsey SM, Fan JH, Yin LY, et al. Association between C-reactive protein, incident liver cancer, and chronic liver disease mortality in the Linxian Nutrition Intervention Trials: a nested case-control study. Cancer Epidemiol Biomark Prev. 2015;24(2):386–92.

48. Nascimento MM, Bruchfeld A, Suliman ME, Hayashi SY, Pecoits R, Manfro RC, et al. Effect of hepatitis C serology on greactive protein in a cohort of Brazilian hemodialysis patients. Braz J Med Biol Res. 2005;38(5):783–8.

49. Kalabay L, Nemesanszky E, Csepregi A, Pusztay M, David K, Horvath G, et al. Paradoxical alteration of acute-phase protein levels in patients with chronic hepatitis C treated with IFN-alpha 2b. Int Immunol. 2004;16(1):51–4.

50. Floris-Moore M, Howard AA, Lo YT, Schoenbaum EE, Arnsten JH, Klein RS. Hepatitis C infection is associated with lower lipids and high-sensitivity C-reactive protein in HIV-infected men. Aids Patient Care STDS. 2007;21(7):479–91.

51. Hernández-Gea V, Ghiassi-Nejad Z, Rozenfeld R, Gordon R, Fiel MI, Yue Z, et al. Autophagy releases lipid that promotes fibrogenesis by activated hepatic stellate cells in mice and in human tissues. Gastroenterology. 2012;142(4):938–46.

52. Anstee QM, Targher G, Day CP. Progression of NAFLD to diabetes mellitus, cardiovascular disease or cirrhosis. Nat Rev Gastroenterol Hepatol. 2013;10(6):330–44.

53. Musso G, Gambino R, De Michieli F, Biroli G, Premoli A, Pagano G, et al. Nitrosative stress predicts the presence and severity of nonalcoholic fatty liver at different stages of the development of insulin resistance and metabolic syndrome: possible role of vitamin A intake. Am J Clin Nutr. 2007;86(3):661–71.

2

Detection of bacterial DNA by in situ hybridization in patients with decompensated liver cirrhosis

Shingo Usui[1*], Hirotoshi Ebinuma[1,2], Po-Sung Chu[1], Nobuhiro Nakamoto[1*], Yoshiyuki Yamagishi[1,3], Hidetsugu Saito[1,4] and Takanori Kanai[1]

Abstract

Background: Spontaneous bacterial peritonitis (SBP) is often difficult to diagnose because bacteria in ascites cannot be detected accurately by conventional culture. In situ hybridization (ISH) was previously developed for rapid detection of genes from bacteria phagocytized by neutrophils. SBP may develop after bacteria enter into the systemic circulation following bacterial translocation. Therefore, we performed ISH to identify bacteria in blood samples collected from patients with decompensated liver cirrhosis (LC).

Methods: In this retrospective study, peripheral blood samples were collected from 60 patients with decompensated LC, and bacteria were detected by both blood culture and ISH. Moreover, 35 patients underwent paracentesis for diagnosis of SBP.

Results: Eight of 35 patients were diagnosed with SBP by polymorphonuclear neutrophil counts, and one patient was diagnosed with bacterascites. Seven of the nine patients showed positive results for ISH, whereas bacteria were detected in only two cases by blood culture. Thirty-seven of 60 cases (62%) showed positive results for ISH, whereas only six samples (10%) were positive by blood culture analysis. Compared with the 23 cases of negative ISH, the 37 cases of positive ISH showed a higher frequency of fever, higher Child-Pugh scores, and lower albumin levels.

Conclusions: Detection of bacteria by ISH suggested that bacterial translocation, which cannot be proven by conventional culture, occurred in these patients, and that ISH could be helpful for the early diagnosis of some types of infection and prevention of SBP in these patients.

Keywords: Spontaneous bacterial peritonitis, Bacterial translocation, Liver cirrhosis, In situ hybridization, Blood culture

Background

Patients with decompensated liver cirrhosis (LC) often suffer from various complications, such as hepatic encephalopathy, jaundice, gastroesophageal varices, and ascites. Spontaneous bacterial peritonitis (SBP), which was first reported by Conn and Fessle in 1971, is associated with a poor prognosis [1–4]. Early diagnosis and antibiotic treatment are necessary for management of SBP [4, 5]. However, it is difficult to diagnose SBP because

bacteria in ascites or blood cannot be detected accurately by conventional culture in a timely manner. Polymorphonuclear neutrophil (PMN) counts in ascites are useful for diagnosis of SBP, and empirical antibiotic therapy should be started immediately after the diagnosis of SBP without knowledge of the causative bacteria [5].

The use of in situ hybridization (ISH) for detection of genes from bacteria phagocytized by neutrophils in ascites may have applications in the diagnosis of SBP [6]. ISH was developed to detect bacteria rapidly in patients with suspected bacterial infection [7] and can be applied to identify bacterial genes in neutrophils directly under a microscope after collection of blood samples from patients. Enomoto et al. reported that ISH is highly

* Correspondence: usui@a3.keio.jp; nobuhiro@z2.keio.jp
[1]Division of Gastroenterology and Hepatology, Department of Internal Medicine, Keio University School of Medicine, 35 Shinanomachi, Shinjuku-ku, Tokyo 160-8582, Japan
Full list of author information is available at the end of the article

sensitive for detection of bacteria in ascites from patients with SBP [6]. Indeed, SBP may develop following bacterial translocation, during which enteric bacteria cross the intestinal epithelial cells, reach mesenteric lymph nodes [8], and enter into the systemic circulation [9]. Therefore, we hypothesized that patients with SBP may already exhibit systemic bacterial inflammation.

Accordingly, in this study, we attempted to detect bacteria in blood samples from patients with decompensated LC by ISH, and evaluated the utility of ISH compared with conventional blood culture in these patients.

Methods
Patients
Patients admitted to Keio University Hospital from April 2008 to March 2011 and who underwent ISH were included in this retrospective study. We performed ISH a total of 110 times in 94 patients. Twenty-five cases were patients without liver disease, and 13 cases were patients without cirrhosis. Sixty of 72 patients had ascites and were diagnosed with decompensated LC. Blood samples from 60 patients diagnosed with decompensated LC were simultaneously examined by ISH and blood culture. Moreover, 35 patients with mild or severe ascites underwent paracentesis to diagnose SBP by PMN counts of no less than 250/μL in ascitic samples, and ascitic samples were investigated with the blood samples simultaneously (Fig. 1). This study was approved by the ethics committee of our university hospital.

ISH
ISH was performed using a commercial kit provided by Fuso Pharmaceuticals (Osaka, Japan). In ISH, the probes used to detect bacterial genomes for *Staphylococcus*

aureus (SA), *S. epidermidis* (SE), *Pseudomonas aeruginosa* (PA), *Enterococcus faecalis* (EF), and a group of enterobacteria (*Escherichia coli*, *Enterobacter cloacae*, and *Klebsiella pneumoniae* [EK]) were previously established [7]. These pathogens are frequent causes of bacterial infections in patients with SBP [4, 10].

ISH was performed using blood samples from patients. Briefly, heparinized blood samples from patients were centrifuged (150×*g* for 10 min); leukocytes were collected after hemolysis with hypotonic buffer and resuspended in phosphate-buffered saline (PBS) at a concentration of 5×10^4 cells/μL. A sample of the cellular suspension (5–10 μL) was spread onto a glass slide and air-dried. The slide was fixed in Carnoy's solution for 20 min and permeabilized; bacterial DNA was denatured. Digoxygenin (Dig)-labeled probes and anti-Dig-alkaline phosphatase (ALP) were used for detection. Intracellular Dig-labeled hybridized signals were detected by anti-Dig-ALP. To visualize the signals, color development was achieved using nitro blue tetrazolium (NBT)-5-bromo-4-chloro-3-indolyl phosphate (BCIP) as a substrate for ALP. Positive signals in the cell cytoplasm were observed under a microscope. Blue-colored dots in neutrophils, representing phagocytic bacteria, were assumed to represent a positive result.

Blood and ascitic cultures
All blood and ascitic samples were collected into both aerobic and anaerobic blood culture bottles. Blood and ascitic culture bottles were sent to the reference microbiology laboratory of our hospital for processing. The blood culture system BD Bactec FX (Nippon Becton Dickinson, Tokyo, Japan) was used for the detection of pathogens. Samples were incubated at 37 °C for 5 days.

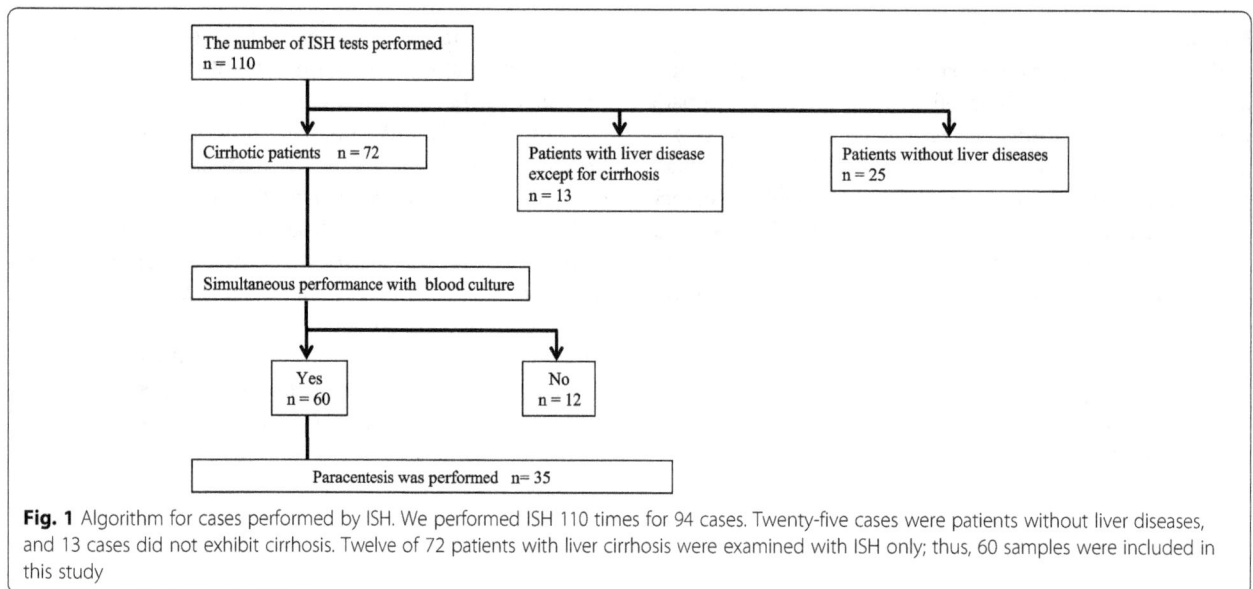

Fig. 1 Algorithm for cases performed by ISH. We performed ISH 110 times for 94 cases. Twenty-five cases were patients without liver diseases, and 13 cases did not exhibit cirrhosis. Twelve of 72 patients with liver cirrhosis were examined with ISH only; thus, 60 samples were included in this study

Isolates of microorganisms were identified using a Bactec FX system.

Statistical analysis

Comparisons of the frequencies between the two groups were analyzed by McNemar's tests. Baseline data for patients with LC were statistically evaluated. Variables were expressed as the mean ± standard deviation (SD), and differences between two groups were evaluated by Student's t-tests, and three groups by ANOVA.

Results

Patient background

Table 1 shows the characteristics of the 60 patients included in this study. ISH and conventional blood cultures were performed in 60 patients with ascites out of 72 decompensated LC patients. The median age was 62 years, and the patients were predominantly male (male:female = 35:25). The causes of cirrhosis were hepatitis B virus infection (n = 4), hepatitis C virus infection (n = 18), alcohol (n = 21), and other factors (n = 17). All patients had ascites, and their Child-Pugh scores were no less than 8. The Child-Pugh classifications were B and C, and the mean score was 9.97 ± 1.55. The median total bilirubin value was 2.85 mg/dL, and the maximum value was 29.2 mg/dL. The mean albumin and creatinine values were 2.41 ± 0.47 mg/dL and 1.18 ± 0.71 g/dL, respectively. The median Model For End-Stage Liver Disease (MELD) score was 15. Patients with diabetes were those who were diagnosed as such by fasting blood glucose or oral glucose tolerance test and treated with insulin or hypoglycemic drugs.

Comparison between ISH and blood cultures in patients undergoing paracentesis

Eight cases were diagnosed with SBP based on PMN counts. The diagnosis of SBP was based on elevated PMN counts ($\geq 250/\mu L$) in 35 cases undergoing paracentesis (Fig. 2). ISH results were positive in six of eight SBP cases, whereas only one case was positive for blood culture. One patient who was positive for ascitic culture was also positive for ISH but negative for blood culture. In seven ascitic culture-negative cases, five were positive for ISH, and one was positive for blood culture. One patient was diagnosed with bacterasites and showed positive results for both ISH and blood culture. Of note, 14 of 27 patients who were not diagnosed with SBP by PMN counts of ascites were positive for ISH, and three out of 14 patients later proved to be positive for blood culture, suggesting that ISH might be useful to diagnose bacterial infection in decompensated LC patients earlier than conventional ways. We did not find any cases who were negative for ISH but positive for ascitic cultures or blood cultures.

Differences in detection rates between ISH and blood culture

Of the 60 cases who underwent both ISH and blood culture, six were positive for bacteremia by blood culture (10.0%), whereas 37 were positive by ISH (61.7%; $p < 0.001$; Table 2). The rate of positive detection by ISH was significantly higher than that by blood culture. All positive cases by blood culture were positively detected by ISH, and no cases were negative for ISH but positive for blood culture.

Clinical features and detection of ISH

Thirty of the 60 patients had fever. Among the patients with fever, 23 cases (76.7%) were positive for ISH analysis, and six (20.0%) were positive for blood cultures. Among the patients without fever, 14 cases (46.7%) were positive for ISH analysis, but none was positive for blood cultures. In 47 C-reactive protein (CRP)-positive cases (≥ 1 mg/dL), 30 (63.8%) and four (8.5%) cases were positive for ISH analysis and blood cultures, respectively. The rates of positive results between ISH and blood cultures differed significantly, suggesting that ISH may detect bacteria more sensitively than conventional blood culture (Table 3). Among 24 patients with antibiotic use, oral or intravenous antibiotic treatment was given to 22 patients for confirmed or suspected bacterial infections with unidentified origin. Two patients received an oral

Table 1 Baseline characteristics of patients with cirrhosis who underwent ISH

	Mean ± SD or median value (range)
Age (years)	62 (29–84)
Sex (male/female)	35/25
Etiology (HBV/HCV/alcohol/others)	4/18/21/17
Child-Pugh classification (B/C)	23/37
Child-Pugh score	9.97 ± 1.55
Total bilirubin (mg/dL)	2.85 (0.3–29.2)
Albumin (g/dL)	2.41 ± 0.47
Prothrombin time (INR)	1.38 (0.97–2.38)
Creatinine (mg/dL)	1.18 ± 0.71
White blood cell counts (/μL)	6350 (2000–27,800)
Platelet counts (× 10³/μL)	78.5 (20–760)
C-reactive protein (mg/dL)	2.42 (0.12–15.53)
MELD score	15 (7–34)
Esophageal varices (+/−)	36/24
Hepatocellular carcinoma (+/−)	19/41
Abdominal pain (+/−)	4/56
Diabetes mellitus (+/−)	17/43

Valuables are the mean ± standard deviations (SDs) or median (range)
HBV: hepatitis B virus, HCV: hepatitis virus

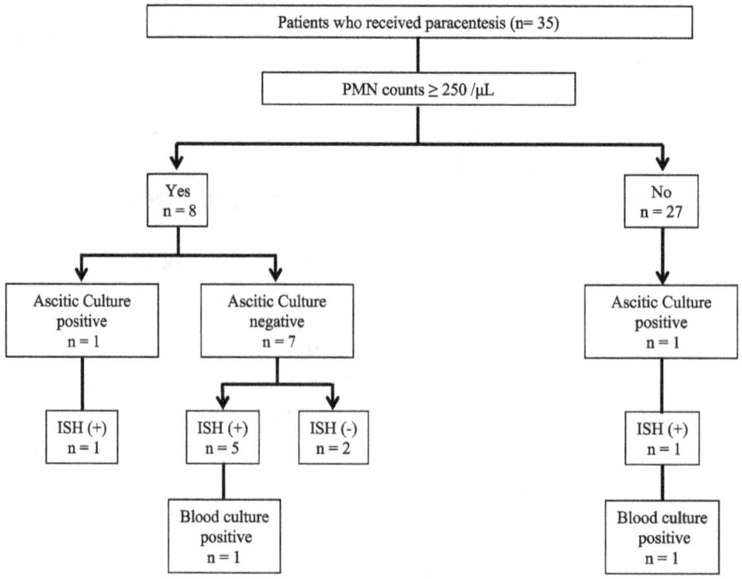

Fig. 2 Algorithm of patients who received paracentesis. Eight of 35 patients were diagnosed with spontaneous bacterial peritonitis (SBP). Six cases of SBP (75.0%) were positive for bacteremia by ISH, but only one patient (12.5%) was positively identified by blood bottle culture

aminoglycoside bactericidal antibiotic called kanamycin for prevention of SBP. It is possible that using antibiotics in these patients possibly affected the sensitivity of blood culture.

Moreover, we compared the clinical characteristics between ISH/blood culture positive (+/+), ISH positive-blood culture negative (+/−), and both negative (−/−) patients (Table 4). There were significant differences in the frequency of clinical symptom of fever between the three groups ($p < 0.05$), suggesting that ISH or the combination of ISH and blood culture is useful for the early diagnosis of bacterial infection. Further study in a larger sample size is needed to validate the results.

Detection of bacterial groups by ISH
Table 5 shows the DNA probes used for detection of bacteria in ISH and the number of positive cases by each probe. The EK probe was positive in almost all cases (81%). Eight cases showed positive ISH results for the EK probe and another probe simultaneously.

Discussion
In this study, we successfully employed ISH to detect pathogens in the blood from patients with decompensated LC in whom blood culture results were negative for bacterial infection. These findings suggested that bacterial translocation cannot be always detected by conventional blood culture because SBP is known to occur after bacterial translocation, defined as the passage of bacteria from the intestine or colon through the intestinal epithelial cells and entrapment in the mesenteric lymph nodes [8, 11]. After bacterial translocation, bacteria are thought to enter the systemic bloodstream and access ascitic fluid, which exhibits low bactericidal capacity [9, 12–14]. Bacterial translocation has been demonstrated in some studies in both human and animal models of LC [15, 16]. However, it is unclear how SBP develops from bacterial translocation because this event cannot be detected easily by conventional blood

Table 3 Positive detection rates by ISH and blood cultures according to clinical manifestations

	No	ISH positive	Blood culture Positive	P value
Total	60	37 (61.7%)	6 (10.0%)	< 0.001
Fever	30	23 (76.7%)	6 (20.0%)	< 0.001
No fever	30	14 (46.7%)	0 (0.0%)	–
CRP ≥ 1 mg/dL	47	30 (63.8%)	4 (8.6%)	< 0.001
CRP < 1 mg/dL	13	7 (53.8%)	2 (15.4%)	0.0253
Antibiotic use	24	15 (62.5%)	2 (8.3%)	< 0.001

Statistical significance was determined by McNemar's test

Table 2 Differences in detection rates between blood culture and ISH

		Blood culture		Total
		Positive	Negative	
ISH	Positive	6 (10.0%)	31 (51.7%)	37 (61.7%)
	Negative	0 (0%)	23 (38.3%)	23 (38.3%)
Total		6 (10.0%)	54 (90.0%)	60 (100%)

Table 4 Comparison of clinical manifestations among positive (+/+), ISH positive-blood culture negative (+/−), and fully negative (−/−) patients

ISH/blood culture	(+/+)	(+/−)	(−/−)	P value
No.	6	31	23	
Fever (+)	6 (10 0%)	17 (55%)	7 (30%)	< 0.001
CRP (mg/dL)	3.40 ± 1.44	3.98 ± 0.63	2.92 ± 0.75	N.S.
Child-Pugh score	11.3 ± 0.6	10.1 ± 0.3	9.4 ± 0.3	0.020
MELD score	18.0 ± 2.6	17.4 ± 1.1	15.6 ± 1.3	N.S.
Total bilirubin (mg/dL)	7.62 ± 2.97	6.85 ± 1.30	4.34 ± 1.51	N.S.
Albumin (g/dL)	2.17 ± 0.19	2.33 ± 0.08	2.58 ± 0.10	N.S.(0.066)
Prothrombin time (INR)	1.49 ± 0.11	1.40 ± 0.05	1.38 ± 0.06	N.S
Platelet counts (× 10^3/μL)	68.8 ± 45.2	99.7 ± 19.9	134.7 ± 23.1	N.S.
Diabetes mellitus (+)	4 (67%)	9 (29%)	4 (17%)	0.049
HCC (+)	4 (67%)	7 (23%)	8 (35%)	N.S.
Esophageal varix (+)	4 (67%)	18 (58%)	14 (61%)	N.S.

culture [11]. Such et al. reported that bacterial DNA can be detected simultaneously in blood and ascitic fluid [17, 18], using a polymerase chain reaction (PCR)-based method. Although this method may provide evidence of the relationship between bacterial translocation and SBP, no studies have compared PCR-based methods with blood culture. Therefore, we hypothesized that ISH could be applied to decompensated LC patients to detect bacteria and may be helpful for selecting patients who may have an infection earlier and determining the proper antibiotic to use if bacteria are present in the systemic bloodstream after bacterial translocation.

ISH was first developed to enable early diagnosis of sepsis within 1 day, using ISH of the bacterial genomes existing in neutrophils after phagocytosis. This method was reported to be four times as sensitive as blood culture for detection of bacteria in patients with sepsis [7]. The other advantages of the ISH method are that it can eliminate potential contamination and is not affected by antibiotic use, as it analyzes pathogens already captured into neutrophils by phagocytosis. Thus, the probability

of false-positive results is low with this procedure. Enomoto et al. developed a new probe mixture, designated a global bacteria (GB) probe, which was capable of detecting all relevant bacterial strains. Using ISH, this probe showed positive results in 10 of 11 SBP cases and negative results in none of 40 non-SBP cases in ascites [6]. Bacteria causing SBP are frequently gram-negative rods, such as *Escherichia coli* and *K. pneumoniae*, or can be *Streptococcus* species [10]. Such et al. studied bacterial DNA to show that *Escherichia coli* were the most frequently identified bacteria [18]. This is consistent with our results demonstrating that *Enterobacteria* were frequently detected. Therefore, even five specific probes without the global bacteria probe may be useful for detection of bacteria in patients with decompensated LC. These results suggest that early detection of specific bacteria causing SBP and early therapeutic intervention using appropriate antibiotics are additional advantages of ISH for patients with LC and SBP. However, further studies are needed to confirm this assumption. Additionally, blood cultures beyond ISH tests are thought to be necessary for such patients because bacteria other than the five species probed by ISH may be detected and because drug susceptibility tests cannot be performed by ISH.

Interestingly, in our study, some clinical parameters were related to the results of ISH tests, including the presence of fever and Child-Pugh scores. These results may also be related to the occurrence of bacterial translocation. Cirera et al. detected enteric organisms increasingly from mesenteric lymph nodes in patients with or without cirrhosis according to the Child-Pugh score: 3.4% in A, 8.1% in B, and 30.8% in C [15]. Bacteria in neutrophils were detected in 47% of patients without

Table 5 Bacterial strains detected by ISH

Bacteria	ISH probe	Number of positive cases
Escherichia coli		
Enterobacter cloacae	EK	30 (81.1%)
Klebsiella pneumoniae		
Enterococcus faecalis	EF	6 (16.2%)
Staphylococcus aureus	SA	5 (13.5%)
Pseudomonas aeruginosa	PA	4 (10.8%)
Staphylococcus epidermidis	SE	0 (0.0%)

fever and in 54% of patients whose CRP levels were below 1 mg/dL in our study. Surprisingly, bacterial translocation may already be present in asymptomatic patients with LC having ascites. Evans et al. reported that 3.5% of all outpatients with cirrhosis had SBP, and 1.9% of these patients had bacterascites [19]. Moreover, several studies have also demonstrated that more severe liver failure is associated with lower CRP levels [20, 21]. Administration of antibiotics may be considered to prevent further deterioration of sepsis or SBP in decompensated LC patients positive for ISH; these patients have no clinical symptoms at this point.

Recent reports have shown that serum albumin functions to maintain oncotic pressure and has immunomodulatory and antioxidant effects. Albumin infusions were found to reduce the incidence of renal failure and mortality in patients with SBP [22, 23]. Patients with positive results by ISH had higher Child-Pugh scores and showed a tendency of lower serum albumin levels (Table 4). If hypoalbuminemia indicates immunological deterioration in patients with decompensated LC, patients who are positive for ISH may be required to receive albumin infusions early in addition to antibiotics.

The limitations of this study include the small number of subjects. Obviously, a larger controlled study will be needed to validate the results and confirm the usefulness of ISH.

Conclusions

In conclusion, bacterial translocation, which often occurs in ascitic patients with LC, cannot be proven by methods such as conventional blood cultures. ISH may be helpful to select patients who are suspected of having an infection, including SBP, and to manage treatment in a timely manner, although additional studies are required.

Abbreviations
CRP: C-reactive protein; EF: *Enterococcus faecalis*; EK: a group of enterobacteria; HCC: hepatocellular carcinoma; ISH: in situ hybridization; LC: liver cirrhosis; MELD: Model For End-Stage Liver Disease; PA: *Pseudomonas aeruginosa*; PCR: polymerase chain reaction; PMN: polymorphonuclear neutrophil; SA: *Staphylococcus aureus*; SBP: spontaneous bacterial peritonitis; SE: *Staphylococcus epidermidis*

Acknowledgements
We thank Dr. Yoshio Kobayashi, Ms. Yuko Sumitani, and Mr. Akio Matsuhisa for their helpful and insightful suggestions and technical assistance.

Funding
This work did not receive any funding.

Authors' contributions
SU: study concept and design, acquisition of data, analysis and interpretation of data, statistical analyses, drafting of the manuscript; HE: study concept and design, acquisition of data, analysis and interpretation of data, critical revision of the manuscript for important intellectual content; P-S C: acquisition of data, analysis and interpretation of data, critical revision of the manuscript for important intellectual content; NN: acquisition of data, analysis and interpretation of data, drafting of the manuscript; YY: acquisition of data, analysis and interpretation of data, critical revision of the manuscript for important intellectual content; HS: study concept and design, drafting of the manuscript; TK: study concept and design, critical revision of the manuscript for important intellectual content; All authors read and approved the final manuscript, and agreed to be accountable for all aspects of the works.

Consent for publication
Not applicable

Competing interests
The authors have no financial or nonfinancial competing interests to declare.

Author details
[1]Division of Gastroenterology and Hepatology, Department of Internal Medicine, Keio University School of Medicine, 35 Shinanomachi, Shinjuku-ku, Tokyo 160-8582, Japan. [2]Department of Internal Medicine, International University of Health and Welfare Mita Hospital, 1-4-3 Mita, Minato-ku, Tokyo 108-8329, Japan. [3]Department of Internal Medicine, Tokyo Dental College Suidobashi Hospital, 2-9-18 Misakicho, Chiyoda-ku, Tokyo 101-0061, Japan. [4]Faculty of Pharmacy, Keio University, 1-5-30 Shiba-kohen, Minato-ku, Tokyo 105-8512, Japan.

References
1. Conn HO, Fessel JM. Spontaneous bacterial peritonitis in cirrhosis: variations on a theme. Medicine (Baltimore). 1971;50:161–97.
2. Garcia-Tsao G. Current management of the complications of cirrhosis and portal hypertension: variceal hemorrhage, ascites, and spontaneous bacterial peritonitis. Gastroenterology. 2001;120:726–48.
3. Solà E, Solé C, Ginès P. Management of uninfected and infected ascites in cirrhosis. Liver Int. 2016;36(Suppl 1):109–15.
4. Dever JB, Sheikh MY. Review article: spontaneous bacterial peritonitis-bacteriology, diagnosis, treatment, risk factors and prevention. Aliment Pharmacol Ther. 2015;41:1116–31.
5. European Association for the Study of the Liver. EASL clinical practice guidelines on the management of ascites, spontaneous bacterial peritonitis, and hepatorenal syndrome in cirrhosis. J Hepatol. 2010;53:397–417.
6. Enomoto H, Inoue S, Matsuhisa A, Aizawa N, Imanishi H, Saito M, et al. Development of a new in situ hybridization method for the detection of global bacterial DNA to provide early evidence of a bacterial infection in spontaneous bacterial peritonitis. J Hepatol. 2012;56:85–94.
7. Shimada J, Hayashi I, Inamatsu T, Ishida M, Iwai S, Kamidono S, et al. Clinical trial of in-situ hybridization method for the rapid diagnosis of sepsis. J Infect Chemother. 1999;5:21–31.
8. Wiest R, Lawson M, Geuking M. Pathological bacterial translocation in liver cirrhosis. J Hepatol. 2014;60:197–209.
9. Bellot P, Francés R, Such J. Pathological bacterial translocation in cirrhosis: pathophysiology, diagnosis and clinical implications. Liver Int. 2013;33(1):31–9.
10. Koulaouzidis A, Bhat S, Saeed AA. Spontaneous bacterial peritonitis. World J Gastroenterol. 2009;15:1042–9.
11. Wiest R, Garcia-Tsao G. Bacterial translocation (BT) in cirrhosis. Hepatology. 2005;41:422–33.
12. Zapater P, Francés R, González-Navajas JM, de la Hoz MA, Moreu R, Pascual S, et al. Serum and ascitic fluid bacterial DNA: a new independent prognostic factor in noninfected patients with cirrhosis. Hepatology. 2008; 48:1924–31.
13. Suliman MA, Khalil FM, Alkindi SS, Pathare AV, Almadhani AA, Soliman NA. Tumor necrosis factor-α and interleukin-6 in cirrhotic patients with spontaneous bacterial peritonitis. World J Gastrointest Pathophysiol. 2012;3:92–8.
14. Sheer TA, Runyon BA. Spontaneous bacterial peritonitis. Dig Dis. 2005;23:39–46.
15. Cirera I, Bauer TM, Navasa M, Vila J, Grande L, Taurá P, et al. Bacterial translocation of enteric organisms in patients with cirrhosis. J Hepatol. 2001;34:32–7.
16. Guarner C, Runyon BA, Young S, Heck M, Sheikh MY. Intestinal bacterial overgrowth and bacterial translocation in cirrhotic rats with ascites. Hepatol. 1997;26:1372–8.

17. Francés R, Zapater P, González-Navajas JM, Muñoz C, Caño R, Moreu R, et al. Bacterial DNA in patients with cirrhosis and noninfected ascites mimics the soluble immune response established in patients with spontaneous bacterial peritonitis. Hepatology. 2008;47:978–85.

18. Such J, Frances R, Munoz C, Zapater P, Casellas JA, Cifuentes A, et al. Detection and identification of bacterial DNA in patients with cirrhosis and culture-negative, nonneutrocytic ascites. Hepatology. 2002;36:135–41.

19. Evans LT, Kim WR, Poterucha JJ, Kamath PS. Spontaneous bacterial peritonitis in asymptomatic outpatients with cirrhotic ascites. Hepatology. 2003;37:897–901.

20. Fernández J, Gustot T. Management of bacterial infections in cirrhosis. J Hepatol. 2012;56(Suppl 1):S1–12.

21. Mackenzie I, Woodhouse J. C-reactive protein concentrations during bacteraemia: a comparison between patients with and without liver dysfunction. Intensive Care Med. 2006;32:1344–51.

22. Garcia-Martinez R, Caraceni P, Bernardi M, Arroyo V, Jalan R. Albumin: pathophysiologic basis of its role in the treatment of cirrhosis and its complications. Hepatology. 2013;58:1836–46.

23. Guevara M, Terra C, Nazar A, Solà E, Fernández J, Pavesi M, et al. Albumin for bacterial infections other than spontaneous bacterial peritonitis in cirrhosis. A randomized, controlled study. J Hepatol. 2012;57:759–65.

3

Streptococcus agalactiae infective endocarditis complicated by multiple mycotic hepatic aneurysms and massive splenic infarction

Pietro Achilli[1], Angelo Guttadauro[2*], Paolo Bonfanti[3], Sabina Terragni[2], Luca Fumagalli[4], Ugo Cioffi[5], Francesco Gabrielli[2], Matilde De Simone[5] and Marco Chiarelli[4]

Abstract

Background: The burden of disease caused by Streptococcus agalactiae has increased significantly among older adults in the last decades. Group B streptococcus infection can be associated with invasive disease and severe clinical syndromes, such as meningitis and endocarditis.

Case presentation: We present the case of a 56-year-old man who developed multiple mycotic aneurysms of the right hepatic artery and massive splenic infarction as rare complications of Streptococcus agalactiae infective endocarditis. The patient underwent urgent right hepatic artery ligation and splenectomy. The postoperative course was complicated by an episode of hemobilia due to the rupture of a partially thrombosed mycotic aneurysm into the biliary tree. Thus, selective radiological embolization of the left hepatic artery branches was necessary.

Conclusion: To our knowledge, this is the first case reported of infected aneurysms of visceral arteries caused by Group B streptococcus infection. Clinical and laboratory findings were non-specific, while imaging features with computed tomography scan and angiography were highly suggestive. In our case, early recognition, culture-specific intravenous antibiotics and urgent surgical treatment combined with interventional radiology played a decisive role in the final result.

Keywords: Hepatic artery aneurysm, Splenic infarction, Infective endocarditis, Streptococcus agalactiae

Background

Streptococcus agalactiae, known as Group B streptococcus (GBS), is a Gram-positive coccus commonly associated with infective disease of pregnant women and newborns [1]. Recent large studies suggest an increasing incidence of invasive GBS disease among non-pregnant adults in Western countries [2, 3]. Common presentations of GBS disease in adults include soft-tissue and skin infection, pneumonia, urinary tract infection and severe clinical syndromes, such as meningitis and endocarditis. We present the first case of GBS endocarditis in a healthy adult patient complicated by multiple mycotic aneurysms (MAs) of hepatic artery and massive splenic infarction (SI).

Case presentation

A 56-year-old man was referred to our emergency department with a 10 days history of pyrexia, productive cough and appetite loss. He reported an adverse reaction to penicillin and he had no history of intravenous drug abuse. Physical examination showed coarse crackles in lower right lung field, and patient's laboratory workup was remarkable for elevated C-reactive protein (CRP) (16 mg/dl) and leukocytosis (16.000/mm^3) with neutrophilia of 88%. Chest X-ray showed right lobar consolidation. The patient was admitted to our hospital based on a diagnosis of community-acquired pneumonia. Blood samples for hemocultures were collected and empirical

* Correspondence: angelo.guttadauro@unimib.it
2Department of Surgery, University of Milan-Bicocca, Istituti Clinici Zucchi, Via Zucchi, 24, 20900 Monza, Italy
Full list of author information is available at the end of the article

therapy with levofloxacin (500 mg/day) was undertaken (day 1). Considering the worsening of the patient's general conditions, a computed tomography (CT) scan of abdomen and thorax was performed: the diagnostic imaging revealed left pleural effusion, extensive SI caused by thrombosis of the splenic artery and a hyperdense round lesion of the right hepatic lobe suspected for hepatic aneurysm (1.4 cm × 1.1 cm) (Fig. 1a). Blood cultures, taken on day 1, were positive for penicillin-sensible GBS and the patient immediately underwent a transthoracic and transesophageal echocardiography finding an infective vegetation (1.0 cm × 1.5 cm) on the mitral valve associated with mitral chordae tendineae rupture and severe regurgitation. Intravenous antibiotic therapy was consequently switched to intravenous vancomycin (2 g/day) and emergency mitral valve repair with artificial chordal replacement was performed (day 12). During post-acute cardiac rehabilitation program the patient developed jaundice and laboratory tests showed a total bilirubin of 7.4 mg/dl and elevation of alkaline phosphatase and γ-glutamyl transferase (day 20). A new emergent abdomen CT scan found an enlarging MA of the right hepatic artery of 2.4 cm × 2.0 cm of size and a 2.7 cm × 3.0 cm intrahepatic aneurysm in segment VIII, causing displacement of the portal vein and compression of the right biliary duct (Fig. 1b). Furthermore, CT images detected three smaller left hepatic artery aneurysms located in segment IV and confirmed massive SI. Thus, multiple hepatic MAs associated with GBS endocarditis was diagnosed. The patient was immediately submitted to surgical intervention, which consisted in ligation of the right hepatic artery and splenectomy. Initial postoperative course was favorable with reduction of conjugated bilirubin level. A duplex ultrasonography performed 4 days after surgery demonstrated complete thrombosis of the proximal right hepatic artery aneurysm, partial thrombosis of the aneurysm in segment VIII and no further enlargement of the small aneurysms of the left hepatic artery. However, on day 28, an episode of melena associated with low hemoglobin count emerged. The patient underwent esophagogastroduodenoscopy and colonoscopy, which did not show any gastrointestinal bleeding. On day 42, because of progressive decrease of hemoglobin level, a multislice abdomen CT angiography was performed (Fig. 2a). The radiological findings were consistent with hemobilia due to a suspected rupture of the partially thrombosed MA of segment VIII into the biliary tree. On the following day, the patient underwent a selective angiography of the coeliac axis, which revealed blood supply to the segment VIII MA from intra-parenchymal branches of the left hepatic artery. The patient was then successfully treated with transcatheter coil embolization, resulting in complete obliteration of the residual segment VIII MA and of the three segment IV small aneurysms (Fig. 2b). The post-procedural course was uneventful and the patient was discharged on day 58, after 10 weeks of antibiotic therapy. A follow-up CT angiography was performed 8 weeks later,

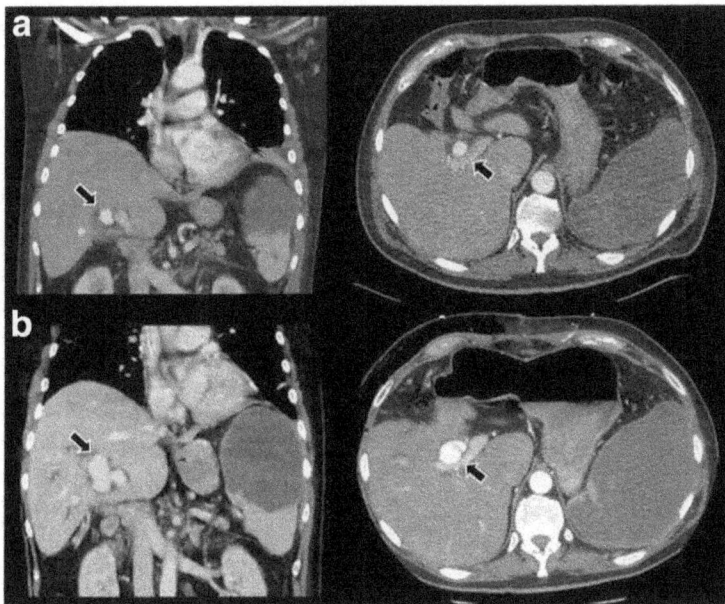

Fig. 1 Abdominal CT taken on day 3 (**a**) shows MA of the proximal right hepatic artery of 1.4 cm × 1.1 cm (*arrow*). Moreover the diagnostic imaging discloses a nonenhancing hypodense area of the spleen consistent with SI. Abdominal enhanced CT taken on day 20 (**b**) reveals an enlargement of the previously detected MA of the proximal right hepatic artery (*arrow*) and the development of a new large MA of the VIII segment (*arrow*). The radiological findings confirm SI

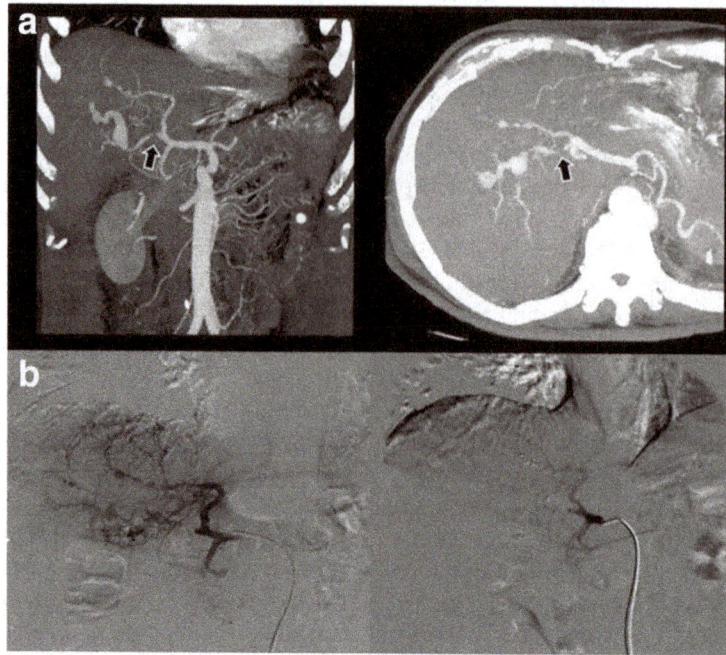

Fig. 2 Multislice abdomen CT angiography taken on day 42 (**a**) showing ligation of the right hepatic artery (*arrow*) and three small MAs of the IV hepatic segment. The radiological images demonstrate residual blood flow in the right hepatic MAs. Selective angiography of the coeliac axis (**b**) demonstrates arterial branches from the left hepatic artery providing blood supply to the right hepatic MAs

showing complete embolization of the residual MAs without any evidence of bile duct dilatation. The patient remained asymptomatic at follow-up of 12 months, with no signs of relapse of biliary obstruction or gastrointestinal bleeding (Fig. 3).

Discussion

Streptococcus agalactiae has been traditionally recognized as a cause of sepsis and meningitis in newborns and pregnant women [1, 2]. Today, given the decline of

neonatal GBS disease in Western countries, as a result of effective intrapartum prophylaxis, the majority of all invasive GBS infections occur in adult people [2, 3]. There are many underlying conditions that can lead to an increased risk for invasive GBS disease, including diabetes, cancer, congestive heart failure, chronic obstructive pulmonary disease and cirrhosis [3, 4]. Clinical manifestations of GBS infection in adults are quite varied [4–6]. Arthritis and upper respiratory tract infections are more frequently reported in adults (< 70 years) while

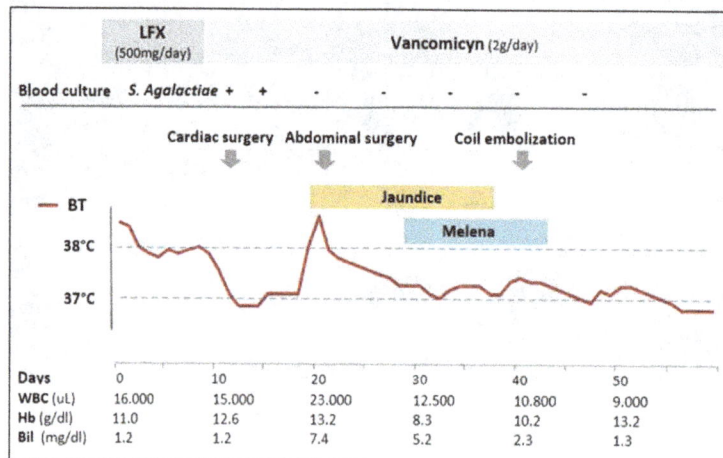

Fig. 3 Clinical timeline of the case. BT: body temperature; WBC: white blood cell count; Hb: hemoglobin; Bil: total bilirubin level; LFX: levofloxacin

skin infections, pneumonia and urinary tract infection are more common among the elderly (>70 years) [5]. Infective endocarditis (IE) caused by GBS infection is uncommon [4, 5, 7]. It represents one of the most severe presentation of GBS infection and it is associated with a high mortality rate [8]. Regarding antibiotic therapy, the combination of β-lactam antibiotic with aminoglycoside can be considered the treatment of choice [7, 9, 10]. In our case, considering the allergy to penicillin of our patient, we successfully used vancomycin as an alternative to β-lactam antibiotic [7, 9]. The peculiar feature of our case consisted in the development of two simultaneous complications such as SI and multiple MAs of the hepatic artery, as a consequence of septic emboli from valvular vegetations.

SI is a relatively uncommon diagnosis. Infarction of the spleen is usually due to the occlusion of the splenic artery secondary to thrombosis or embolism. SI causes include hematologic diseases (sickle cell disease, polycythemia vera), hypercoagulability disorders (antiphospholipid syndrome, cancer) and embolic events (atrial fibrillation, infective endocarditis) [11, 12]. Complications include splenic abscess, pseudocysts and hemorrhage [13]. Clinical presentation of SI consists in left upper quadrant pain irradiated to the shoulder, often associated with anemia and leukocytosis; fever, splenomegaly and left pleural effusion are common findings in SI [11–13]. Lactate dehydrogenase serum levels are frequently elevated [11, 12]. The most sensitive imaging modality is the contrast-enhanced CT, which can show wedged shape hypodense areas in the spleen, splenomegaly with perisplenic fluids and left-sided pleural effusion [11]. When SI is diagnosed, all possible etiologies should be considered and a scrutiny on the source of emboli should be carried out. Intravenous antibiotic therapy based on cultures results is the mainstay of the treatment [11, 12]. Splenectomy is rarely required and surgery is usually considered in case of complications or when medical treatment is ineffective [11, 13]. Unusually our patient did not report any abdominal tenderness or pain at time of diagnosis, while anemia, leukocytosis and pleural effusion were present. In our report the indication for splenectomy was the persistence of septic condition and the need of urgent surgery for hepatic aneurysm.

MA is a rare disease characterized by elusive clinical presentation and high mortality rate [14]. The diffusion of antibiotic therapy in the clinical practice has reduced the incidence of MAs: actually infected aneurysms comprise 1-2.5% of all aortic aneurysms [15]. The typical feature of this pathologic entity is the destruction of the arterial wall caused by bacterial infection leading to vessel dilatation. The etiology of MA is mainly ascribed to septic embolism of vasa vasorum originating from valvular vegetations in the setting of infective endocarditis;

direct colonization of damaged atherosclerotic arterial wall during bacteremia is considered a rare pathogenetic mechanism [16]. Most frequently, MAs occur in abdominal aorta, peripheral arteries, especially femoral artery, and cerebral arteries. Infected aneurysms of visceral arteries are relatively infrequent and generally show an aggressive clinical course with significant mortality [14]. Multidetector CT angiography is considered the pivotal imaging modality in the characterization of MA, showing contrast-enhancing saccular dilatation of the artery with central or eccentric lumen [14]. The most frequent infective agents related to the development of these aneurysms in post-antibiotic era are *Staphylococcus aureus* and Salmonella spp.; β-hemolytic group A Streptococci, Streptococcus pneumoniae and Haemophilus influenzae were more common in the past decades [14, 16]. GBS infection rarely causes MAs and only seven other cases are described in the literature: six of them involving the thoracic or abdominal aorta and one the femoral artery. To our knowledge, this is the first case reported of mycotic aneurysm of visceral arteries caused by *Streptococcus agalactiae*. Hepatic artery MA is usually asymptomatic, but in a minority of cases right upper quadrant pain, jaundice and digestive bleeding may be present [16]. The management of infected aneurysms of hepatic arteries consists in surgical treatment or in endovascular embolization [17]. Although only small series are published, urgent treatment (surgical or radiologic) is generally recommended in symptomatic patients or when aneurysm is larger than 2 cm: these conditions are associated with a higher risk of rupture than atherosclerotic aneurysms [17]. Surgical option is preferable in patients with low surgical risk and proximal aneurysms; embolization should be considered in case of intrahepatic lesions or in high-risk surgical candidates [16]. Antibiotics, possibly tailored on culture sensitivity, are invariably indicated and should be continued for at least 6-8 weeks postoperatively [14]. In our case, we opted for urgent surgical intervention considering the high risk of rupture of the proximal right hepatic aneurysm, proved by its rapid enlargement (from 1.4 to 2.4 cm within 17 days), the sudden increase of bilirubin level and the development of new lesions. In addition, a concomitant splenectomy was required and consequently the open procedure seemed to be the best choice. Unfortunately, the surgical ligation of the right hepatic artery did not result in a complete obliteration of the aneurysms and subsequently endovascular embolization became necessary. This was due to collateral arterial branches from the left hepatic artery that provided blood supply to the right hepatic aneurysms. After selective radiological embolization of the left hepatic artery branches of IV segment, anemia and jaundice were resolved.

Conclusion

We reported the first case of multiple hepatic MAs associated with massive SI, caused by GBS infection in a healthy adult patient. While clinical and laboratory findings were not specific, imaging features with CT scan and angiography were highly suggestive. In our case, early recognition, culture-specific intravenous antibiotics and urgent surgical treatment combined with interventional radiology were crucial factors to the final result.

Abbreviations

CRP: C-reactive protein; CT: Computed tomography; GBS: Group B streptococcus; IE: Infective endocarditis; MA: Mycotic aneurysm; SI: Splenic infarction

Acknowledgments

None.

Funding

Not applicable.

Authors' contributions

PA and MC contributed equally to drafting and writing of the manuscript; AG, PB, UC, MDS, FG and LF revised infective and surgical content of this manuscript; AG and ST supervised the manuscript preparation; LF provided the radiologic images and descriptions. All authors have read and approved the final version of the manuscript.

Consent for publication

Written informed consent was obtained from the patient for publication of this Case report and any accompanying images. A copy of the written consent is available on request.

Competing interests

The authors declare that they have no competing interests.

Author details

[1]University of Milan - Fondazione IRCCS Ca' Granda Ospedale Maggiore Policlinico, Via Sforza 35, 20122 Milan, Italy. [2]Department of Surgery, University of Milan-Bicocca, Istituti Clinici Zucchi, Via Zucchi, 24, 20900 Monza, Italy. [3]Infectious Diseases Unit - A. Manzoni Hospital, Via dell'Eremo 9/11, 23900 Lecco, Italy. [4]Department of Surgery, Ospedale Alessandro Manzoni, Lecco, Via dell'Eremo 9/11, 23900 Lecco, Italy. [5]Department of Surgery, University of Milan, Milan, Italy.

References

1. Schrag SJ, Zywicki S, Farley M, et al. Group B streptococcal disease in the era of intrapartum antibiotic prophylaxis. N Engl J Med. 2000;342:15–20.
2. Phares CR, Lynfield R, Farley MM, et al. Epidemiology of invasive group B streptococcal disease in the United States, 1999-2005. JAMA. 2008; 299:2056–65.
3. Skoff TH, Farley MM, Petit S, et al. Increasing burden of invasive group B streptococcal disease in nonpregnant adults, 1990-2007. Clin Infect Dis. 2009;49:85–92.
4. Blancas D, Santin M, Olmo M, et al. Group B streptococcal disease in nonpregnant adults: incidence, clinical characteristics, and outcome. Eur J Clin Microbiol Infect Dis. 2004;23:168–73.
5. Trivalle C, Martin E, Martel P, et al. Group B streptococcal bacteriemia in the elderly. J Med Microbiol. 1999;47:649–52.
6. Edwards MS, Baker CJ. Group B streptococcal infections in elderly adults. Clin Infect Dis. 2005;41:839–47.
7. Baddour LM, Wilson WR, Bayer AS, et al. Infective endocarditis in adults: diagnosis, antimicrobial therapy, and management of complications. A scientific statement for healthcare professionals from the American Heart Association. Circulation. 2015;132:1435–86.
8. Sambola A, Miro JM, Tornos MP, et al. Streptococcus Agalactiae infective endocarditis: analysis of 30 cases and review of the literature,1962-1998. Clin Infect Dis. 2002;34:1576–84.
9. Habib G, Lancellotti P, Antunes MJ, et al. 2015 ESC guidelines for the management of infective endocarditis: the task force for the management of infective endocarditis of the European Society of Cardiology (ESC). Eur Heart J. 2015;36:3075–128.
10. Kang D-H, Kim Y-J, Kim S-H, et al. Early surgery versus conventional treatment for infective endocarditis. N Engl J Med. 2012;366:2466–73.
11. Antopolsky M, Hiller N, Salameh S, Goldshtein B, Stalnikowicz R. Splenic infarction: 10 years of experience. Am J Emerg Med. 2009;27:262–5.
12. Lawrence YR, Pokroy R, Berlowits D, et al. Splenic infarction: an update on William Osler's observations. IMAJ. 2010;12:362–5.
13. Beeson MS. Splenic infarct presenting as acute abdominal pain in an older patient. J Emerg Med. 1996;14:319–22.
14. Lee WK, Mossop PJ, Little AF, et al. Infected (mycotic) aneurysms: spectrum of imaging appearances and management. Radiographics. 2008;28:1853–68.
15. Ledochowski S, Jacob X, Friggeri A. A rare case of Streptococcus Agalactiae mycotic aneurysm and review of the literature. Infection. 2014;42:569–73.
16. Chaudhari D, Saleem A, Patel P, et al. Hepatic artery mycotic aneurism associated with staphylococcal endocarditis with successful treatment: case report with review of the literature. Case Report Hepatol. 2013; 10.1155/2013/610818. Epub 2013 May 12.
17. Abbas MA, Fowl RJ, Stone WM, et al. Hepatic artery aneurysm: factors that predict complications. J Vasc Surg. 2003;38:41–5.

4

Cirrhosis related functionality characteristic of the fecal microbiota as revealed by a metaproteomic approach

Xiao Wei[1], Shan Jiang[1], Yuye Chen[2], Xiangna Zhao[1], Huan Li[1], Weishi Lin[1], Boxing Li[1], Xuesong Wang[1], Jing Yuan[1*] and Yansong Sun[1*]

Abstract

Background: Intestinal microbiota operated as a whole and was closely related with human health. Previous studies had suggested close relationship between liver cirrhosis (LC) and gut microbiota.

Methods: To determine the functional characteristic of the intestinal microbiota specific for liver cirrhosis, the fecal metaproteome of three LC patients with Child-Turcotte-Pugh (CTP) score of A, B, and C, and their spouse were first compared using high-throughput approach based on denaturing polyacrylamide gel electrophoresis and liquid chromatography–tandem mass spectrometry in our study.

Results: A total of 5,020 proteins (88 % from bacteria, 12 % form human) were identified and annotated based on the GO and KEGG classification. Our results indicated that the LC patients possessed a core metaproteome including 119 proteins, among which 14 proteins were enhanced expressed and 7 proteins were unique for LC patients compared with the normal, which were dominant at the function of carbohydrate metabolism. In addition, LC patients have unique biosynthesis of branched chain amino acid (BCAA), pantothenate, and CoA, enhanced as CTP scores increased. Those three substances were all important in a wide array of key and essential biological roles of life.

Conclusions: We observed a highly comparable cirrhosis-specific metaproteome clustering of fecal microbiota and provided the first supportive evidence for the presence of a LC-related substantial functional core mainly involved in carbohydrate, BCAA, pantothenate, and CoA metabolism, suggesting the compensation of intestinal microbiota for the fragile and innutritious body of cirrhotic patients.

Keywords: Cirrhosis, Metaproteome, Fecal microbiota, BCAA,

Background

Human intestinal tract is colonized by a complex and intimate microbial community that is maintained from early to late adulthood [1]. Human intestinal microbiota was an important organ which has been neglected for a long time. A lot of evidence has suggested that intestinal microbiota works as a whole and plays an important role in human health [2].

Cirrhosis is a condition in which the liver failed to work properly due to long-term damage. The anatomy and physiological functions of liver and intestinal microbiota share a close relationship as a result of enterohepatic circulation. As the cirrhosis worsen, it was usually accompanied with intestinal inflammation, which may affect the prognosis significantly [3]. Previous studies had revealed the important influence of gut microbiota dysbiosis on the complications of advanced liver cirrhosis (such as spontaneous bacterial peritonitis and hepatic encephalopathy) [4] and on the induction and progress of liver damage at early cirrhosis (such as alcoholic hepatitis and nonalcoholic fatty liver disease) [5]. It has been identified that extensive differences in the microbiota community and metabolic potential existed in the fecal microbiota of cirrhotic patients, and the prevalence of

* Correspondence: yuanjing6216@163.com; sunys@qq.com
[1]Institute of Disease Control and Prevention, Academy of Military Medical Sciences, No. 20 Dongda Street, Fengtai District, 100071 Beijing, China
Full list of author information is available at the end of the article

potentially pathogenic bacteria, such as *Enterobacteria-ceae* and *Streptococcaceae*, with the reduction of beneficial populations such as *Lachnospiraceae* in patients with cirrhosis may affect prognosis [3, 6]. In addition, The functional diversity was significantly reduced in the fecal microbiota of cirrhotic patients compared with in the controls. At the module or pathway levels, the fecal microbiota of the HBLC patients showed enrichment in the metabolism of glutathione, branched-chain amino acid, nitrogen, and lipid, whereas there was a decrease in the level of aromatic amino acid, bile acid and cell cycle related metabolism [3]. These high-throughput analyses lay the groundwork for predicting the protein potential of the intestinal microbiota. However, the functional and metabolic associations between intestinal microbiota and cirrhosis in humans are still lacking.

The rapidly increasing catalogue of proteins from intestinal origin provides a platform for high-throughput functional characterization [7]. In the past 20 years, more and more interests were focused on fecal microbiota, partly due to the fast emerging sequencing technique. Given that proteins are much more actual and stable, proteome-based analyses can be expected to provide a more accurate and real view of the functionality of the intestinal microbiota. The LC-MS/MS method has a higher level of proteome coverage, and is more efficient and accurate to analyze differential global protein expression quantitatively and qualitatively. So far there have been several reports related with the use of metaproteomics to characterize complex bacterial ecosystems [8, 9]. 2015, Hernández E et al. collected intestinal microbiota proteins from two adult patients receiving 14-days β-lactam therapy, seven obese and five lean adolescents, followed by metaproteome measurements, to assess the functional differences and metabolic effects in human gastrointestinal tract related with antibiotic treatment and obesity [10]. 2012, Pérez-Cobas AE carried out the multi-omic research on fecal samples from one patient subjected to a β-lactam intravenous therapy, which suggested that antibiotics may ultimately alter the energy metabolism balance in human gastrointestinal tract [11]. 2012, faecal samples were collected from 3 healthy female subjects over a period of six to twelve months to research the composition and stability of human intestinal metaproteome [12]. 2006, Klaassens ES et al. collected fecal samples from two infants at different ages to characterize the complex intestinal bacterial structure, and illustrated the feasibility of metaproteomic approach in analyzing complex mciroecosystem [13].

In this work, human intestinal microbiota was regarded as a whole to analyze. A high-throughput LC-MS/MS measurement were used to detect the metaproteomic changes in the intestinal microbiota of LC patients. This is the first culture-independent metaproteomic analysis in the gastrointestinal tract from cirrhotic patients.

Our findings may provide a more comprehensive understanding of fecal microbiota in patients with cirrhosis, and generate novel perspectives on the progress and prognosis of cirrhosis.

Methods
Fecal samples
The Child-Turcotte-Pugh (CTP) scoring system was used to assess the severity of cirrhosis. Three LC patients (CTP score of A, B, C) and their corresponding spouse, in the age range of 50–60 and with a body mass index (BMI) = 18.5–24.9 kg m^{-2}, were enrolled in this study. Cirrhosis was diagnosed according to the gold standard of biopsy in all patients. Cases that had other complications (such as peritonitis or hepatic encephalopathy) were excluded in this study. All healthy individuals had normal liver biochemistry test results with no evidence of hepatic or other diseases. None of the subjects had food preferences, or received antibiotics, probiotics, steroids or other hormones (including oral, intramuscular or intravenous injection) for at least 3 months before enrolment. Each object was asked to provide a fresh stool sample, which were subjected to metaproteome extraction immediately. This study was approved by the Institutional Review Board of Affiliated Hospital of Academy of Military Medical Sciences. All participants signed an informed consent form prior to entering the study. The study conformed to the ethical guidelines of the 1975 Declaration of Helsinki.

Protein extraction
Faecal samples were resuspended in PBS and vortexed to homogenize the sample. Proteins were precipitated in pre-chilled TCA (trichloroacetic acid)-acetone (50 g TCA dissolved in 500 ml acetone) at -20 °C for 2 h. After centrifugation at 20,000 × g for 30 min, the protein pellet was washed with pre-chilled acetone and ultrasonicated in lysis buffer (8 M urea, 30 mM HEPES (4-(2-Hydroxyethyl)-1-piperazineethanesulfonic acid), 1 mM PMSF (Phenylmethanesulfonyl fluoride), 2 mM EDTA (Ethylene Diamine Tetraacetie Acid), 10 mM DTT (DL-Dithiothreitol)). After centrifugation at 20,000 × g for 30 min, the supernatant were reduced with 10 mM DTT at 56 °C for 1 h, and alkylated with 55 mM IAM (iodoacetamide) at room temperature for 1 h in the dark. The treated proteins were precipitated in pre-chilled acetone at −20 °C for 3 h. After centrifugation at 20,000 × g for 30 min, the protein pellet was resuspended and ultrasonicated in pre-cooled 50 % TEAB (tetraethylammonium bromide) buffer with 0.1 % SDS, and then centrifuged at 20,000 × g to pellet the undissolved substance. The protein concentrations were measured by Bradford assay.

1 D gel electrophoresis and in-gel protein digestion

To reduce the complexity of the protein extract, a 1D gel fractionation according to molecular weight was carried out. Equal volumes of protein solutions were mixed with 4 × Laemmli buffer and Biorad reducing agent and run on NuPAGE 4–12 % Bis-Tris gels (Invitrogen) at a constant voltage of 80 V for 20 min followed by 200 V for 30 min. Gels were stained with PageBlue (Fermentas). Gel pieces were washed and proteins reduced, alkylated and tryptically digested overnight as described previously [14].

LC-MS/MS measurements

Peptide samples were analyzed by LC-MS/MS on a quadrupole-Orbitrap mass spectrometer (Q-Exactive; Thermo Fisher, Germany) equipped with a 15 cm (length) by 75 μm (inside diameter) column packed with 5 μm C18 medium (150A, Thermo Fisher) which was remained at 21 °C throughout the analysis. Mobile phase A was MilliQ water with 0.1 % (v/v) formic acid. Mobile phase B was 99.9 % (v/v) acetonitrile and 0.1 % acetic acid. Gradient was run from 0 % B to 30 % B over 40 min and then to 80 % B for 15 min. An electrospray voltage of 1.8 kV was applied. By data-dependent acquisition, the mass spectrometer was programmed to acquire tandem mass spectra from the top 20 ions in the full scan from 350 to 2,000 m/z. Dynamic exclusion was set to 15 s, singly charged ions were excluded, the isolation width was set to 2 m/z. The full MS resolution was set to 70,000, and the MS/MS resolution to 17,500. Normalized collision energy was set to 28, automatic gain control to 1e6, maximum fill MS to 20 ms, maximum fill MS/MS to 60 ms, and the under fill ratio to 0.1 %. Each sample was repeated triply.

Protein identificaton

Peptide identification were performed using Mascot v2.3.01 (Matrix Science Ltd.) (http://www.matrixscience.com) licensed in-house (http://www.proteomics.cn) [15]. Monoisotopic peptide masses were used to search the databases, allowing a peptide mass accuracy of 30 ppm and fragment ion tolerance of 0.2 Dalton. Both methionine oxidation and cysteine carboxyamidomethylation were considered in the process. For protein identification, peptide masses were searched against the publically available database for Uniprot-Human database and Uniprot-Bacteria database. For unambiguous identification of proteins, more than five peptides must be matched and the sequence coverage must be greater than 15 %.

Bioinformatic analysis

Microbial proteins which had at least one peptide identification in each individual were defined. Functional classification of identified proteins was performed by BLASTPGP [16] searching against the databases of Cluster of Orthologous Groups database (COGs, ftp://ftp.ncbi.nih.gov/pub/COG/COG2014/static/lists/listCOGs.html) [17]. The COG associated with the best BLAST hit (≤1E-10 cutoff) was assigned to the query protein. The identified COGs were mapped on the KEGG metabolic pathways and visualized with the online application of iPath [18]. The spectra those proteins were identified with were taken to sum on COG level per all measurements and were used to rank the COGs according to spectra number. Sequences which did not hit any specific COG were subjected to BLAST search against the NCBI non-redundant database. The cellular localizations of the proteins were predicted by PSORTb version 3.0 [19]. Prediction of signal peptides was carried out with SignalP Version 4.1 [20]. The metaproteomic data from three LC patients (CTP score of A, B, C) were compared with their corresponding spouse, respectively.

Results

Identification of proteins and metabolic pathways in the fecal metaproteome

Three LC patients with CTP score of A, B, C (coded as AP, BP, CP) and their corresponding spouse (coded as AN, BN, CN) were enrolled in this study. Characteristics of the subjects were given in Table 1. Unprocessed fecal material from those subjects were used not only to

Table 1 Characteristics of the patients and controls

Terms	AP	AN	BP	BN	CP	CN
Age	52	50	59	56	51	50
Gender	Male	Female	Male	Female	Male	Female
BMI index	24.1	24.3	25.3	25.1	24.9	25.0
Total bilirubin (μmol/L)	6.6	—	11.8	—	36.3	—
Albumin (g/L)	37.1	—	30.5	—	26.2	—
Stage of hepatic encephalopathy	0	—	0	—	1	—
Ascites degree	No	—	Moderate	—	Severe	—
Prothrombin time prolonged (seconds)	0	—	2	—	2.1	—
CTP	A	—	B	—	C	—

reappear the intestinal microbial proteome characteristics, but also to allow detection of human proteins. Fecal metaproteome were extracted and subjected to 1D-gel (Fig. 1a). A total of over 100,000 spectra were generated by the collection of LC-MS/MS. The raw data has been uploaded to the public websites (http://www.iprox.org/my/index, user ID: reviewer 719, password: 6s6kd6lp). In this study, a total of 5,020 proteins were identified with two or more peptide identifications, including 4,401 (88 %) from bacteria proteins and 619 (12 %) from human proteins (Fig. 1b). Results from the annotation to Uniprot-Bacteria database suggested that almost equal and 600 proteins were identified from AP and AN, and 1100 and 1102 proteins identified from BP and CP respectively, almost twice more than their controls. Results of the fecal metaproteome assigned to Uniprot-Human database suggested a relatively stable expression and an average of 100 proteins were identified from each sample (Fig. 1c). Annotation results of bacterial proteins and human proteins from each sample were shown in Additional file 1: Table S1 and Additional file 2: Table S2. To retrieve further functional information, we annotated these proteins based on the GO and KEGG classification and the overall number of proteins identified were shown in Table 2.

Core metaproteome specific for LC patients

To obtain the LC-related common microbial core proteome, we selected proteins that were found in all the three patients. A total of 119 proteins fulfilled this criterion and their description and functional characteristics were shown in Additional file 3: Table S3. The common and core metaproteome could be grouped into 18 COGs and the most predominant functional categories were J (translation), G (carbohydrate transport and metabolism), C (energy production and conversion), F (nucleotide transport and metabolism), and E (amino acid transport and metabolism) (Fig. 2). Nearly 19 % proteins could be assigned to carbohydrate transport and metabolism, and 8 % assigned to amino acid transport and metabolism, reflecting the high metabolic activity of the intestinal microbiota from LC patients. Among those 119 core proteins, 14 proteins enhanced their expression levels and 7 proteins were specific for LC patients compared with the normal, which were described as below.

Differential fecal microbial metabolism and proteins in LC patients

Fourteen KEGG pathway maps were detected to have different metabolic capacities in the fecal microbiota between

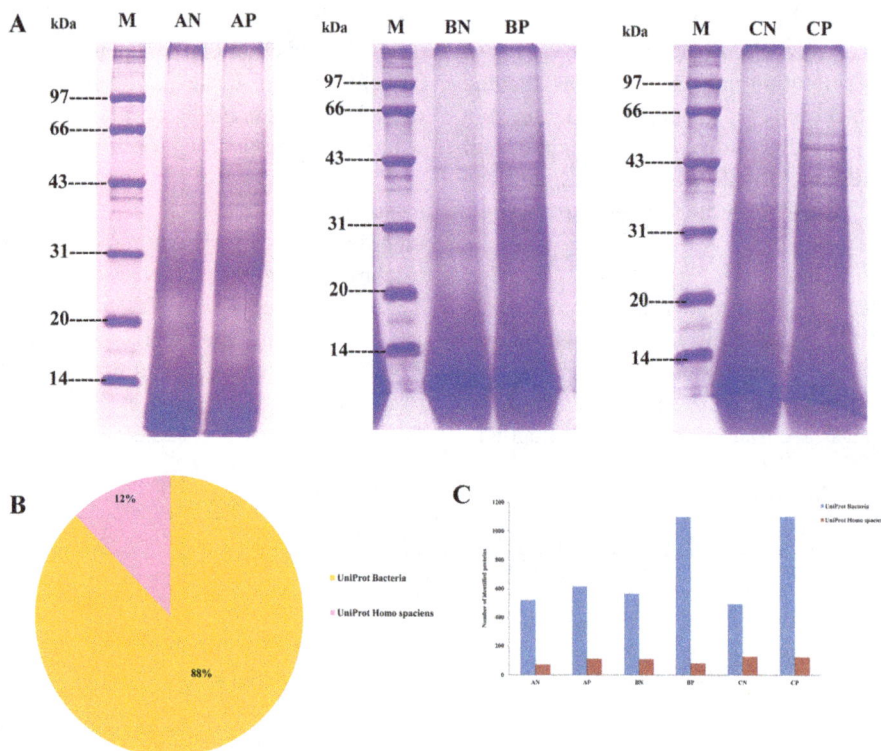

Fig. 1 Electrophoresis maps and annotation results of the fecal metaproteome from six subjects. a The 1D-gel showing the protein pattern from fecal metaproteome of six subjects. b Proportion of proteins allocated to uniprot-bacteria and uniprot-human databases. In this study, a total of 5,020 proteins were identified with two or more peptide identifications, in which 88 % from bacteria proteins and 12 % from human proteins. c Number of proteins allocated to uniprot-bacteria and uniprot-human databases in each sample

Table 2 Overall number of proteins identified from patients and the normal

	Uniprot-Bacteria		Uniprot-Human	
	Patients	Normal	Patients	Normal
Total Protein Number	2,819	1,582	314	305
GO (Cellular Component)				
Number of GO[a]	93	81	171	190
Number of Proteins[b]	1,213	594	87	98
GO (Biological Process)				
Number of GO[a]	1,004	781	867	1,082
Number of Proteins[b]	1,890	954	75	92
GO (Molecular Function)				
Number of GO[a]	861	596	230	248
Number of Proteins[b]	2,173	1,092	91	110
KEGG				
Number of KEGG[a]	127	100	106	123
Number of Proteins[b]	1,697	865	80	80

[a]Number of GO terms or KEGG pathways identified
[b]Number of proteins identified and assigned to corresponding GO terms or KEGG pathways

patients and the normal, including eleven pathways enhanced and three pathways weakened in patients (Additional file 4: Table S4). In the same metabolic pathway, different proteins were identified in different samples, suggesting that the intestinal microbiota have abundant species diversity and protein complexity. In five metabolic pathways, we detected same proteins in different samples, most of which were assigned to carbohydrate metabolism. One of the most predominant pathways was glycolysis/gluconeogenesis, showing high redundancies among microbiota; all the glycolytic/gluconeogenic enzymes could be identified in patients, highlighting the enhanced material metabolism capacity in intestinal microbiota of LC patients.

Fourteen proteins were detected to have enhanced expression level in all the three patients compared with the normal (Table 3), which could be grouped into four COGs (J: Translation, G: Carbohydrate transport and metabolism, E: Amino acid transport and metabolism, O: Posttranslational modification, protein turnover, chaperones), suggesting the enhanced material transport and metabolism function in fecal microbiota from LC patients.

Compatible with the important sugar degradation potential of the gut microbiota, various proteins involved in carbohydrate transport and metabolism were identified and enhanced in patients, including transketolase, transaldolase, xylose isomerase, and glyceraldehyde

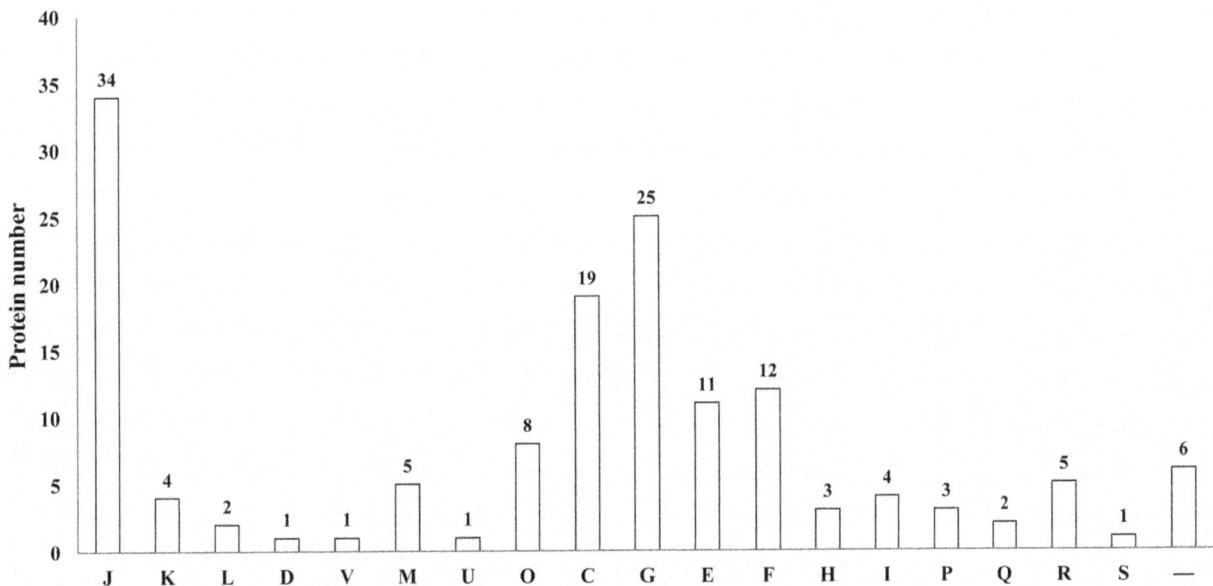

Fig. 2 Functional category of the common and core metaproteome from LC patients. The common and core metaproteome could be grouped into 19 COGs and the most predominant functional categories were J, G, C, F, and E. Categories were taken from the TIGR-CMR (www.tigr.org) and the abbreviation was used to mark the categories. J, translation; K, transcription; L, replication, recombination, and repair; D, cell cycle control, mitosis, and meiosis; V, defense mechanisms; M, cell wall/membrane biogenesis; U, intracellular trafficking and secretion; O, post-translational modification, protein turnover, chaperones; C, energy production and conversion; G, carbohydrate transport and metabolism; E, amino acid transport and metabolism; F, nucleotide transport and metabolism; H, coenzyme transport and metabolism; I, lipid transport and metabolism; P, inorganic ion transport and metabolism; Q, secondary metabolite biosynthesis, transport, and catabolism; R, general function prediction only; S, function unknown; —, not in Clusters of Orthologous Groups (COG)

Table 3 Characteristics of proteins with enhanced expression level in the fecal microbiota from LC patients or specific for patients' intestinal microbiota compared with the normal

Proteins with enhanced expression level in the fecal microbiota from LC patients

No.	Description	Gene name	Length	MW [Da]	KO	COG	Subcellular location	Signal peptide prediction	GO	Functonal Category[a]
1	Chaperone protein DnaK	dnaK	620	66,266	k04043	COG0443	Cytoplasmic	Absence	GO:0006457 GO:0000166 GO:0005524 GO:0051082	O
2	Glutamate dehydrogenase	proS	604	66,842	k01881	COG0442	Cytoplasmic	Absence	GO:0006520 GO:0055114 GO:0016491 GO:0016639	J
3	Elongation factor G	fusA	709	78,383	k02355	COG0480	Cytoplasmic	Absence	GO:0006412 GO:0006414 GO:0000166 GO:0003746 GO:0003924 GO:0005525 GO:0005622 GO:0005737	J
4	Transketolase	tkt	702	75,877	k00615	COG0021	Cytoplasmic	Absence	GO:0008152 GO:0003824 GO:0004802 GO:0016740 GO:0046872	G
5	50S ribosomal protein L25	rplY	206	21,815	k02897.	COG1825	Cytoplasmic	Absence	GO:0006412 GO:0003723 GO:0003735 GO:0008097 GO:0019843 GO:0005840 GO:0030529	J
6	Glyceraldehyde 3-phosphate dehydrogenase	BMOU_0196	351	37,881	—	—	Cytoplasmic	Absence	GO:0006006 GO:0055114 GO:0016491 GO:0016620 GO:0050661 GO:0051287	—
7	Glycine-tRNA ligase	glyQS	446	52,295	k01880	COG0423	Cytoplasmic	Absence	GO:0006412 GO:0006418 GO:0006426 GO:0000166 GO:0004812 GO:0004820 GO:0005524	J

Table 3 Characteristics of proteins with enhanced expression level in the fecal microbiota from LC patients or specific for patients' intestinal microbiota compared with the normal (*Continued*)

No.	Protein	Gene			KO	COG	Location		GO	
8	60 kDa chaperonin	groL	541	56,837	k04077	COG0459	Cytoplasmic	Absence	GO:0016874 GO:0046983 GO:0005737	O
9	Elongation factor Tu	tuf	399	43,936	k02358.	COG0050	Cytoplasmic	Absence	GO:0006412 GO:0006414 GO:0000166 GO:0003746 GO:0003924 GO:0005525 GO:0005622 GO:0005737	J
10	Xylose isomerase	xylA	449	50,765	k01805	COG2115	Cytoplasmic	Absence	GO:0005975 GO:0006098 GO:0042732 GO:0000287 GO:0009045 GO:0016853 GO:0046872 GO:0005737	G
11	ABC transporter substrate-binding protein	BBPC_1795	430	47,488	K10117	COG1653	Cytoplasmic	Absence	GO:0006810 GO:0005215	G
12	Elongation factor Ts	tsf	283	29,835	k02357	COG0264	Cytoplasmic	Absence	GO:0006412 GO:0006414 GO:0003746 GO:0005622 GO:0005737	J
13	Transaldolase	tal	367	39,871	k00616	COG0176	Cytoplasmic	Absence	GO:0005975 GO:0006098 GO:0003824 GO:0004801 GO:0016740 GO:0005737	G
14	ABC transporter substrate-binding protein	BBPC_1231	550	59,251	K15580	COG4166	Cytoplasmic	Absence	GO:0055085 GO:0043190	E

Table 3 Characteristics of proteins with enhanced expression level in the fecal microbiota from LC patients or specific for patients' intestinal microbiota compared with the normal *(Continued)*

Proteins specific for patients' intestinal microbiota compared with the normal

1	Ketol-acid reductoisomerase	ilvC	350	38,768	—	—	Cytoplasmic	Absence	GO:0008652, GO:0009082, GO:0009097, GO:0009099, GO:0055114, GO:0004455, GO:0016491, GO:0016853	—
2	Phosphoglycerate kinase	pgp	401	41,995	K00927	COG0126	Cytoplasmic	Absence	GO:0006096, GO:0016310, GO:0000166, GO:0004618, GO:0005524, GO:0016301, GO:0016740, GO:0005737	G
3	50S ribosomal protein L4	rplD	221	23,761	K02926	COG0088	Unknown	Absence	GO:0006412, GO:0003723, GO:0003735, GO:0019843, GO:0005840, GO:0030529	J
4	Ribose-phosphate pyrophosphokinase	prs	337	36,843	K00948	COG0462	Cytoplasmic	Absence	GO:0006015, GO:0009165, GO:0016310, GO:0000166, GO:0000287, GO:0004749, GO:0005524, GO:0016301, GO:0016740, GO:0046872, GO:0005737	F E
5	Probable thiol peroxidase	tpx	171	18,391	K11065	COG2077	Periplasmic	Absence	GO:0005623, GO:0045454, GO:0055114, GO:0098869, GO:0004601, GO:0008379, GO:0016209, GO:0016491, GO:0016684, GO:0005623	O

Table 3 Characteristics of proteins with enhanced expression level in the fecal microbiota from LC patients or specific for patients' intestinal microbiota compared with the normal (Continued)

6	30S ribosomal protein S4	rpsD	208	23,719	K02986	COG0522	Cytoplasmic	Absence	GO:0006412 GO:0003723 GO:0003735 GO:0019843 GO:0005622 GO:0005840 GO:0015935 GO:0030529	J
7	50S ribosomal protein L3	rplC	213	22,687	K02906	COG0087	Cytoplasmic	Absence	GO:0006412 GO:0003723 GO:0003735 GO:0019843 GO:0005622 GO:0005840 GO:0030529	J

[a]Categories were taken from the TIGR-CMR (www.tigr.org) and the abbreviation was used to mark the categories. J Translation, O Posttranslational modification, protein turnover, chaperones, G Carbohydrate transport and metabolism, E Amino acid transport and metabolism, F Nucleotide transport and metabolism; —: not in COGs

3-phosphate dehydrogenase, which were grouped into the KEGG pathway of map 00030 (Pentose phosphate pathway), map 00040 (Pentose and glucuronate interconversions), map 00051 (Fructose and mannose metabolism), map 00010 (Glycolysis/Gluconeogenesis), as well as map 01110 (Biosynthesis of secondary metabolites). The abundance of bacterial proteins devoted to the utilization of carbohydrates testified for their importance as metabolic substrates in the intestinal tract.

The most significantly differential protein was glyceraldehyde 3-phosphate dehydrogenase (EC1.2.1.12), which catalyzes the oxidative phosphorylation of glyceraldehyde 3-phosphate (G3P) to 1,3-bisphosphoglycerate (BPG) using the cofactor NAD. This protein is involved in step 1 of the subpathway, part of carbohydrate degradation and glycolysis pathway, that synthesizes pyruvate from D-glyceraldehyde 3-phosphate. 3-phosphoglycerate kinase assists in the transformation of 3-phospho-D-glycerate to 3phospho-D-glyceroyl phosphate by consumption of ATP.

Another significantly differential protein was glutamate dehydrogenase (GDH). Moreover, detailed analysis of these peptides revealed GDH to show a high level of redundancy in the intestinal tract since we could identify it as a major protein in a large variety of bacterial families, including *Bacteroidaceae*, *Streptococcaceae*, *Ruminococcaceae* and *Bifidobacteriaceae* (Additional file 1: Table S1). It is known that GDH not only links the nitrogen and the carbon-cycle via the incorporation of ammonia into 2-ketoglutarate, but also have another metabolic role and act as an electron sink [12]. This pathway, which operates in several strict anaerobes to assure a low level of free electrons, resulting in the net conversion of pyruvate and ammonia into alanine while consuming NAD(P)H that can be generated via a ferredoxin NAPDH oxidoreductase [12]. This potential role of intestinal GDH as an electron sink requires the activity of aminotransferases, many of which were identified in the metaproteome, including branched-chain amino acid aminotransferase, aminotransferase class-V family protein, phosphoserine aminotransferase, taurine–pyruvate aminotransferase, aspartate/tyrosine/aromatic aminotransferase, glucosamine–fructose-6-phosphate aminotransferase, acetylornithine aminotransferase, N-succinyldiaminopimelate aminotransferase, histidinol-phosphate aminotransferase, 4-aminobutyrate aminotransferase, which were all specially enhanced in BP and CP patients.

Unique fecal microbial proteins and metabolism for LC patients

To identify the fecal microbiota proteins specific for patients, we selected proteins that were found only in all the three patients but absent in the normal. A total of seven proteins fulfill the criterion. Charicteristics of

unique fecal microbial proteins for LC patients were shown in Table 3.

Additionally, Two KEGG pathways, map 00290 (Valine, leucine and isoleucine biosynthesis) and map 00770 (Pantothenate and CoA biosynthesis) were common in the fecal microbiota from the three patients and absent in normal. As the patients' condition worse, the number of specific enzymes from the two metabolic pathways were remarkably increased, and the metabolic pathways were enhanced. In patient CP, the specific enzymes from map 00290 and map 00770 were almost covered the whole metabolic pathway (Fig. 3). LC patients have an enhanced function of branched-chain amino acid (BCAA) and vitamin metabolism, which were in accordance with the metagenomic results from Wei [21].

The most unique enzymes detected were ketol-acid reductoisomerase (EC 1.1.1.86) and dihydroxy-acid dehydratase (EC 4.2.1.9). Degradation of BCAA involved the branched-chain alpha-keto acid dehydrogenase complex. Those two enzymes were both important in the KEGG pathways of map 00290 and map 00770 and have the protein interactions of neighborhood and coexpression.

Ketol-acid reductoisomerase (EC 1.1.1.86), specific in fecal microbiota from patients, were key enzyme from metabolic pathway of valine, leucine and isoleucine biosynthesis and pantothenate and CoA biosynthesis. This enzyme can catalyse the reduction of 2-ethyl-2-hydroxy-3-oxobutanoate to 2,3-dihydroxy-3-methylpentanoate. This protein is involved in step 2 of the subpathway that synthesizes L-valine from pyruvate and L-isoleucine from 2-oxobutanoate, which are part of the pathway of L-valine biosynthesis and L-isoleucine biosynthesis, respectively. The chemical reactions and pathways resulting in the formation of valine, 2-amino-3-methylbutanoic acid and isoleucine, (2R*, 3R*)-2-amino-3-methylpentanoic acid. In addition, this enzyme is involved in step 2 of the subpathway that synthesizes patothenate from pyruvate, which are part of the pathway of Pantothenate and CoA biosynthesis.

Dihydroxy-acid dehydratase (EC 4.2.1.9), specific in the fecal microbiota from BP and CP, catalyzes third step in the common pathway leading to biosynthesis of branched-chain amino acids and is important in the KEGG pathway of map 00290 and map 00770. This protein is involved in step 3 of the subpathway that synthesizes L-isoleucine from 2-oxobutanoate and L-valine from pyruvate, which are part of the pathway of L-valine biosynthesis and L-isoleucine biosynthesis, respectively.

Branched-chain-amino-acid transaminase (EC 2.6.1.42), specific in the fecal microbiota from BP and CP, belongs to the class-IV pyridoxal-phosphate-dependent aminotransferase family. Branched-chain-amino-acid transaminase can catalyze the transfer of an alpha-amino group from an amino acid to an alpha-keto acid leading to

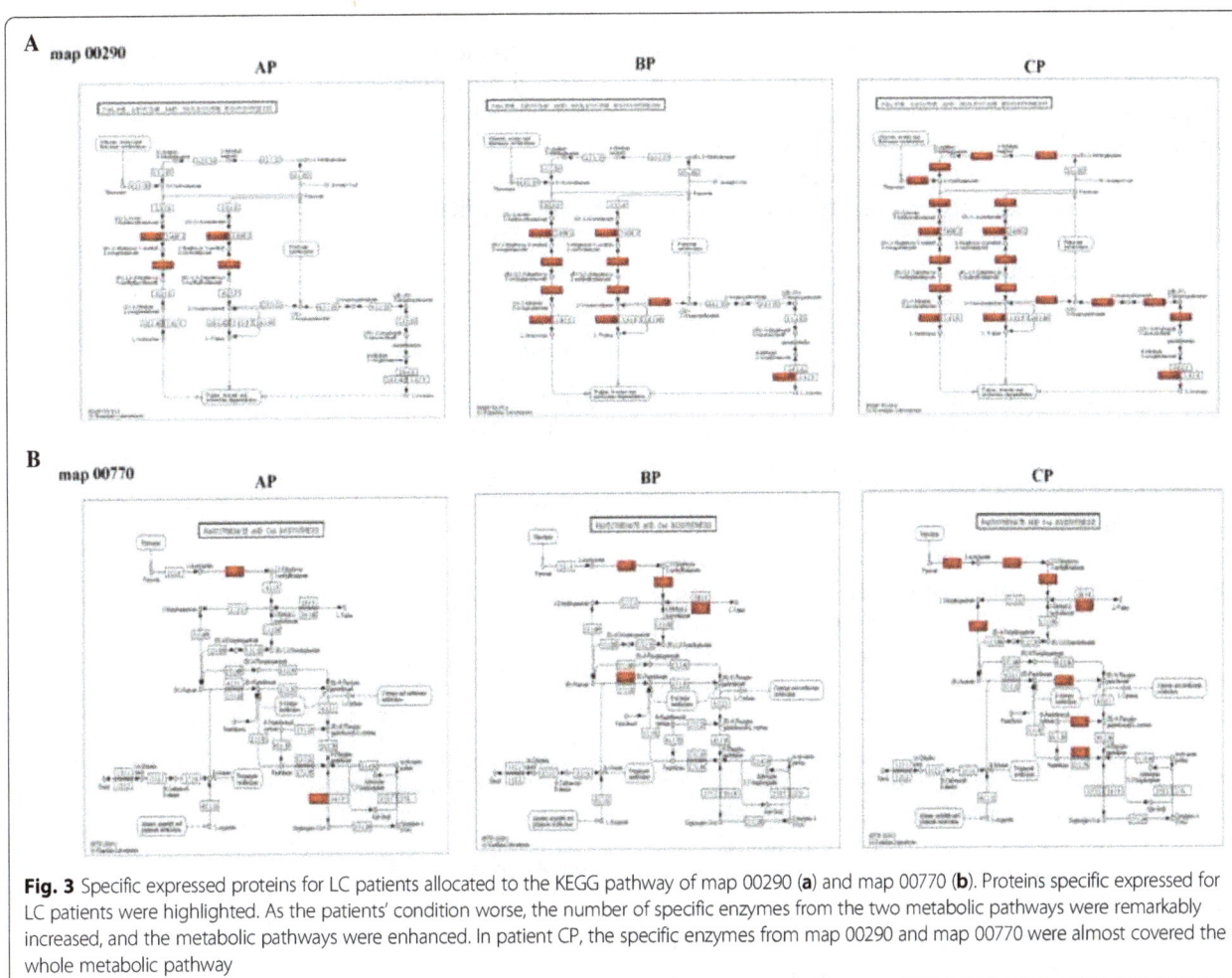

Fig. 3 Specific expressed proteins for LC patients allocated to the KEGG pathway of map 00290 (**a**) and map 00770 (**b**). Proteins specific expressed for LC patients were highlighted. As the patients' condition worse, the number of specific enzymes from the two metabolic pathways were remarkably increased, and the metabolic pathways were enhanced. In patient CP, the specific enzymes from map 00290 and map 00770 were almost covered the whole metabolic pathway

biosynthesis of branched-chain amino acids and is important in the KEGG pathway of map 00290 and map 00770. The amino group is usually covalently bound by the prosthetic group pyridoxal phosphate.

Non-bacterial proteins

The vast majority of the identified proteins, approximately 87.7 %, were of microbial origin. Moreover, in total, 619 human proteins, excluding possible contaminants [22], were identified as representing host cell activity along the digestive tract. In general, the identified human proteins were mostly involved in carbohydrates and proteins digestion, maintaining mucosal barrier function, and providing energy resources for intestinal microbes.

Discussion

In any microbiome environment, expression of microbiota proteins were all closely affected by the microenvironment and bacteria-host interactions [23]. However, culture-based research was unable to reappear the real condition of microbiome in the environment and the insufficient microbiome sequence information confounded identification of the proteins [12]. Currently, people were focusing more and more interests on metaproteomics approaches to monitor the disease related functional products of the microbiota [13], and the ongoing protein library analysis enabled meaningful identification in time [2, 24]. For the first time, extraction of metaproteome from LC patients and tentative identification using LC-MS/MS were carried out in this study. To retrieve further functional information, we annotated these proteins based on the GO and KEGG classification and analyzed the characteristic of the intestinal microbiota from LC patients at the expression level.

As revealed by the protein identification searched against the publically available database for Uniprot-Bacteria database, nearly equal proteins were identified from AP and AN, however, almost twice proteins were identified from BP and CP compared with the normal, implying that as the disease processed, the changes in intestinal microenvironment caused by cirrhosis compelled fecal microbiota to enhance their growth activity and protein expression to survival.

A LC-related core metapoteome including 119 proteins was described in this study. Majority of the proteins could be assigned to carbohydrate and amino acid transport and metabolism, reflecting the active metabolic ability of the intestinal microbiota from LC patients. Among those 119 core proteins, 14 proteins, involved in carbohydrate transport and metabolism, enhanced their expression levels in the fecal microbiota from LC patients, which further illustrated that human gut bacteria encountered a broad spectrum of carbohydrate substrates.

Fourteen KEGG pathway maps were detected to have different metabolic capacities in the fecal microbiota between patients and the normal, including eleven pathways enhanced and three pathways weakened in patients. In the same metabolic pathway, different proteins were identified in different samples, suggesting the abundant species diversity and protein complexcity, that is why we got rid of species boundaries and regarded fecal microbiota as a whole in this study.

Seven proteins were identified as the unique fecal microbial proteins for LC patients compared with the normal. Correspondingly, two KEGG pathways, map 00290 (Valine, leucine and isoleucine biosynthesis) and map 00770 (Pantothenate and CoA biosynthesis), were unique in the fecal microbiota from LC patients. More interestingly, as the patients' condition worse, the patients-specific enzymes were almost covered the whole metabolic pathway. Valine, leucine and isoleucine were all BCAA, which were among the nine essential amino acids for humans. Pantothenate was an essential nutrient for human and used to synthesize CoA, as well as to synthesize and metabolize proteins, carbohydrates, and fats. Pantothenate, in the form of CoA, is also required for acylation and acetylation, which, for example, are involved in signal transduction and enzyme activation and deactivation, respectively [25, 26]. CoA was important in energy metabolism for pyruvate to enter the TCA cycle as acetyl-CoA, and for α-ketoglutarate to be transformed to succinyl-CoA in the cycle, as well as in the biosynthesis of many important compounds such as fatty acids, cholesterol, and acetylcholine [26]. BCAA and pantothenate were both important in a wide array of key biological roles. LC patients were weak fitness and as a result the peripheral tissues need to increase their consumption of a variety of nutrients including carbohydrates, BCAA and vitamins. The specific expression of bacterial proteins devoted to map 00290 and map 00770 testified the compensation for the fragile health and need for nutrition.

Conclusions

Altogether, we observed a first and highly comparable cirrhosis-specific metaproteome clustering of fecal microbiota. Our findings provided a supportive evidence for the presence of a LC-related substantial metaproteome core which enhanced the expression level involved in sugar transport and degradation, as well as BCAA, pantothenate and CoA biosynthesis. Our results suggested that the fecal microbiota not only had strong adaptability to the intestinal microenvironment, but also could compensate for the fragile and innutritious body of cirrhotic patients.

Additional files

Additional file 1: Table S1. Protein identification with peptide masses searched against the publically available database for Uniprot-Bacteria database.

Additional file 2: Table S2. Protein identification with peptide masses searched against the publically available database for Uniprot-Human database.

Additional file 3: Table S3. Core metaproteome of intestinal microbiota from LC patients.

Additional file 4: Table S4. Fourteen KEGG pathway maps detected to have different metabolic capacities in the fecal microbiota between patients and the normal.

Abbreviations

BCAA: Branched-chain amino acid; BMI: Body mass index; CTP: Child-Turcotte-Pugh; DTT: DL-Dithiothreitol; EDTA: Ethylene Diamine Tetraacetie Acid; G3P: Glyceraldehyde 3-phosphate; GDH: Glutamate dehydrogenase; HEPES: 4-(2-Hydroxyethyl)-1-piperazineethanesulfonic acid; IAM: Iodoacetamide; LC: Liver cirrhosis; PMSF: Phenylmethanesulfonyl fluoride; TCA: Trichloroacetic acid; TEAB: Tetraethylammonium bromide

Acknowledgements
Not applicable.

Funding
This work was supported by a grant from the National Natural Science Foundation of China (81400592) to X.W. and (31370093) to J.Y., Mega-projects of Science and Technology Research of China (Grant 2011ZX10004-001), the German Academic Exchange Service/Federal Ministry of Education and Research to C.U.R (Grant D/09/04778), and a grant from the National High Technology Research and Development Program of China (863 Program; grant no. SS2014AA022210).

Authors' contributions
YS, JY, and XW designed research; XW, SJ, HL, and WL performed research; XW, SW, BL, and XZ contributed new reagents or analytic tools; XW, SJ, and YC analyzed data; XW, YC, and YS wrote the paper. All authors read and approved the final manuscript.

Competing interests
The authors declare that they have no competing interests.

Consent for publication
All authors approve to publish this paper on BMC gastroenterology.

Author details
[1]Institute of Disease Control and Prevention, Academy of Military Medical Sciences, No. 20 Dongda Street, Fengtai District, 100071 Beijing, China. [2]Hospital of Traditional Chinese Medicine, Liquan 713200, Shanxi, China.

References

1. Turnbaugh PJ, Ley RE, Hamady M, Fraser-Liggett CM, Knight R, Gordon JI. The human microbiome project. Nature. 2007;449:804–10.
2. Gill SR, Pop M, Deboy RT, Eckburg PB, Turnbaugh PJ, Samuel BS, et al. Metagenomic analysis of the human distal gut microbiome. Science. 2006;312:1355–9.
3. Usami M, Miyoshi M, Yamashita H. Gut microbiota and host metabolism in liver cirrhosis. World J Gastroenterol. 2015;21:11597–608.
4. Garcia-Tsao G, Wiest R. Gut microflora in the pathogenesis of the complications of cirrhosis. Best Pract Res Clin Gastroenterol. 2004;18:353–72.
5. Benten D, Wiest R. Gut microbiome and intestinal barrier failure–the "Achilles heel" in hepatology? J Hepatol. 2012;56:1221–3.
6. Chen Y, Yang F, Lu H, Wang B, Chen Y, Lei D, et al. Characterization of fecal microbial communities in patients with liver cirrhosis. Hepatol Baltim Md. 2011;54:562–72.
7. Zoetendal EG, Rajilic-Stojanovic M, de Vos WM. High-throughput diversity and functionality analysis of the gastrointestinal tract microbiota. Gut. 2008;57:1605–15.
8. Ram RJ, Verberkmoes NC, Thelen MP, Tyson GW, Baker BJ, Blake RC, et al. Community proteomics of a natural microbial biofilm. Science. 2005;308:1915–20.
9. Wilmes P, Bond PL. The application of two-dimensional polyacrylamide gel electrophoresis and downstream analyses to a mixed community of prokaryotic microorganisms. Environ Microbiol. 2004;6:911–20.
10. Hernández E, Bargiela R, Diez MS, Friedrichs A, Pérez-Cobas AE, Gosalbes MJ, et al. Functional consequences of microbial shifts in the human gastrointestinal tract linked to antibiotic treatment and obesity. Gut Microbes. 2013;4:306–15.
11. Ferrer M, Martins dos Santos VAP, Ott SJ, Moya A. Gut microbiota disturbance during antibiotic therapy: a multi-omic approach. Gut Microbes. 2014;5:64–70.
12. Kolmeder CA, de Been M, Nikkilä J, Ritamo I, Mättö J, Valmu L, et al. Comparative metaproteomics and diversity analysis of human intestinal microbiota testifies for its temporal stability and expression of core functions. PLoS One. 2012;7:e29913.
13. Klaassens ES, de Vos WM, Vaughan EE. Metaproteomics approach to study the functionality of the microbiota in the human infant gastrointestinal tract. Appl Environ Microbiol. 2007;73:1388–92.
14. Shevchenko A, Tomas H, Havlis J, Olsen JV, Mann M. In-gel digestion for mass spectrometric characterization of proteins and proteomes. Nat Protoc. 2006;1:2856–60.
15. Albrethsen J, Knol JC, Piersma SR, Pham TV, de Wit M, Mongera S, et al. Subnuclear proteomics in colorectal cancer: identification of proteins enriched in the nuclear matrix fraction and regulation in adenoma to carcinoma progression. Mol Cell Proteomics MCP. 2010;9:988–1005.
16. Altschul SF, Madden TL, Schäffer AA, Zhang J, Zhang Z, Miller W, et al. Gapped BLAST and PSI-BLAST: a new generation of protein database search programs. Nucleic Acids Res. 1997;25:3389–402.
17. Tatusov RL, Galperin MY, Natale DA, Koonin EV. The COG database: a tool for genome-scale analysis of protein functions and evolution. Nucleic Acids Res. 2000;28:33–6.
18. Letunic I, Yamada T, Kanehisa M, Bork P. iPath: interactive exploration of biochemical pathways and networks. Trends Biochem Sci. 2008;33:101–3.
19. Yu NY, Wagner JR, Laird MR, Melli G, Rey S, Lo R, et al. PSORTb 3.0: improved protein subcellular localization prediction with refined localization subcategories and predictive capabilities for all prokaryotes. Bioinforma Oxf Engl. 2010;26:1608–15.
20. Petersen TN, Brunak S, von Heijne G, Nielsen H. SignalP 4.0: discriminating signal peptides from transmembrane regions. Nat. Methods. 2011;8:785–6.
21. Wei X, Yan X, Zou D, Yang Z, Wang X, Liu W, et al. Abnormal fecal microbiota community and functions in patients with hepatitis B liver cirrhosis as revealed by a metagenomic approach. BMC Gastroenterol. 2013;13:175.
22. Bragulla HH, Homberger DG. Structure and functions of keratin proteins in simple, stratified, keratinized and cornified epithelia. J Anat. 2009;214:516–59.
23. Qin J, Li R, Raes J, Arumugam M, Burgdorf KS, Manichanh C, et al. A human gut microbial gene catalogue established by metagenomic sequencing. Nature. 2010;464:59–65.
24. Manichanh C, Rigottier-Gois L, Bonnaud E, Gloux K, Pelletier E, Frangeul L, et al. Reduced diversity of faecal microbiota in Crohn's disease revealed by a metagenomic approach. Gut. 2006;55:205–11.
25. Spry C, van Schalkwyk DA, Strauss E, Saliba KJ. Pantothenate utilization by Plasmodium as a target for antimalarial chemotherapy. Infect Disord Drug Targets. 2010;10:200–16.
26. Bernal V, Masdemont B, Arense P, Cánovas M, Iborra JL. Redirecting metabolic fluxes through cofactor engineering: Role of CoA-esters pool during L(-)-carnitine production by Escherichia coli. J Biotechnol. 2007;132:110–7.

5

Comparison of risk adjustment methods in patients with liver disease using electronic medical record data

Yuan Xu[1,2], Ning Li[1*], Mingshan Lu[2,3], Elijah Dixon[2,4], Robert P. Myers[2,5], Rachel J. Jolley[2] and Hude Quan[2]

Abstract

Background: Risk adjustment is essential for valid comparison of patients' health outcomes or performances of health care providers. Several risk adjustment methods for liver diseases are commonly used but the optimal approach is unknown. This study aimed to compare the common risk adjustment methods for predicting in-hospital mortality in cirrhosis patients using electronic medical record (EMR) data.

Methods: The sample was derived from Beijing YouAn hospital between 2010 and 2014. Previously validated EMR extraction methods were applied to define liver disease conditions, Charlson comorbidity index (CCI), Elixhauser comorbidity index (ECI), Child-Turcotte-Pugh (CTP), model for end-stage liver disease (MELD), MELD sodium (MELDNa), and five-variable MELD (5vMELD). The performance of the common risk adjustment models as well as models combining disease severity and comorbidity indexes for predicting in-hospital mortality was compared using c-statistic.

Results: Of 11,121 cirrhotic patients, 69.9% were males and 15.8% age 65 or older. The c-statistics across compared models ranged from 0.785 to 0.887. All models significantly outperformed the baseline model with age, sex, and admission status (c-statistic: 0.628). The c-statistics for the CCI, ECI, MELDNa, and CTP were 0.808, 0.825, 0.849, and 0.851, respectively. The c-statistic was 0.887 for combination of CTP and ECI, and 0.882 for combination of MELDNa score and ECI.

Conclusions: The liver disease severity indexes (i.e., CTP and MELDNa score) outperformed the CCI and ECI for predicting in-hospital mortality among cirrhosis patients using Chinese EMRs. Combining liver disease severity and comorbidities indexes could improve the discrimination power of predicting in-hospital mortality.

Keywords: Risk adjustment, Electronic medical record, Liver disease, In-hospital mortality

Background

Risk adjustment methods have increasingly been used for a large range of researches, such as health outcomes studies and health care provider performance assessment. In the past few decades, numerous risk adjustment models have been developed for both general medical inpatients as well as disease-specific inpatients, including disease groupers, disease severity indexes, and comorbidity indexes [1]. For liver disease patients, four risk adjustment instruments are commonly used to predict in-hospital mortality: Charlson comorbidity index (CCI) [2], Elixhauser comorbidity index (ECI) [3], Child-Turcotte-Pugh (CTP) [4, 5], and model for end-stage liver disease (MELD) [6, 7].

CCI was originally developed based on medical charts to estimate 1-year mortality of patients with breast cancer and was validated in another 10-year follow-up cohort [3]. Since then, the index has been most widely used for risk adjustment [8, 9]. In 1998 Elixhauser et al. introduced a new comorbidity algorithm based on United States administrative health data to define the 31 conditions for predicting health outcomes including in-hospital mortality, hospital cost and length of stay [3]. Liver disease studies have shown that ECI performed better than CCI in administrative health data [9–12].

* Correspondence: liningya@ccmu.edu.cn
[1]Beijing YouAn Hospital, Capital Medical University, Beijing, China
Full list of author information is available at the end of the article

Hepatologists use CTP or MELD frequently to predict short-term prognoses or outcomes such as in-hospital mortality, post-surgery mortality or procedure related complications in patients with chronic liver diseases given both instruments are readily applicable at bedside. CTP contains five clinical measures and could be used either as CTP classifications (3 classes for 10 levels of risk) or as a summary score. CTP included two subjective measures (degree of ascites and encephalopathy) which lead to the issue of inter-rater variation. MELD score, on the other hand, does not employ any subjective measure and includes three laboratory test results instead. MELD was initially used to evaluate the risk of death after transjugular intrahepatic portosystemic shunt for patients with cirrhosis, and later used for predicting mortality before or after liver transplantation for patients with end-stage liver diseases [6, 7]. MELD score is regarded more objective and reproducible than CTP and replaced CTP in organ allocation systems such as United Network for Organ Sharing for patients waiting for liver transplantation [13, 14].

The choice of these four risk adjustment methods often depends on data availability. CCI and ECI can be constructed using administrative health data [9, 10, 12, 15–19], while MELD and CTP are used in primary clinical data [20–24]. As a result, performance of these risk adjustment models has not been compared on the same liver patient population. It remains unclear what is the best risk adjustment approach for liver disease.

As a result of rapid development and wide use of electronic medical record (EMR) in China in recent years, an enormous amount of EMR data is being collected [25, 26]. Additionally, liver diseases, including viral hepatitis, cirrhosis, and primary liver cancer (PLC), are highly prevalent in China [27]. About 97 million people are hepatitis B carriers [28]; at least 20 million patients have chronic hepatitis B with or without cirrhosis and/or PLC [27, 28]. Between 2006 and 2010, about 1.2% of inpatients in general hospitals in Beijing were admitted due to cirrhosis (mainly hepatitis cirrhosis) [29]. Therefore, Chinese hospital EMR data provides a unique chance to conduct the comparison study of different risk adjustment methods in the content of liver disease.

To the best of our knowledge, this is the first study that compares the performance of common risk adjustment models in predicting in-hospital mortality for the same large inpatient population with cirrhosis.

Methods
Data source and study population
The data used in our study was derived from the EMR of Beijing YouAn hospital, one of the leading teaching hospitals specialized in liver diseases in China and treating over 300,000 patients from all over China each year. In 2008, the EMR system was officially implemented in YouAn hospital and inpatient documentation completely switched from paper charts to EMR. For each patient, the EMR contains a front summary page, as well as sections with detailed information on admission, discharge, surgery/procedure, death, laboratory test results, radiology test results, pathology report, physician's notes, hospitalization billing records, and electronic prescription. Among these sections, laboratory test results, electronic prescriptions, and billing records are completely structured without any free text. The front page, admission and discharge records, and radiology test results, however, are only semi-structured and contain both structured drop-down lists and free-text fields. The hospital assigned a unique identification number to each patient; all sections of EMRs are linked using the identification number.

The study population included patients with cirrhosis hospitalized at Beijing YouAn hospital between January 1st, 2010 and September 30th, 2014, who were at least 18 years old and consented to use their EMRs for research (nearly all patients provided consent), and excluded patients with missing in-hospital mortality status. We excluded 145 (1.3%) patients due to missing information on in-hospital mortality (the missing was likely caused by physicians' unintentional incomplete documentation) and 180 (1.6%) patients who underwent liver transplantation, given this group of patients were much more complicated in contrast to other patients. In total, 11,122 adult cirrhosis patients were analyzed. This study was approved by the YouAn Hospital Research Board of Ethics and the Health Research Ethics Board at University of Calgary (Ethic committee's reference number: REB14-0815).

Outcome and independent variables
The outcome measure was in-hospital mortality that was recorded in the EMR. Liver disease variables were defined using our previously developed and validated EMR case definitions [30]. The validation study showed that most of the case definitions had high validity (positive predictive value over 80%). Using the validated case definitions, we defined the following variables: cirrhosis, PLC, hepatitis, hepatic encephalopathy (HE) and ascites, as well as the Charlson and Elixhauser comorbidities at the time of admission. In addition, the laboratory test results required to construct the CTP and MELD scores were directly extracted from the EMR system. These laboratory test results included the serum level of albumin, total bilirubin, creatinine, sodium (Na), and the international normalized ratio of prothrombin time (PT-INR). For inpatient episode with multiple laboratory tests, results from the tests conducted at or immediately after admission were used. Only 232 patients had missing values of one of above laboratory tests. We assumed these missing values fell in the normal range at admission. Chart review on 30

charts randomly selected out of these 232 patients supported this assumption.

Using EMR data in the latest admission, we defined in-hospital mortality and the laboratory test results. To define chronic diseases (e.g., comorbidities) we included the information in the multiple admissions within 1 year prior to the latest admission date.

Risk adjustment models

Commonly used variants of CCI [10, 12] were tested: the all individual comorbidities of CCI (referred to as CCI), the number of Charlson comorbidities categorized (0, 1, 2, ≥3 comorbidities) (referred to as CCI categorized), the score of CCI (referred to as CCI score), which is the summation of the weighted score of each comorbidity, and the categorized CCI score (0, 1–2, 3–4, ≥5 points) (referred to as CCI score categorized), (See detailed description of the tested models in Table 1). For ECI, models using the individual Elixhauser comorbidities (referred to as ECI), and the number of Elixhauser comorbidities categorized (0, 1, 2, ≥3 comorbidities) (referred to as ECI categorized) [11] were tested (Table 1). Both CCI and ECI contain variables related to liver diseases. We excluded "mild/moderate to severe liver disease" in CCI and the "liver disease" in ECI. PLC was excluded from the variables of "any malignancy", "metastatic solid tumor", and "solid tumor without metastases".

For MELD, three common variants were tested (Table 1), including MELD score (referred to as MELD score) [6], MELD sodium score (referred to as MELDNa score) [31], and five-variable MELD score (referred to as 5vMELD score) [32]. MELD score = $3.78 \times \ln$[serum total bilirubin (mg/dL)] + $11.2 \times \ln$[INR] + $9.57 \times \ln$[serum creatinine (mg/dL)] + 6.43 [6]. To avoid scores below 0 in the logarithm, value less than one is rounded to 1 (e.g., for total bilirubin with 0.75, a value of 1.0 is assigned). MELDNa = MELD score + 1.59 [135 - Na], where Na is bounded between 120 and 135 mmol/L (Na lower than the low limit is assigned with a value of 120 mmol/L, and Na higher than 135 mmol/L is assigned a value of 135 mmol/L) [31]. 5vMELD score = MELDNa + $(5.275 \times$ [4-albumin]) − $(0.136 \times$ MELDNa $\times$ [4 - serum albumin]), where albumin is bounded between 1 and 4 g/dL [32]. Two variants of CTP were tested: CTP classification (referred to as CTP) and CTP score (referred to as CTP score) (Table 1). The CTP score is defined by summing the assigned score for each of the five variables including HE (absence = 1, slight-medium = 2, and refractory = 3), ascites (none = 1, mild = 2, and moderate to severe = 3), total bilirubin (<34 μmol/L = 1, 34–50 μmol/L = 2, and >50 μmol/L = 3), PT-INR (<1.7 = 1, 1.7–2.3 = 2, and > 2.3 = 3), and albumin (>3.5 = 1, 2.8–3.5 = 2, and <2.8 = 3) [5]. Calculating CTP score requires the refined severity of HE and ascites; however, 13.5% patients had unknown severity of HE, and the patients with unknown severity of ascites accounted for 52.6%. We excluded these patients from the CTP score model because we were not able to calculate CTP score for these patients. To include the patients with unknown severity of HE or

Table 1 The description of compared models

Method		Variants	Description
Comorbidity methods	CCI	CCI	Charlson individual comorbidities (binary variables)
		CCI categorized	number of Charlson comorbidities excluding liver disease (0, 1, 2, ≥3)
		CCI score	the score of Charlson comorbidities (weighted score)
		CCI score categorized	the score of CCI categorized as 0, 1–2, 3–4, ≥5
	ECI	ECI	Elixhauser individual comorbidities (binary variables)
		ECI categorized	number of Elixhauser comorbidities (0, 1, 2, ≥3)
Liver specific severity methods	MELD	MELD score	calculated by total bilirubin, PT-INR, and creatinine
		MELDNa score	calculated by MELD score and serum sodium
		5vMELD score	calculated by MELDNa score and serum albumin
	CTP	CTP	the classification of Child-Turcotte-Pugh (including the individual binary variables of hepatic encephalopathy, ascites, total bilirubin, prothrombin time, and albumin)
		CTP score	calculated by summing the weighted score of each CTP variable
Comorbidity + Liver severity		MELDNa score + ECI	the score of MELDNa + individual binary variable of Elixhauser comorbidities
		CTP + ECI	individual binary variables of CTP + individual binary variable of Elixhauser comorbidities

CTP Child-Turcotte-Pugh, *MELD* model for end-stage liver disease, *MELDNa* MELD sodium, *5vMELD* five variable MELD, *CCI* Charlson comorbidity index, *ECI* Elixhauser comorbidity index

ascites, we also categorized HE and ascites into binary variables (presence or absence) in the CTP classification model. In addition, we tested risk adjustment models using combination of CTP, MELDNa scorer and ECI (Table 1). For these models incorporated both comorbidity index and liver disease severity score, we tested the interactions between different risk adjustment instruments.

Statistical analysis

Descriptive analysis was conducted and logistic regression models (as described above) were used to predict in-hospital mortality. The baseline model consisted of age, sex, and admission status (urgently or not). Concordance-statistic (c-statistic) was used to assess the performance of the risk adjustment models [33, 34]. C-statistic of 0.5 means that the ability of discrimination of the model is zero; the discrimination power is regarded as "unacceptable" when c-statistic range from 0.50 to 0.69; or "acceptable" when c-statistic range from 0.70 to 0.79; or "good to excellent" when c-statistic is 0.80 or greater. The 10-fold cross validation [35] was used to calculate the corrected c-statistics to adjust for the number of independent variables in the model considering that c-statistic increases with the number of independent variables. We also conducted bootstrapping (1000 samples) and calculated 95% confidence interval for c-statistics (95% CI) for internal validation of the c-statistic of each model [36].

Probability of death for each patient was calculated by the logistic regression models; patients were ranked and allocated to different risk groups based on the predicted probability of death. The agreement of observed and expected number of death was assessed. Graphs were plotted to show the expected and observed mortality rates across the various risk groups.

In addition, similar analyses were conducted using the subsample of patients with viral hepatitis, alcoholic hepatitis, PLC, decompensated cirrhosis, and no-procedure subgroups (without undergoing hepatectomy, liver transplantations, transcatheter arterial chemoembolization, and endoscopic treatment). All analyses were performed in SAS version 9.4 (Cary, NC).

Results

Of 11,121 cirrhotic patients (Table 2), the median age was 53 (interquartile range: 46–61) years, 69.9% (7773) were male and 11.0% (1219) patients were admitted emergently. The common causes for cirrhosis were hepatitis B (73.1%), alcoholic hepatitis (25.0%), hepatitis C (8.8%), and fatty liver (4.6%). Of the cirrhosis patients, 3824 (34.4%) had PLC (hepatocellular carcinoma account for 96.5%); and 5433 (48.9%) patients did not undergo any major surgeries or procedures (i.e., hepatectomy, liver transplantation, transcatheter arterial chemoembolization, sclerotherapy and variceal banding), radiofrequency

ablation or radiotherapy. Overall the in-hospital mortality was 8.3%.

Outcome measure and independent variables

At time of admission, 25.0% (2764) of the cirrhotic patients were diagnosed with hyponatremia (Na < 135 mmol/L), 19.7% (2190) with high creatinine level (>88.4 umol/L), 9.5% (1051) with abnormal PT-INR (>1.7), 40.98% (4558) with high total bilirubin level (>34.2 umol/L), and 51.7% (5752) with hypoproteinemia (albumin < 2.8 g/dL). At time of admission, 18.6% (2069) of the cirrhotic patients had HE, and 58.3% (6478) had ascites. The most common five comorbidities were diabetes uncomplicated (35.6%), hypertension (complicated and uncomplicated) (28.5%), alcohol abuse (25.0%), fluid and electrolyte disorder (15.4%) and peptic ulcer disease (11.1%).

In general, in-hospital mortality was higher among male patients, older patients, urgently admitted patients, patients with abnormal clinical variables, patients with a certain comorbidity (except for acquired immune deficiency syndrome and peripheral vascular disease), or patients with higher MELD, MELDNa or 5vMELD score than their counterparts (see Table 3). As number of Charlson or Elixhauser comorbitites increased, so did in-hospital mortality. A similar pattern was found with the number of abnormal CTP variables.

Performance of risk adjustment models

The c-statistics and its 95% confidence intervals (CI) of the risk adjustment models predicting in-hospital mortality for overall cirrhotic patients were presented in Table 4, while those for the subgroups of cirrhotic patients (viral hepatitis, alcoholic hepatitis, PLC, decompensated cirrhosis, and non-procedure) were presented in Table 5.

For model with age, sex and admission status as the baseline model, c-statistic was 0.628 (95% CI: 0.609–0.650). All risk adjustment models with comorbidities, MELD or CTP significantly outperformed the baseline model, with c-statistics ranging from 0.785 to 0.887. For models with variable of the number of comorbidities (0, 1, 2 and ≥3), the c-statistic obviously dropped from 0.825 (95% CI: 0.749–0.848) to 0.794 (95% CI: 0.743–0.841) for ECI; and from 0.809 (95% CI: 0.792–0.822) to 0.786 (95% CI: 0.771–0.801) for CCI. The CCI score categorized model had very similar c-statistic with the CCI score model (0.786 versus 0.785). The c-statistic for MELD score model (0.818, 95% CI: 0.805–0.833) was significantly lower than MELDNa score model (0.849, 95% CI: 0.838–0.861) and 5vMELD score model (0.845, 95% CI: 0.833–0.858). The performance of the CTP is very similar with the MELDNa score (c-statistics 0.851 versus 0.849, p = 0.073). The performance of CTP score was significantly lower than CTP (c-statistics: 0.793, 95%

Table 2 Characteristics of patients with cirrhosis (N = 11,121)

Characteristics	Median (interquartile range) or frequency
Na (mmol/L)	138.4 (135.0–140.0)
Creatinine (umol/L)	66.3 (54.5–81.9)
PT-INR	1.2 (1.0–1.4)
Total bilirubin (umol/L)	27.2 (17.1–59.3)
Albumin (g/dl)	34.7 (29.4–40.0)
CTP score[a]	5.0 (5.0–6.0)
MELD score	8.0 (7.0–11.0)
MELDNa score	10.0 (8.0–14.0)
5vMELD score	13.0 (9.0–18.0)
Charlson comorbidity score	1 (0–2)
LOS (day)	13 (5–26)
Age (year)	
18–44	2576 (23.2%)
45–64	6785 (61.0%)
≥ 65	1761 (15.8%)
Male	7773 (69.9%)
Urgent admission	1219 (11.0%)
Na < 135 mmol/L	2764 (24.9%)
Creatinine > 88.4 umol/L	2190 (19.7%)
PT-INR	
< 1.7 (normal range)	10071 (90.6%)
1.7–2.2	724 (6.5%)
> 2.2	327 (2.9%)
Total bilirubin (umol/L)	
< 34.2 (normal range)	6564 (59.0%)
34.2–51.3	1328 (11.9%)
> 51.3	3230 (29.0%)
Albumin (g/dl)	
> 3.5 (normal range)	5370 (48.3%)
2.8–3.5	3660 (32.9%)
< 2.8	2092 (18.8%)
Hepatic encephalopathy[b]	
Grade I-II	455 (4.1%)
Grade III-IV (or refractory)	109 (1.0%)
Severity unknown	1505 (13.5%)
Ascites[b]	
Mild	522 (4.7%)
Moderate to sever	103 (0.9%)
Severity unknown	5853 (52.6%)
CTP classification[b]	
A (CTP score 5–6)	3952 (35.5%)
B (CTP score 7–9)	1002 (9.0%)
C (CTP score 10–15)	80 (0.7%)

Table 2 Characteristics of patients with cirrhosis (N = 11,121) (Continued)

Number of abnormal CTP variables	
0	2803 (25.2%)
1	2255 (20.3%)
2	2390 (21.5%)
≥ 3	3674 (33.0%)
Number of Charlson comorbidities	
0	3580 (32.2%)
1	4564 (41.0%)
2	2212 (19.9%)
≥ 3	766 (6.9%)
Number of Elixhauser comorbidities	
0	2595 (23.3%)
1	3239 (29.1%)
2	2355 (21.2%)
≥ 3	2933 (26.4%)
Charlson comorbidities	
Myocardial infarction	62 (0.6%)
Cerebrovascular disease	371 (3.3%)
Dementia	6 (0.1%)
Renal disease	1228 (11.0%)
Any malignancy[c]	645 (5.8%)
Charlson and Elixhauser shared comorbidities	
Congestive heart failure	25 (0.2%)
Peripheral vascular disease	7 (0.1%)
Chronic pulmonary disease	191 (1.7%)
Rheumatologic disease	62 (0.6%)
Peptic ulcer disease	1234 (11.1%)
Diabetes complicated	130 (1.2%)
Diabetes uncomplicated	3957 (35.6%)
Hemiplegia or paraplegia	8 (0.1%)
Metastatic solid tumor[c]	275 (2.5%)
AIDS	40 (0.4%)
Elixhauser comorbidities[d]	
Cardiac arrhythmias	447 (4.0%)
Valvular disease	30 (0.3%)
Hypertension uncomplicated	2008 (18.1%)
Hypertension complicated	1156 (10.4%)
Hypothyroidism	95 (0.9%)
Lymphoma	20 (0.2%)
Solid tumor without metastasis[c]	178 (1.6%)
Coagulopathy	5 (0.04%)
Blood loss anemia	335 (3.0%)
Deficiency anemia	959 (8.6%)
Depression	41 (0.4%)

Table 2 Characteristics of patients with cirrhosis (N = 11,121) (Continued)

Fluid and electrolyte disorders	1707 (15.4%)
Alcohol abuse	2780 (25.0%)
Psychoses	19 (0.2%)
Renal failure	236 (2.1%)

IQR interquartile range, Na serum sodium, PT-INR international normalized ratio of prothrombin time, LOS length of stay in hospital, CTP Child-Turcotte-Pugh, MELD model for end-stage liver disease, MELDNa MELD sodium, 5vMELD five variable MELD, AIDS acquired immune deficiency syndrome

[a]CTP score was not available for patients with unknown severity of HE or ascites

[b]The sum of proportion of the categories is less than 100% because there were missing values on ascites and hepatic encephalopathy

[c]Excluded primary liver cancer

[d]The obesity, weight loss, pulmonary circulatory disorders, other neurological disorders and drug abuse were excluded due to 0% prevalence

CI: 0.736–0.844 versus 0.851, 95% CI: 0.839–0.864). In summary, for the overall cirrhotic patients, among the risk adjustment models, c-statistics increased in a consistent order from the CCI, ECI, MELDNa score, to CTP. The comparison result using bias-corrected c-statistic was slightly different (order from low to high performance: CCI, ECI, CTP to MELDNa score). The corrected c-statistics for CTP and MELDNa score models were very similar (0.847 versus 0.849).

Results on model performance within patient's subgroups (those with viral hepatitis, alcoholic hepatitis, PLC, decompensated cirrhosis, and no-procedure subgroups) remained the same: c-statistics increased in a consistent order from the CCI, ECI to MELDNa score (or CTP). Compared with models employing only single risk adjustment model, c-statistic of models that combined both liver disease severity and comorbidity indexes was shown to be better. Model combining CTP and ECI improved the c-statistic compared with the CTP model (c-statistics: 0.887 versus 0.851, $p < 0.0001$). Similarly, model that combined ECI and MELDNa score outperformed model that includd MELDNa score only (c-statistics: 0.882 versus 0.849, $p < 0.0001$).

Figure 1 presents the observed and expected mortality across model-defined risk groups for the six models (CCI, ECI, MELDNa score, CTP, ECI + MELDNa score, and ECI + CTP) in the overall sample. The "spread-out" of the expected mortality generated from combined models (i.e., CI + MELDNa score and ECI + CTP) was much wider than the models with only comorbidities, MELD or CTP.

Discussion

To the best of our knowledge, this is the first study that compared the performance of common risk adjustment methods in predicting in-hospital mortality for patients with cirrhosis, using large Chinese EMR data. The EMR data provided comprehensive information on both comorbidities as well as disease specific clinical information for large inpatient sample, presenting researchers a valuable opportunity to assess performance of various risk adjustment models on the same patient population. Our large sample also statistically empowered precision of the assessment. Overall, our study highlighted: 1) liver specific scores of CTP and MELDNa performed better than comorbidity methods of CCI and ECI; 2) combination of liver disease severity and comorbidity indexes (such as CTP + ECI or MELDNa score + ECI) significantly improved performance of in-hospital mortality prediction; and 3) these findings were consistent across subtypes of liver diseases.

Comparison of risk adjustment methods

We assessed the performance of risk adjustment models in predicting in-hospital mortality for patients with cirrhosis, using a single model or a combination of two models among ECI and CTP (or MELDNa score). All models significantly outperformed the baseline model with age, sex, and admission status. These results provided support of the use of these models as risk adjustment instruments for liver disease. While all models were shown to have reasonable predictive power, liver disease severity indexes (CTP and MELDNa score) were shown to be better than the comorbidity indexes (CCI and ECI). Moreover, comparing with individual comorbidity or liver disease severity index, combined models (e.g., CTP + ECI or MELDNa + ECI) demonstrated higher performance in predicting in-hospital mortality.

Between the two comorbidity indexes tested, ECI was found to be more predictive than CCI among all cirrhotic patients as well as for all the subgroups. This result was consistent with findings in the existing risk adjustment literatures for liver disease that used administrative data [9, 16, 18, 37]. The better performance of ECI could be explained by that ECI identified substantially more conditions than CCI, which contributed to a higher c-statistic [16, 37]. In our study, we used a category of number of comorbidities presence as one independent variable for ECI and CCI. This method showed similar c-statistics for ECI and CCI (0.794 versus 0.786).

Among the liver disease severity indexes tested, the discrimination ability of CTP was consistently shown to be higher than MELD and 5vMELD scores, and close to MELDNa score among all of the subgroups. This proved the appropriateness of ongoing use of CTP in practice to predict in-hospital mortality in cirrhotic patients. However, refined degree of HE and ascites may not be available in many datasets, making it impossible to use CTP as a risk adjustment instrument. The construction of MELDNa score only requires routine laboratory test results, which makes MELDNa score more reproducible, reliable and easier to apply [20–22]. More importantly,

Table 3 Crude in-hospital mortality by study variables ($N = 11{,}121$)

Variables		Mortality % (n)	P-value[1]
Age (year)	18–44	4.9 (125)	<0.0001
	45–64	8.0 (543)	
	≥65	14.3 (252)	
Sex	male	9.1 (704)	<0.0001
	female	6.5 (216)	
Admission status	non-urgent	6.3 (627)	<0.0001
	urgent	24.0 (293)	
Hepatic encephalopathy	no	4.0 (360)	<0.0001
	yes	27.1 (560)	
Ascites	no	1.8 (85)	<0.0001
	yes	12.9 (835)	
PT-INR	<1.7	6.2 (628)	<0.0001
	1.7–2.3	23.2 (168)	
	>2.3	37.9 (124)	
Total bilirubin (umol/L)	<34.2	4.1 (271)	<0.0001
	34.2–51.3	7.1 (94)	
	>51.3	17.2 (555)	
Albumin (g/dl)	>35	3.2 (170)	<0.0001
	28–35	10.0 (367)	
	<28	18.3 (383)	
Creatinine (umol/L)	≤88.4	5.0 (445)	<0.0001
	>88.4	21.7 (475)	
Na	≥135	4.4 (364)	<0.0001
	<135	20.1 (556)	
MELD score	<7.0	1.9 (54)	<0.0001
	7.0–8.0	3.6 (100)	
	8.0–10.0	7.0 (195)	
	>10.0	20.5 (571)	
MELDNa score	<8.0	0.7 (19)	<0.0001
	8.0–10.0	2.7 (74)	
	10.0–14.0	6.6 (184)	
	>14.0	23.1 (643)	
5vMELD score	<9.0	0.5 (15)	<0.0001
	9.0–13.0	2.3 (65)	
	13.0–18.0	8.0 (223)	
	>18.0	22.2 (617)	
CTP classification	A (CTP score 5–6)	0.9 (34)	<0.0001
	B (CTP score 7–9)	3.2 (32)	
	C (CTP score 10–15)	11.3 (9)	
Number of abnormal CTP variables	0	0.5 (13)	<0.0001
	1	2.3 (52)	
	2	6.2 (147)	
	≥3	19.3 (708)	

Table 3 Crude in-hospital mortality by study variables ($N = 11{,}121$) (Continued)

Myocardial infarction	no	8.2 (902)	<0.0001
	yes	29.0 (18)	
Cerebrovascular disease	no	7.9 (846)	<0.0001
	yes	20.0 (74)	
Renal disease	no	5.9 (586)	<0.0001
	yes	27.2 (334)	
Any malignancy[a]	no	8.0 (841)	<0.0001
	yes	12.2 (79)	
Congestive heart failure	no	8.3 (10)	<0.0001
	yes	40.0 (10)	
Chronic pulmonary disease	no	8.1 (888)	<0.0001
	yes	16.8 (32)	
Rheumatologic disease	no	8.3 (913)	0.39
	yes	11.3 (7)	
Peptic ulcer disease	no	8.1 (801)	0.06
	yes	9.6 (119)	
Diabetes complicated	no	8.3 (907)	0.47
	yes	10.0 (13)	
Diabetes uncomplicated	no	5.2 (374)	<0.0001
	yes	13.8 (546)	
Hemiplegia or paraplegia	no	8.3 (919)	0.66
	yes	12.5 (1)	
Metastatic solid tumor	no	7.8 (844)	<0.0001
	yes	27.6 (76)	
Cardiac arrhythmias	no	7.9 (840)	<0.0001
	yes	17.9 (80)	
Valvular disease	no	8.3 (916)	0.31
	yes	13.3 (4)	
Hypertension uncomplicated	no	7.8 (708)	<0.0001
	yes	10.6 (212)	
Hypertension complicated	no	7.9 (784)	<0.0001
	yes	11.8 (136)	
Hypothyroidism	no	8.3 (911)	0.67
	yes	9.5 (9)	
Lymphoma	no	8.3 (918)	0.78
	yes	10.0 (2)	
Solid tumor without metastasis[a]	no	8.1 (886)	0.31
	yes	19.2 (34)	
Coagulopathy	no	8.3 (918)	0.01
	yes	40.0 (2)	
Blood loss anemia	no	7.6 (818)	<0.0001
	yes	30.5 (102)	
Deficiency anemia	no	7.4 (755)	<0.0001
	yes	17.2 (165)	

Table 3 Crude in-hospital mortality by study variables ($N = 11,121$) (Continued)

Depression	no	8.2 (913)	<0.0001
	yes	17.1 (7)	
Fluid and electrolyte disorders	no	5.5 (519)	<0.0001
	yes	23.5 (401)	
Psychoses	no	8.3 (918)	0.72
	yes	10.5 (2)	
Renal failure	no	7.4 (803)	<0.0001
	yes	49.6 (117)	
AIDS	no	8.3 (920)	0.06
	yes	0.0 (0)	
Peripheral vascular disease	no	8.3 (920)	0.43
	yes	0.0 (0)	
Alcohol abuse	no	7.49 (625)	<0.0001
	yes	10.62 (295)	
Number of Charlson comorbidities	0	2.6 (92)	<0.0001
	1	6.0 (272)	
	2	14.2 (315)	
	≥3	31.5 (241)	
Charlson comorbidity score categorized	0	2.6 (92)	<0.0001
	1–2	6.2 (310)	
	3–4	16.75 (325)	
	≥5	30.4 (193)	
Number of Elixhauser comorbidities	0	2.1 (54)	<0.0001
	1	3.9 (126)	
	2	7.4 (175)	
	≥3	19.3 (565)	

IQR interquartile range, Na serum sodium, PT-INR International normalized ratio of prothrombin time, CTP Child-Turcotte-Pugh, MELD model for end-stage liver disease, MELDNa MELD sodium, 5vMELD five variable MELD, AIDS acquired immune deficiency syndrome
[1]P-value of Chi-square exact test is for each contingency table (mortality by each predictor)
[a]Excluded primary liver cancer

Table 4 C-statistics (95% CI) for predicting in-hospital mortality of the compared risk adjustment methods[a] in the overall cirrhosis patients ($N = 11,121$)

Model	Mean c-statistic (95% CI)[b]	Bias-corrected c-statistic[c]
CCI	0.809 (0.792–0.822)	0.816
CCI categorized	0.786 (0.771–0.801)	0.784
CCI score	0.785 (0.769–0.799)	0.787
CCI score categorized	0.786 (0.770–0.801)	0.783
ECI	0.825 (0.749–0.848)	0.827
ECI categorized	0.794 (0.743–0.841)	0.773
MELDNa score	0.849 (0.838–0.861)	0.849
5vMELD score	0.845 (0.833–0.858)	0.847
MELD score	0.818 (0.805–0.833)	0.817
CTP	0.851 (0.839–0.864)	0.847
CTP score	0.793 (0.736–0.844)	0.803
MELDNa score + ECI	0.882 (0.826–0.898)	0.882
CTP + ECI	0.887 (0.846–0.901)	0.885

CI confidence interval, CCI Charlson comorbidity index, ECI Elixhauser comorbidity index, CTP Child-Turcotte-Pugh, MELD model for end-stage liver disease, MELDNa MELD sodium, 5vMELD five variable MELD
[a]Age, sex and admission status were included in all regression models
[b]1000 samples bootstrapping mean c-statistic and 95% CI
[c]10-fold cross validation corrected c-statistic

our results showed that the performance of MELDNa score were very close to or better than that of CTP. This indicates that using MELDNa score instead of CTP might simplify the analysis without compromising the predictive accuracy.

MELDNa and 5vMELD scores had similar performance in predicting in-hospital mortality. 5vMELD score was generated through adding serum albumin level to MELDNa score. The additional variable in 5vMELD did not significantly improve its predictability of in-hospital mortality. The possible reason is that albumin level

Table 5 C-statistics (95% CI)[a] of the logistic regression models[b] in the subgroups of cirrhotic patients

Model	Viral hepatitis	PLC	Alcoholic hepatitis	Decompensated	No-procedure[c]
Number of cases (%)	8132 (73.1)	3824 (34.4)	2778 (25.0)	7183 (64.6)	5433 (48.9)
CCI	0.807 (0.789–0.825)	0.788 (0.764–0.812)	0.791 (0.761–0.817)	0.788 (0.771–0.805)	0.796 (0.778–0.815)
ECI	0.821 (0.756–0.846)	0.828 (0.805–0.849)	0.837 (0.809–0.860)	0.807 (0.786–0.825)	0.834 (0.817–0.852)
MELDNa score	0.848 (0.835–0.863)	0.846 (0.828–0.861)	0.853 (0.833–0.873)	0.827 (0.810–0.841)	0.845 (0.831–0.860)
CTP	0.856 (0.842–0.869)	0.869 (0.851–0.885)	0.847 (0.827–0.867)	0.822 (0.806–0.838)	0.852 (0.837–0.867)
MELDNa score + ECI	0.878 (0.836–0.897)	0.888 (0.871–0.903)	0.896 (0.876–0.914)	0.863 (0.846–0.877)	0.889 (0.876–0.902)
CTP + ECI	0.887 (0.847–0.905)	0.907 (0.891–0.920)	0.897 (0.878–0.914)	0.864 (0.848–0.877)	0.892 (0.878–0.904)

CI confidence interval, CCI Charlson comorbidity index, ECI Elixhauser comorbidity index
CTP Child-Turcotte-Pugh, MELDNa model for end-stage liver disease and sodium
[a]1000 samples bootstrapping mean c-statistic and 95% CI
[b]Age, sex and admission status were included in all regression models
[c]Procedure refers to the major procedures such as the hepatectomy, liver transplantation, transcatheter arterial chemoembolization, endoscopic treatment (i.e., sclerotherapy and variceal banding), and radiofrequency ablation and radiotherapy

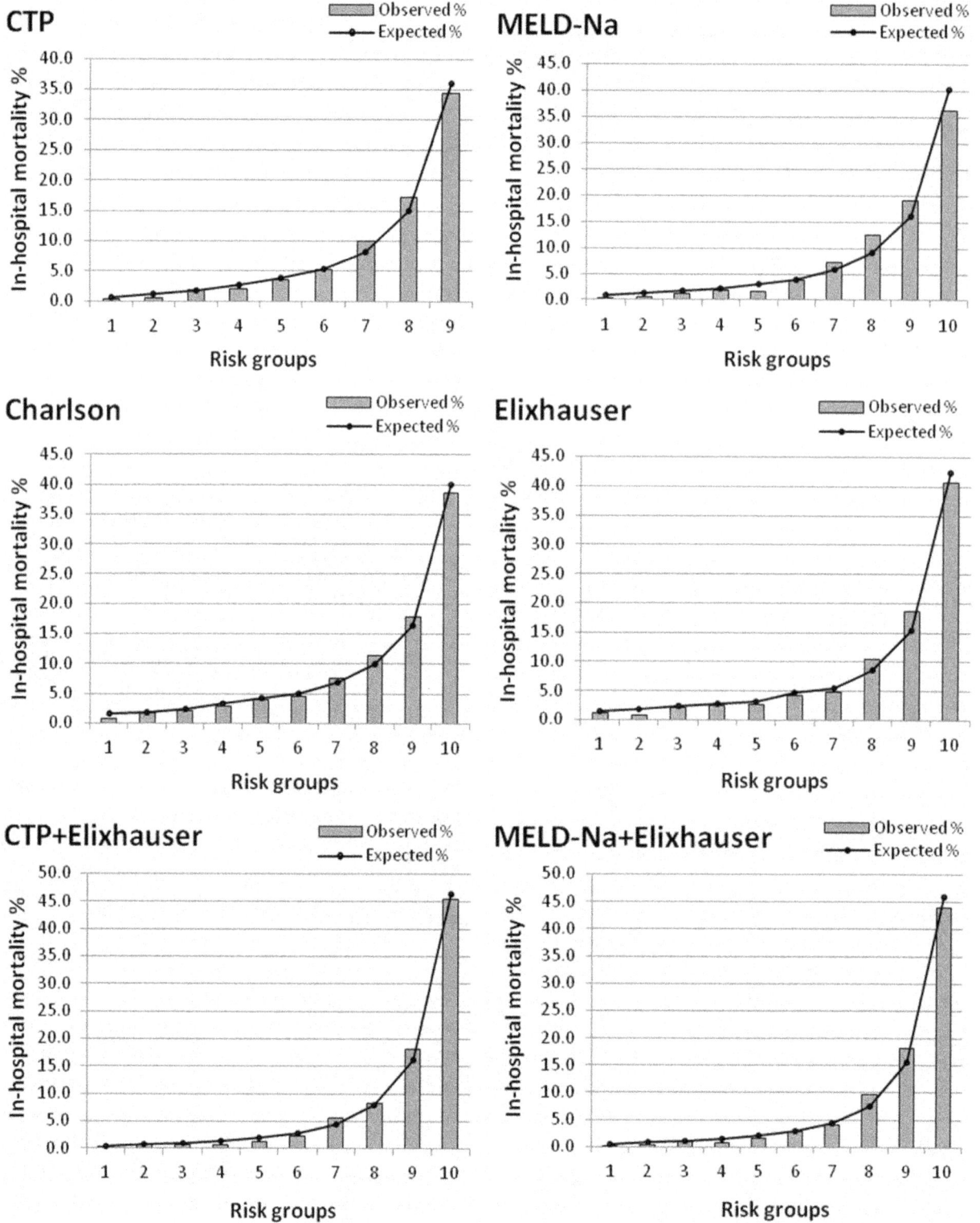

Fig. 1 Expected and observed mortality in various risk groups for patients with cirrhosis. CTP: Child-Turcotte-Pugh; MELDNa: model for end-stage liver disease and sodium

measured during hospitalization did not reflect the patient's severity of disease because albumin was commonly administrated in inpatients with cirrhosis.

Overall, the liver disease severity indexes (MELD score and CTP) outperformed the comorbidity indexes (CCI and ECI) on prediction of in-hospital mortality. The possible reason is that the most recent laboratory test results within one hospitalization episode could reflect the severity of liver disease at the occurrence of hospitalization outcome (mortality). We conducted sensitivity analysis to address this explanation. We calculated MELDNa score at near discharge time and fitted model to predict in-hospital mortality. The c-statistic for MELDNa model increased significantly from 0.849 (95% CI: 0.838–0.861) for near admission time to 0.912 (95% CI: 0.903–0.921) for near discharge time. This supported our hypothesis that the performance of risk adjustment instruments improves when they are constructed based on information collected close to the outcome event.

The model incorporated MELDNa score and Elixhauser comorbidities obtained significantly higher predictive ability compared to the MELDNa score model. This indicated that to increase predictive probability of mortality during hospitalization, physicians should not only consider the MELDNa score but also presence of comorbidities. Further research is required to develop summary score and cut-off value to predict individual patient's outcome.

Limitations

Our study has several limitations. First, we used data derived from one hospital EMRs, and the generalizablility of the results may be a concern. However, generally the c-statistics of the compared risk adjustment methods were consistent with results from other studies in existing literatures [9–12, 15, 20–23]. Second, we only analyzed inpatient EMR data and were unable to assess patients' outcome after discharge. Third, the odds ratios of certain predictors were not reliable due to low prevalence. The possible reason for the low prevalence of these diseases is that the data is from a hospital specialized in liver disease. However, the purpose of this study is to compare the performance of the common risk adjustment instruments. Lastly, the missing values on certain variables were common. In our EMRs, presence of ascites was well recorded but degree of ascites was often missing (more than 50%). Exclusion of these patients from the CTP score model could under-estimate the c-statistic. Other study also reported that severity of HE and ascites was commonly missing [22].

Conclusion

The liver specific scoring instruments of CTP and MELDNa outperformed the ECI and CCI methods for predicting in-hospital mortality among patients with cirrhosis using Chinese EMRs. Combining severity and comorbidities could improve the statistical power of predicting in-hospital mortality. These risk adjustment methods should be further evaluated for predicting long-term outcomes.

Abbreviations
5vMELD: Five-variable MELD; CCI: Charlson comorbidity index; CTP: Child-Turcotte-Pugh; ECI: Elixhauser comorbidity index; EMR: Electronic medical record; HE: Hepatic encephalopathy; MELD: Model for end-stage liver disease; MELDNa: MELD sodium; Na: Sodium; PT-INR: International normalized ratio of prothrombin time

Acknowledgements
Not applicable.

Funding
Dr. Xu was supported by the Ward of the 21st Century (W21C) and Western Regional Training Centre (WRTC). Dr. Quan is supported by Alberta Innovation-Health Solution. Dr. Lu is supported by Alberta's Strategy for Patient-Oriented Research Support.

Authors' contributions
YX contributed to study design conceptualization, structuring the EMR definitions, data collection, data mining, statistical analysis, and drafting the manuscript. NL contributed to study design conceptualization, developing and refining the EMR definitions, data collection, results interpretation, and revision of the manuscript. HQ contributed to study design conceptualization, statistical analysis, interpretation and presentation of the results, and revision of the manuscript. ML contributed to statistical analysis, results interpretation, and revision of the manuscript. ED contributed to study design, results interpretation, and revision of the manuscript. RM contributed to study design conceptualization, results interpretation, and revision of the manuscript. RJ contributed to study design, results interpretation, and revision of the manuscript. All authors have read and approved the final version of the manuscript.

Competing interests
The authors declare that they have no competing interests.

Consent for publication
Not applicable.

Author details
[1]Beijing YouAn Hospital, Capital Medical University, Beijing, China. [2]Department of Community Health Sciences, University of Calgary, Calgary, AB, Canada. [3]Department of Economics, University of Calgary, Calgary, AB, Canada. [4]Division of General Surgery, Department of Medicine, University of Calgary, Calgary, AB, Canada. [5]Liver Unit, Division of Gastroenterology and Hepatology, Department of Medicine, University of Calgary, Calgary, AB, Canada.

References
1. Lu M, Sajobi T, Lucyk K, Lorenzetti D, Quan H. Systematic review of risk adjustment models of hospital length of stay (LOS). Med Care. 2015;53:355–65.
2. Charlson ME, Pompei P, Ales KL, MacKenzie CR. A new method of classifying prognostic comorbidity in longitudinal studies: development and validation. J Chronic Dis. 1987;40:373–83.

3.   Elixhauser A, Steiner C, Harris DR, Coffey RM. Comorbidity measures for use with administrative data. Med Care. 1998;36:8–27.

4.   Child CG, Turcotte JG. Surgery and portal hypertension. Major Probl Clin Surg. 1964;1:1–85.

5.   Pugh RN, Murray-Lyon IM, Dawson JL, Pietroni MC, Williams R. Transection of the oesophagus for bleeding oesophageal varices. Br J Surg. 1973;60:646–9.

6.   Malinchoc M, Kamath PS, Gordon FD, Peine CJ, Rank J, ter Borg PC. A model to predict poor survival in patients undergoing transjugular intrahepatic portosystemic shunts. Hepatology. 2000;31:864–71.

7.   Kamath PS, Kim WR, Advanced Liver Disease Study G. The model for end-stage liver disease (MELD). Hepatology. 2007;45:797–805.

8.   Deyo RA, Cherkin DC, Ciol MA. Adapting a clinical comorbidity index for use with ICD-9-CM administrative databases. J Clin Epidemiol. 1992;45:613–9.

9.   Myers RP, Quan H, Hubbard JN, Shaheen AA, Kaplan GG. Predicting in-hospital mortality in patients with cirrhosis: results differ across risk adjustment methods. Hepatology. 2009;49:568–77.

10. Nguyen GC, Segev DL, Thuluvath PJ. Racial disparities in the management of hospitalized patients with cirrhosis and complications of portal hypertension: a national study. Hepatology. 2007;45:1282–9.

11. Myers RP, Papay KD, Shaheen AA, Kaplan GG. Relationship between hospital volume and outcomes of esophageal variceal bleeding in the United States. Clin Gastroenterol Hepatol. 2008;6:789–98.

12. Dixon E, Schneeweiss S, Pasieka JL, Bathe OF, Sutherland F, Doig C. Mortality following liver resection in US medicare patients: does the presence of a liver transplant program affect outcome? J Surg Oncol. 2007;95:194–200.

13. Wiesner RH. Evidence-based evolution of the MELD/PELD liver allocation policy. Liver Transpl. 2005;11:261–3.

14. Myers RP, Shaheen AA, Faris P, Aspinall AI, Burak KW. Revision of MELD to include serum albumin improves prediction of mortality on the liver transplant waiting list. PLoS One. 2013;8:e51926.

15. Quan H, Li B, Couris CM, Fushimi K, Graham P, Hider P, et al. Updating and validating the Charlson comorbidity index and score for risk adjustment in hospital discharge abstracts using data from 6 countries. Am J Epidemiol. 2011;173:676–82.

16. Southern DA, Quan H, Ghali WA. Comparison of the Elixhauser and Charlson/Deyo methods of comorbidity measurement in administrative data. Med Care. 2004;42:355–60.

17. Li B, Evans D, Faris P, Dean S, Quan H. Risk adjustment performance of Charlson and Elixhauser comorbidities in ICD-9 and ICD-10 administrative databases. BMC Health Serv Res. 2008;8:12.

18. Gutacker N, Bloor K, Cookson R. Comparing the performance of the Charlson/Deyo and Elixhauser comorbidity measures across five European countries and three conditions. Eur J Public Health. 2015;25 Suppl 1:15–20.

19. Ladha KS, Zhao K, Quraishi SA, Kurth T, Eikermann M, Kaafarani HM, et al. The Deyo-Charlson and Elixhauser-van Walraven Comorbidity Indices as predictors of mortality in critically ill patients. BMJ Open. 2015;5:e008990.

20. Ochs A, Rossle M, Haag K, Hauenstein KH, Deibert P, Siegerstetter V, et al. The transjugular intrahepatic portosystemic stent-shunt procedure for refractory ascites. N Engl J Med. 1995;332:1192–7.

21. Boursier J, Cesbron E, Tropet AL, Pilette C. Comparison and improvement of MELD and Child-Pugh score accuracies for the prediction of 6-month mortality in cirrhotic patients. J Clin Gastroenterol. 2009;43:580–5.

22. Durand F, Valla D. Assessment of the prognosis of cirrhosis: child-Pugh versus MELD. J Hepatol. 2005;42 Suppl 1:S100–7.

23. Botta F, Giannini E, Romagnoli P, Fasoli A, Malfatti F, Chiarbonello B, et al. MELD scoring system is useful for predicting prognosis in patients with liver cirrhosis and is correlated with residual liver function: a European study. Gut. 2003;52:134–9.

24. Said A, Williams J, Holden J, Remington P, Gangnon R, Musat A, et al. Model for end stage liver disease score predicts mortality across a broad spectrum of liver disease. J Hepatol. 2004;40:897–903.

25. Liu D, Wang X, Pan F, Yang P, Xu Y, Tang X, et al. Harmonization of health data at national level: a pilot study in China. Int J Med Inform. 2010;79:450–8.

26. Lei J, Sockolow P, Guan P, Meng Q, Zhang J. A comparison of electronic health records at two major Peking University Hospitals in China to United States meaningful use objectives. BMC Med Inform Decis Mak. 2013;13:96.

27. Huang H, Hu XF, Zhao FH, Garland SM, Bhatla N, Qiao YL. Estimation of cancer burden attributable to infection in Asia. J Epidemiol. 2015;25:626–38.

28. Liang X, Bi S, Yang W, Wang L, Cui G, Cui F, et al. Epidemiological serosurvey of hepatitis B in China–declining HBV prevalence due to hepatitis B vaccination. Vaccine. 2009;27:6550–7.

29. Bao XY, Xu BB, Fang K, Li Y, Hu YH, Yu GP. Changing trends of hospitalisation of liver cirrhosis in Beijing, China. BMJ Open Gastroenterol. 2015;2:e000051.

30. Xu Y, Li N, Lu M, Myers RP, Dixon E, Walker R, et al. Development and validation of method for defining conditions using Chinese electronic medical record. BMC Med Inform Decis Mak. 2016;16:110.

31. Kim WR, Biggins SW, Kremers WK, Wiesner RH, Kamath PS, Benson JT, et al. Hyponatremia and mortality among patients on the liver-transplant waiting list. N Engl J Med. 2008;359:1018–26.

32. Myers RP, Tandon P, Ney M, Meeberg G, Faris P, Shaheen AA, et al. Validation of the five-variable Model for End-stage Liver Disease (5vMELD) for prediction of mortality on the liver transplant waiting list. Liver Int. 2014; 34:1176–83.

33. Steyerberg EW, Vickers AJ, Cook NR, Gerds T, Gonen M, Obuchowski N, et al. Assessing the performance of prediction models: a framework for traditional and novel measures. Epidemiology. 2010;21:128–38.

34. DeLong ER, DeLong DM, Clarke-Pearson DL. Comparing the areas under two or more correlated receiver operating characteristic curves: a nonparametric approach. Biometrics. 1988;44:837–45.

35. Smith GC, Seaman SR, Wood AM, Royston P, White IR. Correcting for optimistic prediction in small data sets. Am J Epidemiol. 2014;180:318–24.

36. Steyerberg EW, Harrell Jr FE, Borsboom GJ, Eijkemans MJ, Vergouwe Y, Habbema JD. Internal validation of predictive models: efficiency of some procedures for logistic regression analysis. J Clin Epidemiol. 2001;54:774–81.

37. Stukenborg GJ, Wagner DP, Connors Jr AF. Comparison of the performance of two comorbidity measures, with and without information from prior hospitalizations. Med Care. 2001;39:727–39.

6

Unexplained chronic liver disease in Ethiopia

Stian Magnus Staurung Orlien[1], Nejib Yusuf Ismael[2,3], Tekabe Abdosh Ahmed[3,4], Nega Berhe[1,5], Trine Lauritzen[6], Borghild Roald[7,8], Robert David Goldin[9], Kathrine Stene-Johansen[10], Anne Margarita Dyrhol-Riise[8,11,12], Svein Gunnar Gundersen[13,14], Marsha Yvonne Morgan[15] and Asgeir Johannessen[1,16*] (iD)

Abstract

Background: Hepatitis B virus (HBV) infection is assumed to be the major cause of chronic liver disease (CLD) in sub-Saharan Africa. The contribution of other aetiological causes of CLD is less well documented and hence opportunities to modulate other potential risk factors are being lost. The aims of this study were to explore the aetiological spectrum of CLD in eastern Ethiopia and to identify plausible underlying risk factors for its development.

Methods: A cross-sectional study was undertaken between April 2015 and April 2016 in two public hospitals in Harar, eastern Ethiopia. The study population comprised of consenting adults with clinical and radiological evidence of chronic liver disease. The baseline evaluation included: (i) a semi-structured interview designed to obtain information about the ingestion of alcohol, herbal medicines and local recreational drugs such as khat (*Catha edulis*); (ii) clinical examination; (iii) extensive laboratory testing; and, (iv) abdominal ultrasonography.

Results: One-hundred-and-fifty patients with CLD (men 72.0%; median age 30 [interquartile range 25–40] years) were included. CLD was attributed to chronic HBV infection in 55 (36.7%) individuals; other aetiological agents were identified in a further 12 (8.0%). No aetiological factors were identified in the remaining 83 (55.3%) patients. The overall prevalence of daily khat use was 78.0%, while alcohol abuse, defined as > 20 g/day in women and > 30 g/day in men, was rare (2.0%). Histological features of toxic liver injury were observed in a subset of patients with unexplained liver injury who underwent liver biopsy.

Conclusion: The aetiology of CLD in eastern Ethiopia is largely unexplained. The widespread use of khat in the region, together with histopathological findings indicating toxic liver injury, suggests an association which warrants further investigation.

Keywords: Hepatotoxicity, Epidemiology, *Catha edulis*, Viral hepatitis, Sub-Saharan Africa

Background

'Chronic liver disease' (CLD) is the term used to describe disordered liver function lasting for six or more months. It results from a process of progressive destruction and regeneration of the liver parenchyma and encompasses a wide range of liver pathologies including: chronic hepatitis, cirrhosis and hepatocellular carcinoma. CLD is a major cause of morbidity and mortality, and was responsible for an estimated 1.3 million deaths worldwide in 2015 [1]. The commonest causes of CLD are chronic infection with hepatitis B (HBV) or C (HCV), alcohol misuse and non-alcoholic fatty liver disease (NAFLD) [2].

Ethiopia is a low-income country in East Africa with a population of nearly 100 million [3]. The prevalence of CLD in Ethiopia is largely unknown but is assumed to be high [4]. The estimated seroprevalence of hepatitis B surface antigen (HBsAg) in Ethiopia is 6.0% [5] and of HCV-antibody (anti-HCV) 3.1% [6]. Although these data are extracted predominantly from institution-based studies and may not be representative of the situation nationwide, chronic HBV infection is thought to be a major cause of CLD in this region [4].

* Correspondence: johannessen.asgeir@gmail.com
[1]Regional Centre for Imported and Tropical Diseases, Oslo University Hospital Ullevål, Oslo, Norway
[16]Department of Infectious Diseases, Vestfold Hospital Trust, Tønsberg, Norway
Full list of author information is available at the end of the article

Community-based, longitudinal studies have been undertaken in several rural areas of Ethiopia, in recent years, using a verbal autopsy method to assign causes of death [7–9]. CLD was the leading cause of death in the age group 15–49 years in Kersa in eastern Ethiopia (13.7%) [9] and in Butajira in central Ethiopia (11.3%) [7]. In contrast, CLD was the cause of death in only 3.5% of adults of the same age in Kilte Awlalo in northern Ethiopia [8]. One suggested explanation for this difference is the relative availability of khat (*Catha edulis*), an indigenous plant which is chewed for its psychotropic effects. Khat chewing has been associated with the development of CLD [10]; its use is widespread in eastern [11] and south-central Ethiopia [12] but much less so in northern parts of the country [13].

One of the most important aspects of CLD prevention is the identification and management of potential risk factors. Public health efforts to reduce the toll of CLD in Ethiopia and other countries in sub-Saharan Africa will be considerably hampered if information on avoidable or treatable risk factors is unavailable. Thus, the aims of this study were to explore the aetiological spectrum of CLD in eastern Ethiopia and to identify plausible underlying risk factors for CLD using a hospital-based cross-sectional design.

Methods
Study setting and participants
A cross-sectional study of indigenous adults, aged ≥18 years, presenting for the first time with features of CLD was undertaken in two governmental hospitals in Harar, eastern Ethiopia between April 2015 and April 2016. CLD was defined as: (i) the presence of clinical features suggestive of decompensated liver disease viz. ascites, jaundice and/or hepatic encephalopathy; and (ii) the presence, on ultrasound, of hepatic parenchyma heterogeneity and/or surface irregularity. Patients presenting with severe acute hepatitis defined as liver injury of < 6 weeks duration, serum alanine aminotransferase (ALT) activity of > 100 U/L and the absence of coarsened echotexture and surface irregularity on ultrasonography, were excluded. Also excluded were patients with liver dysfunction secondary to comorbidities viz. congestive cardiac failure, biliary obstruction and septicaemia. Patients who had previously diagnosed CLD were excluded since they might represent a subgroup with more severe liver disease, or might have altered their risk habits in response to previous medical advice.

Patient assessment
Suitable patients presenting to the regional Hiwot Fana Specialized University Hospital, and the local Jugal Hospital underwent a semi-structured interview by local nurses fluent in their mother tongue. Demographic data

were recorded and potential risk factors for CLD were explored. Information on past and current use of alcohol was obtained and quantified in grams. Daily alcohol consumption of > 20 g in women and > 30 g in men, for a minimum period of 6 months, was classified as alcohol misuse. Information on khat usage was obtained using a visual analogue scale and quantified in grams. The frequency and duration of khat use in years was used to classify lifetime khat exposure as *khat-years*. Approximately 100–300 g of fresh khat leaves are chewed in a typical session [14]; thus, one khat-year was defined as daily use of 200 g of fresh khat for 1 year.

Clinical examination was undertaken using a prespecified proforma.

Laboratory tests
Blood was collected by venous puncture for immediate processing; serum and plasma were separated and stored in aliquots at − 20 °C until transported on ice/dry ice for analysis either in Ethiopia or Norway. Full blood counts were performed using a KX-21 N™ haematology analyser (Sysmex, Kobe, Japan). Standard biochemical tests were analysed using a semi-automatic biochemistry analyser DR-7000D (DIRUI, Changchun, China) and HumaLyzer 3000 (HUMAN, Wiesbaden, Germany). The serum aspartate aminotransferase (AST) to platelet ratio index (APRI) was calculated as $\frac{\frac{AST\ (U/L)}{upper\ reference\ range\ of\ AST\ (U/L)}}{platelet\ count\ (10^9/L)} \times 100$ [15], using a threshold of 0.7 as indicator of significant fibrosis [16]. The Fibrosis-4 (FIB-4) score was calculated as $\frac{age\ (years)\ x\ AST\ (U/L)}{platelet\ count\ (10^9/L)\ x\ \sqrt{ALT\ (U/L)}}$, using a threshold of 3.25 to indicate advanced fibrosis/cirrhosis [17].

HBsAg was measured using the rapid diagnostic test (RDT) Determine™ (Alere, Waltham, MA, USA); anti-HCV was measured using the SD BIOLINE HCV RDT (Standard Diagnostics, Yongin-si, Republic of Korea). Confirmatory testing of HBsAg and anti-HCV was undertaken using enzyme-linked immunosorbent assays (Elisys Uno, HUMAN, Wiesbaden, Germany; or Architect, Abbott Diagnostics, IL, USA). HBV DNA and HCV RNA were measured in patients who tested positive for HBsAg or anti-HCV by polymerase chain reaction using RealTime HBV, m2000 system (Abbott Molecular, Abbott Park, IL, USA). Plasma was analysed for hepatitis D virus (HDV) antigen and HDV-antibody using the ETI-DELTAK-2 and ETI-AB-DELTAK-2 assay (DiaSorin, Turin, Italy), respectively.

Human immunodeficiency virus (HIV) screening was performed using the KHB HIV (1 + 2) Antibody RDT (Shanghai Kehua Bio-Engineering, Shanghai, China) and confirmed using the HIV 1/2 STAT-PAK® RDT (Chembio Diagnostics, Medford, NY, USA). Malaria screening was performed using the SD BIOLINE Malaria Ag P.f/

P.v RDT (Standard Diagnostics) and confirmed by microscopy of blood smears.

Serum was analysed for immunoglobulin G using the IMMAGE® 800 Immunochemistry System (Beckman Coulter, Brea, CA, USA). Serum iron and transferrin concentrations were quantified using ARCHITECT ci16200 (Abbott Diagnostics). Total iron binding capacity (TIBC) was calculated as $25.1 \times$ serum transferrin (g/L) and transferrin saturation as $\frac{\text{serum iron (μmol/L)}}{\text{TIBC (μmol/L)}} \, 100\%$.

Anti-nuclear, anti-mitochondrial and anti-actin antibodies were analysed by the Phadia™250 Laboratory system (Thermo Fisher Scientific, Waltham, MA, USA) using the EliA™ Symphony assay (Phadia, Freiburg, Germany), QUANTA Lite® M2 EP (MIT3) and QUANTA Lite® Actin IgG (Inova Diagnostics, San Diego, CA, USA).

A stool sample was collected and five thick smears processed according to a modified Kato-Katz technique using 41.7-mg templates for detection of the ova of *Schistosoma mansoni* [18].

Patients who, after initial screening, appeared to have unexplained CLD underwent more extensive testing including: measurement of serum alpha-1-antitrypsin and caeruloplasmin concentrations using the IMMAGE® 800 Immunochemistry System (Beckman Coulter); high iron Fe (*HFE*) genotyping, if the serum transferrin saturation was increased above 50%, without obvious explanation; and, screening for visceral leishmaniasis using a recombinant K39-antigen strip test IT-LEISH® (Bio-Rad) and confirmed by Giemsa stained splenic smear.

Urine from all women < 45 years of age was tested for human chorionic gonadotropin (hCG) using a HCG Pregnancy Strip Test (Nantong Egens Biotechnology, Jiangsu, China).

Abdominal imaging

Abdominal ultrasonography was undertaken to a predetermined standard by a local radiologist using a 3.5 MHz convex transducer Flexus SSD-1100 (Aloka, Tokyo, Japan). The diagnosis of CLD was based on the presence of an irregular liver surface and/or liver parenchyma heterogeneity [19]. The presence of schistosomal periportal fibrosis was diagnosed using WHO criteria [20] and re-evaluated by an independent expert.

Determination of the aetiology of the CLD

Historical, clinical, laboratory and imaging data were used to identify the aetiology of the underlying CLD using published criteria (Table 1) [21–25].

Liver biopsy and histopathology

It was intended that all patients in whom the aetiology of the CLD remained unexplained following investigation would be offered a liver biopsy. However, during the period April 2015 to April 2016, no suitably trained personnel were available to undertake this procedure. This situation was eventually resolved and the patients were subsequently contacted and asked to return for liver biopsy. In the interim several of the more decompensated patients had died and as the biopsies were to be performed percutaneously, only those with a normal or marginally elevated prothrombin time were considered suitable [26].

The procedure was performed, under ultrasound guidance, using a sterile Menghini technique with local anaesthetic and a 17G needle Hepafix® (Braun, Melsungen, Germany). Serial four μm sections were cut and stained with haematoxylin and eosin; Gomori (reticulin); van Gieson (collagen); Masson Trichrome (metachromatic); periodic acid-Schiff (PAS), with and without diastase (glycogen); and Perls (iron). Histopathologists in Norway and London independently assessed the histological findings blinded to the clinical information; inflammation and fibrosis were graded and staged using the semi-quantitative, modified Histological Activity Index [27]. Subsequent immunohistochemistry was undertaken using Ki-67 as a proliferation marker (Dako, catalogue number M724, concentration 1/100 with pre-treatment) and activated caspase-3, (Cell Signalling Technology, catalogue number 9664, concentration 1/100 with pre-treatment) as an apoptotic marker. Image analysis to quantify the degree of fibrosis and to calculate the collagen proportionate area (CPA) was carried out on scanned, Sirius Red stained sections [28].

Statistical methods

Statistical analyses were performed in SPSS 23.0 (SPSS Inc., Chicago, IL, USA). Categorical variables were summarized as frequencies, while continuous variables were presented as median and interquartile range (IQR). Comparisons between groups were performed using the Pearson χ^2-test for categorical variables and Mann-Whitney U-test for continuous variables. A *p*-value < 0.05 was considered significant. The *Strengthening the Reporting of Observational studies in Epidemiology* (STROBE) statement guidelines were followed [29].

Ethics

The study was approved by the National Research Ethics Review Committee (Ref. No.: 3.10/829/07 and 3.10/129/2016) in Ethiopia and by the Regional Committees for Medical and Health Research Ethics (Ref. No.: 2014/1146) in Norway. The study was conducted in accordance with the Declaration of Helsinki [30]. Written informed consent was obtained from all participating individuals.

Table 1 Criteria used to assign the aetiology of the liver disease

Aetiology		Criteria used to assign diagnosis
1	Chronic hepatitis B infection	Evidence of CLD on liver ultrasound and positive serum HBsAg.
2	Chronic hepatitis C infection	Evidence of CLD on liver ultrasound and positive serum anti-HCV and positive HCV RNA.
3	Chronic hepatitis D infection	Chronic hepatitis B infection and positive serum anti HDV IgG confirmed by detection of HDV RNA.

4	Primary biliary cholangitis	i. Strongly positive anti-mitochondrial antibodies and
		ii. Cholestatic liver function tests:
		  a. ALP > 1.5 x URR and
		  b. AST < 5 x URR

5	Autoimmune hepatitis[a]	i. Strongly positive anti-nuclear antibodies or anti-actin and ii. Elevated IgG > 1.1 x URR
6	Alcoholic liver disease	i. Clinical and radiological signs of CLD and ii. Daily alcohol consumption > 20 g/day in women and > 30 g/day in men for 6 months or more.
7	Non-alcoholic fatty liver disease	i. Liver ultrasound findings of steatosis and ii. Absence of significant alcohol consumption[b] or other recognised secondary causes of steatosis and iii. BMI > 25 kg/m^2 [c]
8	Haemochromatosis	i. Transferrin saturation > 50% and ii. Genotyping showing C282Y homozygosity or C282Y/H63D heterozygosity or C282Y/S65C heterozygosity on the HFE gene.
9	Wilson's disease	i. Serum caeruloplasmin < 0.140 g/L and ii. Age < 40 years
10	Alpha-1-antitrypsin deficiency	Serum alpha-1-antitrypsin level < 0.85 g/L.
11	Malaria	Positive malaria rapid diagnostic test and positive microscopy.
12	Hepatic schistosomiasis	Presence of ova from *Schistosoma mansoni* in Kato-Katz thick stool smears and typical liver ultrasound findings viz. periportal thickening/'pipestem' fibrosis confirmed by an independent expert.
13	Visceral leishmaniasis	Ultrasound findings of hepatosplenomegaly and positive K39 antigen strip test confirmed by positive splenic smear.
14	Unexplained chronic liver disease	None of the above

Abbreviations: ALP alkaline phosphatase, *anti-HCV* hepatitis C virus antibody, *anti-HDV* hepatitis D virus antibody, *AST* aspartate aminotransferase, *BMI* body mass index, *CLD* chronic liver disease, *HBsAg* hepatitis B surface antigen, *HCV* hepatitis C virus, *HDV* hepatitis D virus, *HFE* high iron Fe, *IgG* immunoglobulin G, *URR* upper reference range
Laboratory reference ranges: ALP (60–306 U/L); AST (14–40 U/L); IgG (0.8–27.8 g/L) [21]
[a]Based on the American Association for the Study of Liver Disease (AASLD) simplified criteria [22] in the absence of histology
[b]Alcohol consumption < 20 g/day in women and < 30 g/day in men
[c]Not a part of the AASLD criteria [23] but adopted to exclude cases of starvation-induced steatosis

Results

Study population

A total of 244 patients with liver disease were admitted to hospital during the study period. Of these, 212 patients presented with a new diagnosis of probable CLD and were evaluated for inclusion. The final study population comprised of 150 cases with newly diagnosed CLD (Fig. 1).

Aetiological spectrum

The aetiology of the liver disease was identified in 67 (44.7%) of the 150 patients and ascribed to chronic HBV infection in 55 (36.7%); hepatic schistosomiasis in four (2.7%); alcohol misuse in three (2.0%); chronic HCV infection in two (1.3%); autoimmune hepatitis in two (1.3%) and visceral leishmaniasis in one (0.7%). No cause was identified in the remaining 83 (55.3%) patients, in whom the liver disease was, therefore, unexplained.

Demography

Overall, there were more men (72.0%) than women; the median age was 30 (IQR 25–40) years (Table 2). The majority of the study subjects were Muslim (92.7%). The overall reported prevalence of daily khat use was 78.0%. Khat use was more common among men than women (92.6% vs. 40.5%; $p < 0.001$); overall khat exposure was also higher in men than women (36 vs. 0.6 khat-years; $p < 0.001$).

Women were more likely to have unexplained CLD than men (71.4% vs. 49.1%; $p = 0.013$). Otherwise there were no significant differences in demographic features between the aetiology known/unknown groups.

Clinical presentation

The majority of the patients presented with clinical features suggestive of hepatic decompensation (Table 3). Patients with unexplained CLD were more likely to

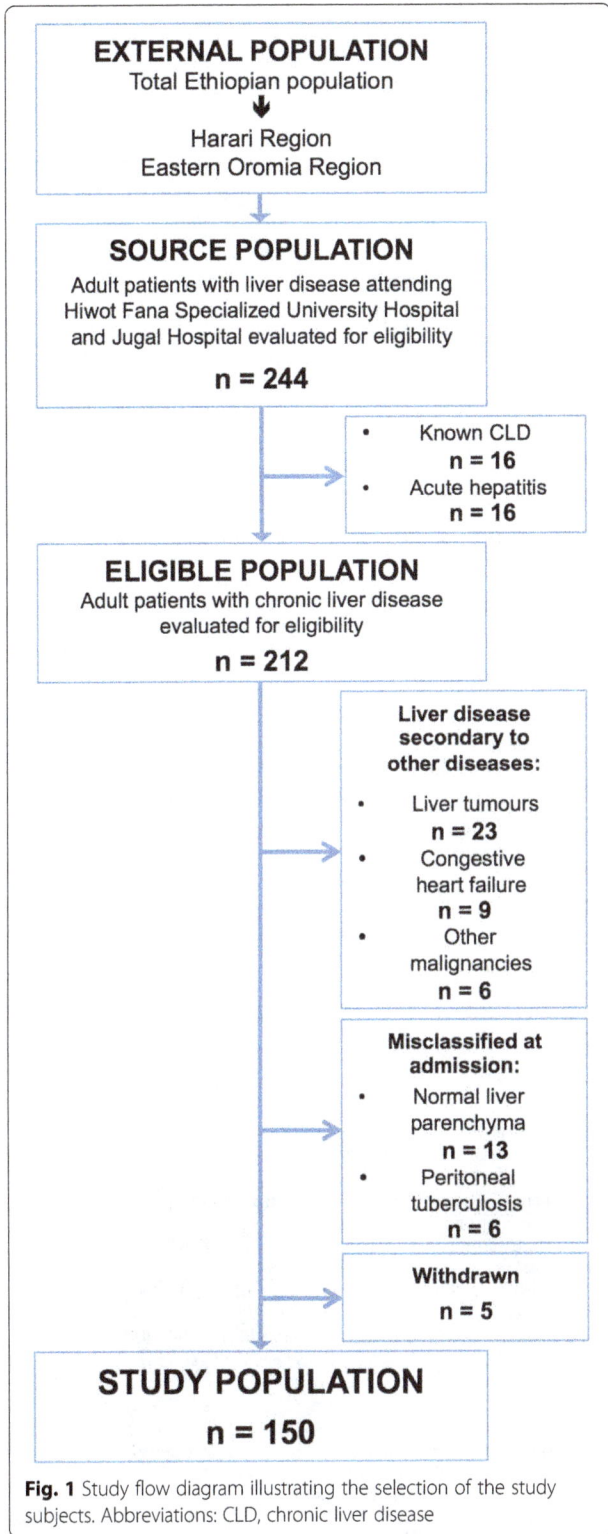

Fig. 1 Study flow diagram illustrating the selection of the study subjects. Abbreviations: CLD, chronic liver disease

Table 2 Demographic features of the study subjects with chronic liver disease, by aetiology

Variable	All patients (n = 150)	Aetiology known (n = 67)	Aetiology unknown (n = 83)
Sex (n, % men)	108 (72.0)	55 (82.1)	53 (63.9)*
Age (years)	30 (25–40)	30 (20–40)	30 (25–40)
Ethnic group			
Oromo	134 (89.3)	59 (88.1)	75 (90.4)
Amhara	9 (6.0)	5 (7.5)	4 (4.8)
Somali	5 (3.3)	2 (3.0)	3 (3.6)
Gurage	2 (1.3)	1 (1.5)	1 (1.2)
Religion			
Islam	139 (92.7)	60 (89.6)	79 (95.2)
Christianity	11 (7.3)	7 (10.4)	4 (4.8)
Occupation			
Farmer	100 (66.7)	46 (68.7)	54 (65.1)
Unemployed	14 (9.3)	5 (7.5)	9 (10.8)
Housewife	11 (7.3)	2 (3.0)	9 (10.8)
Student	8 (5.3)	5 (7.5)	3 (3.6)
Day worker	5 (3.3)	3 (4.5)	2 (2.4)
Public servant	4 (2.7)	1 (1.5)	3 (3.6)
Health professional	2 (1.3)	2 (3.0)	0
Other	6 (4.0)	3 (4.5)	3 (3.6)
Pregnant	3 (2.0)	1 (8.3)	2 (6.7)
Previous blood transfusion	23 (15.3)	9 (13.4)	14 (16.9)
Family history of liver disease	8 (5.3)	4 (6.0)	4 (4.8)
Dietary grain stored underground	53 (35.3)	25 (37.3)	28 (33.7)
Weeks of storage	24 (12–52)	24 (12–52)	24 (12–52)
Traditional herbal medicine	40 (26.7)	16 (23.9)	24 (28.9)
History of alcohol consumption:			
Never	139 (92.7)	61 (91.0)	78 (94.0)
Current	6 (4.0)	5 (7.5)	1 (1.2)
Stopped	5 (3.3)	1 (1.5)	4 (4.8)
Alcohol abuse[a]	3 (2.0)	3 (4.5)	0
History of daily use of khat	117 (78.0)	56 (83.6)	61 (73.5)
Khat-years[b]	20 (3–70)	20 (3–75)	18 (1–60)

Data are presented as number (%) or as median (interquartile range) unless otherwise noted

*$p < 0.05$; significance of the difference between the aetiology known/unknown group

[a]Daily consumption of > 20 g/day in women and > 30 g/day in men for 6 months or more

[b]One khat-year is defined as daily use of 200 g fresh khat for 1 year

present with abdominal swelling than those in whom the aetiology was known (92.8% vs. 76.1%; $p = 0.004$). Otherwise there were no distinguishing clinical features between the aetiology known/unknown groups.

Laboratory findings

Overall, the alterations in laboratory variables were mild (Table 4). A total of 92 (61.7%) patients had an APRI score of > 0.7 while 43 (28.9%) had a FIB-4 score of > 3.25. Patients with unexplained CLD had a lower median serum ALT activity (30 U/L [IQR 21–51] vs. 41 [IQR

Table 3 Clinical characteristics and ultrasound findings in the study subjects with chronic liver disease, by aetiology

Variable	All patients (n = 150)	Aetiology known (n = 67)	Aetiology unknown (n = 83)
Symptoms			
Abdominal swelling	128 (85.3)	51 (76.1)	77 (92.8)*
Epigastric pain	12 (80.0)	56 (83.6)	64 (77.1)
Weight loss	119 (79.3)	54 (80.6)	65 (78.3)
Fever	77 (51.3)	35 (52.2)	42 (50.6)
Arthralgia/myalgia	75 (50.3)[a]	33 (49.3)	42 (51.2)[a]
Nausea	69 (46.3)[a]	30 (45.5)[a]	39 (47.0)
Diarrhoea	64 (42.7)	27 (40.3)	37 (44.6)
Haematemesis	53 (35.3)	27 (40.3)	26 (31.3)
History of jaundice	47 (31.3)	24 (35.8)	23 (27.7)
Clinical findings			
Ascites	138 (92.0)	60 (89.6)	78 (94.0)
Splenomegaly	99 (66.0)	48 (71.6)	51 (61.4)
Jaundice	28 (18.7)	16 (23.9)	12 (14.5)
Caput medusae	25 (16.7)	8 (11.9)	17 (20.5)
Hepatic encephalopathy	16 (10.7)	7 (10.4)	9 (10.8)
Traditional scarring/burning	101 (67.3)	46 (68.7)	55 (66.3)
Ultrasound findings			
Ascites	138 (92.0)	60 (89.6)	78 (94.0)
Smooth liver surface	4 (2.7)	3 (4.5)	1 (1.2)
Mild uneven liver surface	44 (29.3)	15 (22.4)	29 (34.9)
Nodular liver surface	102 (68.0)	49 (73.1)	53 (63.9)
Heterogeneous echotexture	62 (41.3)	22 (32.8)	40 (48.2)
Coarse echotexture	87 (58.0)	44 (65.7)	43 (51.8)
Hepatic steatosis	1 (0.7)	1 (1.5)	0
Periportal fibrosis	21 (14.0)	9 (13.4)	12 (14.5)
In-hospital death	9 (6.0)[a]	4 (6.0)	5 (6.1)[a]

Data are presented as number (%) or as median (interquartile range) unless otherwise noted
[a]One observation missing
*p < 0.05; significance of the difference between the aetiology known/unknown group

Table 4 Laboratory findings in the study subjects with chronic liver disease, by aetiology

Laboratory variable	All patients (n = 150)	Aetiology known (n = 67)	Aetiology unknown (n = 83)
ALT (U/L)	34 (22–55)	41 (24–58)	30 (21–51)*
> URR	60 (40.0)	34 (50.7)	26 (31.3)*
AST (U/L)	44 (28–81)	52 (31–83)	41 (28–78)
> URR	84 (56.0)	41 (61.2)	43 (51.8)
ALP (U/L)	317 (207–416)	315 (250–423)	320 (200–385)
> URR	80 (53.3)	37 (55.2)	43 (51.8)
GGT (U/L)	29 (19–48)	29 (21–47)	29 (18–52)
> URR	30 (20.0)	14 (20.9)	16 (19.3)
Total bilirubin (µmol/L)	19 (10–38)	21 (12–51)	17 (10–31)
> URR	36 (24.0)	20 (29.9)	16 (19.3)
Albumin (g/L)	37 (28–50)	36 (30–50)	37 (27–50)
< LRR	63 (42.0)	27 (40.3)	36 (43.4)
Creatinine (µmol/L)	80 (62–97)	80 (62–97)	71 (62–88)
> URR	23 (15.3)	11 (16.4)	12 (14.5)
< LRR	19 (12.7)	8 (11.9)	11 (13.3)
Platelet count (10⁹/L)	125 (76–206)	123 (71–186)	147 (76–223)
< LRR	75 (50.0)	36 (53.7)	39 (47.0)
IgG (g/L)	23.9 (17.1–32.5)	27.0 (16.7–34.2)	21.6 (17.2–30.6)
> URR	55 (36.7)	31 (46.3)	24 (28.9)
HIV infection[a]	4 (2.7)	1 (1.5)	3 (3.6)
Kato-Katz smear positive	23 (16.5)[b]	13 (21.3)[c]	10 (12.8)[d]
APRI score > 0.7[e]	92 (61.7)[f]	46 (69.7)[f]	46 (55.4)
FIB-4 score > 3.25[g]	43 (28.9)[f]	20 (30.3)[f]	23 (27.7)
APRI score > 0.7 OR FIB-4 score > 3.25	94 (63.1)[f]	46 (69.7)[f]	48 (57.8)

Data are presented as number (%) or as median (interquartile range)
Laboratory reference ranges: ALT (8–40 U/L); AST (14–40 U/L); ALP (60–306 U/L); GGT (7–61 U/L); Bilirubin (3–38 µmol/L); Albumin (35–52 g/L); Creatinine (47–109 µmol/L); Platelet count (126–438 × 10⁹/L); IgG (0.8–27.8 g/L) [21]
[a]One patient with chronic HCV was co-infected with HIV.
[b]Stool sample missing in 11 patients.
[c]Stool sample missing in six patients.
[d]Stool sample missing in five patients.
[e]APRI: (AST (U/L)/URR of AST (U/L))/platelet count (10⁹/L) × 100
[f]One observation missing.
[g]FIB-4: age (years) x AST (U/L)/(platelet count (10⁹/L) x √ALT (U/L))
*p < 0.05; significance of the difference between the aetiology known/unknown group
Abbreviations: ALP alkaline phosphatase, ALT alanine aminotransferase, APRI aspartate aminotransferase to platelets ratio index, AST aspartate aminotransferase, GGT gamma-glutamyltransferase, HCV hepatitis C virus, HIV human immunodeficiency virus, IgG immunoglobulin G, LRR lower reference range, URR upper reference range

24–58]; p = 0.032) and values above the upper reference range (URR) were observed in proportionately fewer patients than amongst those in whom the aetiology was known (31.3% vs. 50.7%; p = 0.016). Otherwise there were no distinguishing laboratory features between the aetiology known/unknown groups.

Abdominal ultrasound findings
The commonest findings on liver ultrasound were an irregular/nodular liver surface (68.0%), coarse liver texture (58.0%) and ascites (92.0%) (Table 3). There were no significant differences in abdominal ultrasound findings between the aetiology known/unknown groups.

Histopathology
Of the 83 patients with unexplained CLD, 15 (18.1%) died during or shortly after admission; 35 (42.2%) could not be contacted; four (4.8%) refused to undergo the procedure, while 24 (28.9%) were unsuitable because of a severe coagulopathy. Thus, only five (6.0%) patients

underwent liver biopsy a median (range) of 33 (20–64) weeks after their initial hospitalization (Table 5); three (Cases 1/2/4) had a history of khat chewing.

Microscopically none of the specimens showed more than mild fibrosis and inflammation (Table 6). Foci of pale stained swollen hepatocytes were identified in Cases 1–4, with no marked zonal distribution; these stained negative for PAS and were thus suggestive of toxic injury (Case 1; Fig. 2a-f). The fifth patient showed no evidence of adaptive parenchymal changes but mild mixed steatosis and focal single cell necrosis (Fig. 2g-h). Although the numbers were modest and the differences small, the proliferation index, apoptotic scores and the CPA tended to be higher among the three patients (Cases 1/2/4) who chewed khat compared to the two who did not (Cases 3/5).

Discussion

This study aimed to explore the aetiological spectrum and underlying risk factors for the development of CLD in eastern Ethiopia. Chronic HBV infection was the major identified risk factor, explaining the development of CLD in roughly one-third of the patients. However, an aetiological factor was identified in less than 10% of the remainder. Thus, in over half of the included cases the aetiology of the liver disease was unexplained.

Of prime importance in this study was the surety of the diagnosis of CLD. The criteria used were stringent and required not only that patients had clinical evidence of decompensated liver disease but also evidence of hepatic parenchyma heterogeneity and/or surface irregularity on ultrasound. The liver function test abnormalities were mild but this is not incompatible with the diagnosis of CLD. Over two-thirds of the patients had APRI and/or FIB-4 scores compatible with a diagnosis of significant fibrosis/cirrhosis. The histological findings in the five patients who underwent liver biopsy would seem at odds with a diagnosis of CLD; however, these patients fulfilled the inclusion criteria at presentation and biopsies undertaken after a considerable delay still showed evidence of ongoing disease. Thus, the fact that the patients included in this study had CLD can be accepted with a high degree of certainty.

The proportion of patients, in the present study, in whom the CLD was aetiologically unexplained is substantially higher than might be expected. In the 1980's more than 50% of cases of CLD worldwide did not have an ascribed cause compared with the current global estimate of approximately 5% [31–33]. Thus, the prevalence of unexplained CLD in this area of eastern Ethiopia is ten-fold higher than would be expected. No observational studies exploring the aetiological spectrum of CLD in eastern Ethiopia or in sub-Saharan Africa are available for comparison.

The seroprevalence of HBsAg in the present population was high while the seroprevalence of anti-HCV was low. There are no representative population-based prevalence studies on viral hepatitis in this part of Ethiopia. However, a recent study of blood donors in eastern Ethiopia found similar seroprevalence rates to those reported here [34].

No data are available on the prevalence of NAFLD in Ethiopia although it is known that Ethiopia has one of the lowest prevalence rates of obesity worldwide [35]. The data that are available from other populations suggest that the overall prevalence of NAFLD in sub-Saharan Africa is low [36]. In a case-control study undertaken in Nigeria, 16.7% of patients with type II diabetes mellitus were found to have NAFLD compared with only 1.2% of non-diabetic control subjects, suggesting that, in comparison with Caucasian, Indian and Asian populations, diabetes may be a more important risk factor for NAFLD in Africa than obesity [37]. None of the patients in the present study was obese; other than one case with alcoholic liver disease, none had significant steatosis on hepatic ultrasound and only one had diabetes. Thus, the prevalence of NAFLD in this study population is likely to be very low.

The prevalence of daily khat use identified in the present study was much higher than previously reported [11, 13]. A regional study in Harar city found that 20.9% of 1890 secondary school students chewed khat daily; the lifetime prevalence of khat chewing was 24.2% [11]. The 2011 Ethiopian Demographic and Health Survey identified an overall prevalence of khat chewing of 15.3%. However, there are significant regional variations in the prevalence from 53.2% in the Harari region in eastern Ethiopia to 1.1% in the Tigray region in northern Ethiopia [13]. Khat use is more widespread amongst Muslims than Christians and amongst men than in women [11, 13], which accords with the findings in the present study.

There are a number of case reports which implicate khat as a factor in the development of both acute [38] and chronic liver disease [39–41]. In addition, khat-related hepatotoxicity has been convincingly demonstrated in animal models [42]. The fact that khat use was similar amongst patients with and without other risk factors indicated that it may act as a sole or an adjuvant cause of liver injury. Although only a limited number of liver biopsies was undertaken, the histological findings of focal parenchymal changes mirror those observed in animal models [42] and are supportive of toxic liver injury. However, the design of this study does not allow a definitive conclusion to be made, and further studies to assess causality are needed.

This study had a number of strengths despite the resource limitations at the Ethiopian sites. First: the

Table 5 Characteristics of the five patients with unexplained chronic liver disease who underwent liver biopsy

No.	Sex	Age (yr)	Alcohol use	Khat use	Main symptoms and signs	Main ultrasound findings	ALT (U/L)	AST (U/L)	ALP (U/L)	Albumin (g/L)	Bilirubin (µmol/L)	APRI score[a]	FIB-4 score[b]	Biopsy delay (wk)
1	Female	26	Never	100 g/day, 10 yr	Abdominal swelling; abdominal pain; nausea; diarrhoea; fatigue Ascites	Heterogenous liver texture Mild uneven liver surface Gross ascites Moderate splenomegaly	15	16	88	50	9	0.20	0.53	20
2	Male	25	Never	200 g/day, 5 yr	Abdominal pain; Diarrhea; arthralgia / myalgia	Heterogenous liver texture Mild uneven liver surface Periportal fibrosis Moderate splenomegaly	15	19	107	46	19	0.74	1.92	33
3	Female	30	Never	Never	Abdominal swelling; abdominal pain Ascites; umbilical hernia; non-specific rash	Heterogenous liver texture Mild uneven liver surface Gross ascites Reduced liver span	43	44	258	20	5	0.68	1.25	64
4	Male	25	36 g/day × 1/ wk., 3 yr	400 g/day × 3/ wk., 5 yr	Abdominal pain; nausea; diarrhea; arthralgia/myalgia Splenomegaly	Heterogenous liver texture Mild uneven liver surface Splenomegaly	100	98	300	58	31	1.34	1.34	22
5	Female	25	Never	Never	Abdominal swelling; fatigue; peripheral oedema. Ascites	Heterogenous liver texture Mild uneven liver surface Gross ascites Reduced liver span	39	62	385	27	17	0.76	1.22	58

Abbreviations: ALP alkaline phosphatase, *ALT* alanine aminotransferase, *APRI* aspartate aminotransferase to platelets ratio index, *AST* aspartate aminotransferase, *URR* upper reference range
Laboratory reference ranges: ALT (8–40 U/L); AST (14–40 U/L); ALP (60–306 U/L); Albumin (35–52 g/L); Bilirubin (3–38 µmol/L)
[a]APRI: (AST (U/L)/URR of AST (U/L)/platelet count (10^9/L) × 100
[b]FIB-4: age (years) x AST (U/L)/(platelet count (10^9/L) x √ALT (U/L))

Table 6 Histopathological findings of the five patients with unexplained chronic liver disease who underwent liver biopsy

No	Sex	Age (yr)	General microscopy	Parenchymal changes	Ishak-score
1	Female	26	Mild portal and lobular hepatitis with sinusoidal lymphocytosis. Variation of hepatic cord thickness. Normal bile ducts and intact liver plate.	Focal adaptive parenchymal changes with diffuse hepatocyte swelling/ clarification. No steatosis or haemosiderosis. Collagen proportionate area: 5% Proliferation index: 8% Apoptosis index: 3%	Fibrosis = 2 Necroinflammation = 2 • piecemeal 0 • lobular 1 • confluent 0 • portal 1
2	Male	25	Normal architecture with normal portal areas, no inflammation. Normal bile ducts and intact liver plate.	Adaptive parenchymal changes with diffuse hepatocyte swelling/ clarification. No steatosis or haemosiderosis. Collagen proportionate area: 6% Proliferation index: 12% Apoptosis index: 5%	Fibrosis = 1 Necroinflammation = 0
3	Female	30	Normal architecture with normal portal areas, no inflammation. Normal bile ducts and intact liver plate.	Mild adaptive parenchymal changes with diffuse hepatocyte swelling/clarification. No steatosis or haemosiderosis. Collagen proportionate area: 3% Proliferation index: 6% Apoptosis index: 1%	Fibrosis = 1 Necroinflammation = 1 • piecemeal 0 • lobular 1 • confluent 0 • portal 0
4	Male	25	Normal architecture with normal portal areas, no inflammation. Normal bile ducts and intact liver plate.	Adaptive parenchymal changes with diffuse hepatocyte swelling/clarification. No steatosis or haemosiderosis. Collagen proportionate area: 8% Proliferation index: 15% Apoptosis index: 6%	Fibrosis = 0 Necroinflammation = 0
5	Female	25	Normal architecture with normal portal areas. Normal bile ducts and intact liver plate	Mild mixed steatosis ≈ 20% Focal single cell necrosis, a few apoptotic hepatocytes, a few parenchymal granulocytes. No adaptive changes. Collagen proportionate area: 3% Proliferation index: 3% Apoptosis index: 2%	Fibrosis = 0 Necroinflammation = 1 • piecemeal 0 • lobular 1 • confluent 0 • portal 0

sample size was large and the prospective inclusion of study subjects provided consistent data sampling throughout the study period. Second: robust clinical, laboratory and ultrasound criteria were used to define CLD. Third: the aetiology of the liver injury was determined following a comprehensive, standardized clinical evaluation, multicentre laboratory testing using high-performance diagnostics, abdominal ultrasound with expert review, and, in a small number, histological examination of liver biopsy material.

The study also has its limitations. First: selection bias cannot be excluded, as an unknown proportion of patients with CLD may not have been seen by the recruiting medical services for a variety of practical, cultural and socioeconomic reasons. Second: liver biopsies were undertaken in only a small number of patients with unexplained CLD; the selection procedure for liver biopsy undoubtedly favoured those with the mildest disease and the time interval between presentation and the procedure was sufficiently long for there to have been some resolution of the liver disease. Nevertheless, the histological findings provided useful confirmatory evidence of toxic liver injury in some. Third: issue could be taken with the criteria used to diagnose schistosomal liver

disease. Positive assignment required a positive stool smear and radiological evidence of periportal thickening/'pipe stem' fibrosis confirmed by expert opinion; thus, the diagnosis may have been underestimated. Fourth: HBV DNA levels were not measured in 95 HBsAg-negative patients and thus the presence of occult HBV could not be ruled out in this subgroup [43]. However, the pathogenetic mechanism of occult HBV infection is still not clear [44] and the role of occult HBV in unexplained CLD is still debated [33]. Approximately 95% of the patients with unexplained CLD in the present study had decompensated disease on presentation but only low-grade abnormalities in the liver transaminase activities. Thus, it is unlikely that occult HBV infection was the underlying cause of the unexplained CLD in this population. Finally: the diagnosis of CLD was not confirmed by advanced imaging, endoscopy or, in the majority, by histological examination of liver biopsy material. Furthermore, certain causes of CLD could not be ruled out due to resource limitations, including: primary sclerosing cholangitis, veno-occlusive disease/Budd-Chiari syndrome and injury from other hepatotoxins.

CLD has recently been reported as the leading cause of death in adults less than 50 years of age in eastern

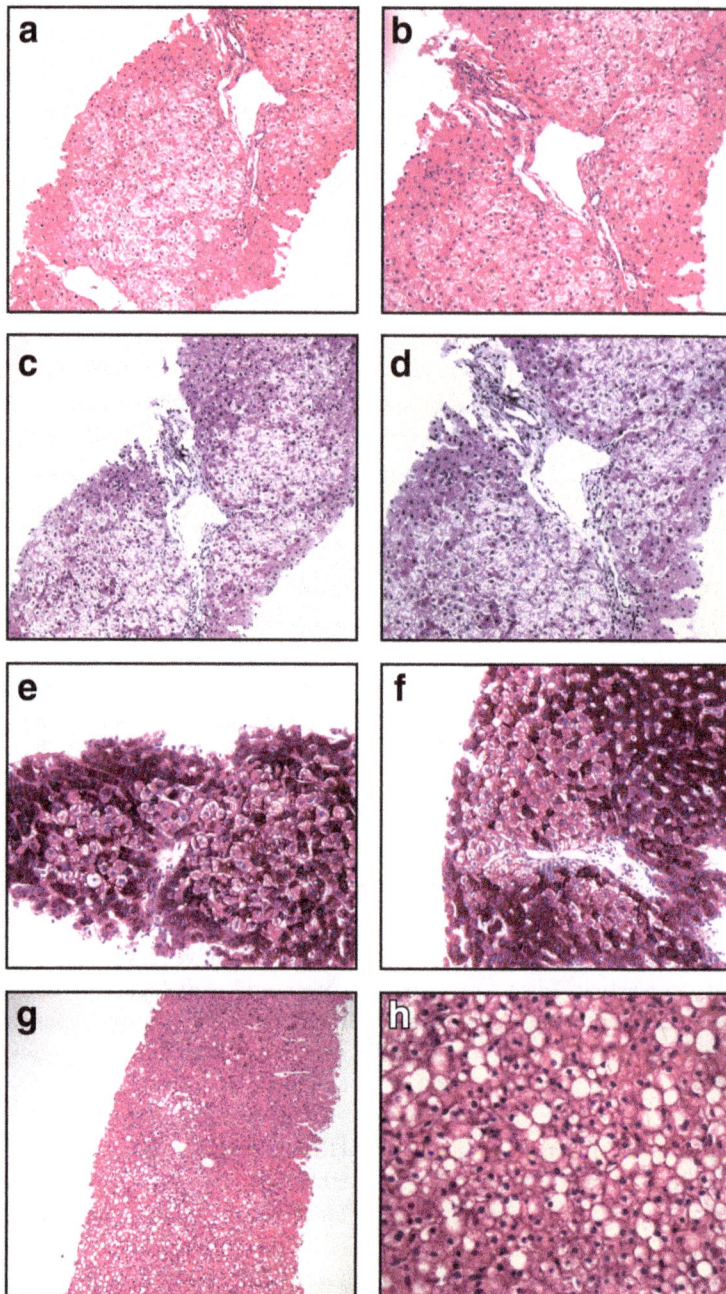

Fig. 2 Liver histology in Ethiopian patients with unexplained chronic liver disease. **a** Case 1: Adaptive parenchymal changes with focal diffuse swollen pale stained hepatocytes stretching through all zones. H&E, 100×. **b** Case 1: Intact liver plate, normal bile ducts and patent central vein. Sinusoidal lymphocytosis. H&E, 200×. **c + d** Case 1: Masson Trichrome stain negative indicated non-cirrhotic liver disease. 100×, 200×. **e + f** Case 1: Swollen hepatocyte clarification negative for periodic acid-Schiff stain in approximately 30%. 200×. **g** Case 5: Mild mixed steatosis. H&E, 100×. **h** Case 5: Mixed macro- and microvesicular steatosis with focal single cell necrosis and sporadic parenchymal granulocytes. H&E, 400×. Abbreviations: H&E, haematoxylin and eosin

Ethiopia [9]. If, as identified in the present study, a high proportion of the CLD is 'unexplained' then it may be difficult, if not impossible, to prevent its occurrence and hence to reduce the burden it imposes. If, however, as suggested in the present study, exposure to the recreational substance khat is of major aetiological importance, then there is an urgent need to further investigate this possibility with analytic studies designed to assess causality. There are campaigns in place to radically reduce the burden of viral liver disease worldwide [45], and this is undoubtedly vital. However, if khat was found to be a major contributor to the development of CLD, then given its widespread use, legal status and social acceptability it would be a much more difficult problem to deal with requiring concerted governmental action in the countries and communities involved.

Conclusions

Chronic HBV infection was found in around one third of patients hospitalized with CLD in eastern Ethiopia. However, in over half of the patients the aetiology of the liver disease was unexplained. The prevalence of khat chewing was much higher in the CLD population than expected, suggesting khat as an effect modifier and/or independent risk factor for development of CLD in this part of the world. Further epidemiological studies, which include appropriate comparison groups, should be undertaken to assess whether khat plays a causal role in the development of CLD.

Abbreviations

ALT: Alanine aminotransferase; anti-HCV: Hepatitis C virus antibody; anti-HDV: Hepatitis D virus antibody; APRI: Aspartate aminotransferase to platelet ratio index; AST: Aspartate aminotransferase; CLD: Chronic liver disease; CPA: Collagen proportionate area; HBsAg: Hepatitis B surface antigen; HBV: Hepatitis B virus; HCV: Hepatitis C virus; HDV: Hepatitis D virus; NAFLD: Non-alcoholic fatty liver disease

Acknowledgements

We are indebted to the patients who participated in the study. We acknowledge the hospital staff at the Jugal Hospital and the Hiwot Fana Specialized University Hospital, in particular the laboratory technicians, radiologists and physicians, and the laboratory technicians at Harari Health Research and Regional Laboratory, the Aklilu Lemma Institute of Pathobiology, the Department of Medical Biochemistry at Drammen Hospital, and the Department of Virology at the Norwegian Institute of Public Health for their dedication and efforts. We also wish to thank the Department of Medical Biochemistry at Oslo University Hospital Rikshospitalet for undertaking the HFE genotyping, the staff at Department of Pathology at Ålesund Hospital for their help with the staining of serial sections from the biopsy specimen, and the pathologists at the International Clinical Laboratories in Addis Ababa for histopathological services. Finally, we are grateful for the support from the Harari Regional Health Bureau and the Haramaya University College of Health and Medical Sciences.

Funding

This study was funded by The Norwegian Research Council, grant number 220622/H10, and the South-Eastern Norway Regional Health Authority, grant number 2011068.

Authors' contributions

AJ, NB and SGG conceived and designed the study with substantial contributions from NYI, TAA, TL and KSJ. SMSO, NYI and TAA were responsible for the inclusion of patients and data collection. TL and KSJ were responsible for the laboratory work, and BR and RDG for the pathological examinations. SMSO, AJ and MYM performed the statistical analysis. SMSO, AJ, MYM and AMDR drafted the first version of the manuscript, and all authors critically revised the manuscript and approved it.

Consent for publication

Not applicable.

Competing interests

The authors declare that they have no competing interest.

Author details

[1]Regional Centre for Imported and Tropical Diseases, Oslo University Hospital Ullevål, Oslo, Norway. [2]Department of Internal Medicine, Hiwot Fana Specialized University Hospital, Harar, Ethiopia. [3]Haramaya University College of Health and Medical Sciences, Harar, Ethiopia. [4]Department of Internal Medicine, Jugal Hospital, Harar, Ethiopia. [5]Aklilu Lemma Institute of Pathobiology, Addis Ababa University, Addis Ababa, Ethiopia. [6]Department of Medical Biochemistry, Vestre Viken Hospital Trust, Drammen, Norway. [7]Department of Pathology, Oslo University Hospital Ullevål, Oslo, Norway. [8]Institute of Clinical Medicine, Faculty of Medicine, Oslo University, Oslo, Norway. [9]Centre for Pathology, Imperial College London, London, UK. [10]Department of Molecular Biology, Norwegian Institute of Public Health, Oslo, Norway. [11]Department of Infectious Diseases, Oslo University Hospital Ullevål, Oslo, Norway. [12]Department of Clinical Science, University of Bergen, Bergen, Norway. [13]Research Unit, Sørlandet Hospital HF, Kristiansand, Norway. [14]Department of Global Development and Planning, University of Agder, Kristiansand, Norway. [15]UCL Institute for Liver & Digestive Health, Division of Medicine, University College London, Royal Free Campus, London, UK. [16]Department of Infectious Diseases, Vestfold Hospital Trust, Tønsberg, Norway.

References

1. GBD 2015 Mortality and Causes of Death Collaborators. Global, regional, and national life expectancy, all-cause mortality, and cause-specific mortality for 249 causes of death, 1980–2015: a systematic analysis for the Global Burden of Disease Study 2015. Lancet. 2016;388:1459–544.
2. Tsochatzis EA, Bosch J, Burroughs AK. Liver cirrhosis. Lancet. 2014;383:1749–61.
3. World Health Organization. WHO African Regional Offices. Ethiopia. Country information. http://www.afro.who.int/countries/ethiopia Accessed 13 Jan 2018.
4. Tsega E, Nordenfelt E, Hansson BG, Mengesha B, Lindberg J. Chronic liver disease in Ethiopia: a clinical study with emphasis on identifying common causes. Ethiop Med J. 1992;30:1–33.
5. Schweitzer A, Horn J, Mikolajczyk RT, Krause G, Ott JJ. Estimations of worldwide prevalence of chronic hepatitis B virus infection: a systematic review of data published between 1965 and 2013. Lancet. 2015;386:1546–55.
6. Belyhun Y, Maier M, Mulu A, Diro E, Liebert UG. Hepatitis viruses in Ethiopia: a systematic review and meta-analysis. BMC Infect Dis. 2016;16:761.
7. Lulu K, Berhane Y. The use of simplified verbal autopsy in identifying causes of adult death in a predominantly rural population in Ethiopia. BMC Public Health. 2005;5:58.
8. Weldearegawi B, Ashebir Y, Gebeye E, Gebregziabiher T, Yohannes M, Mussa S, et al. Emerging chronic non-communicable diseases in rural communities of northern Ethiopia: evidence using population-based verbal autopsy method in Kilite Awlaelo surveillance site. Health Policy Plan. 2013;28:891–8.
9. Ashenafi W, Eshetu F, Assefa N, Oljira L, Dedefo M, Zelalem D, et al. Trend and causes of adult mortality in Kersa health and demographic surveillance system (Kersa HDSS), eastern Ethiopia: verbal autopsy method. Popul Health Metr. 2017;15:22.
10. Al-Motarreb A, Al-Habori M, Broadley KJ. Khat chewing, cardiovascular diseases and other internal medical problems: the current situation and directions for future research. J Ethnopharmacol. 2010;132:540–8.
11. Reda AA, Moges A, Biadgilign S, Wondmagegn BY. Prevalence and determinants of khat (Catha Edulis) chewing among high school students in eastern Ethiopia: a cross-sectional study. PLoS One. 2012;7:e33946.
12. Alem A, Kebede D, Kullgren G. The prevalence and socio-demographic correlates of khat chewing in Butajira, Ethiopia. Acta Psychiatr Scand Suppl. 1999;397:84–91.

13. Haile D, Lakew Y. Khat chewing practice and associated factors among adults in Ethiopia: further analysis using the 2011 demographic and health survey. PLoS One. 2015;10:e0130460.

14. Toennes SW, Harder S, Schramm M, Niess C, Kauert GF. Pharmacokinetics of cathinone, cathine and norephedrine after the chewing of khat leaves. Br J Clin Pharmacol. 2003;56:125–30.

15. Wai CT, Greenson JK, Fontana RJ, Kalbfleisch JD, Marrero JA, Conjeevaram HS, et al. A simple noninvasive index can predict both significant fibrosis and cirrhosis in patients with chronic hepatitis C. Hepatology. 2003;38:518–26.

16. Lin ZH, Xin YN, Dong QJ, Wang Q, Jiang XJ, Zhan SH, et al. Performance of the aspartate aminotransferase-to-platelet ratio index for the staging of hepatitis C-related fibrosis: an updated meta-analysis. Hepatology. 2011;53:726–36.

17. Sterling RK, Lissen E, Clumeck N, Sola R, Correa MC, Montaner J, et al. Development of a simple noninvasive index to predict significant fibrosis in patients with HIV/HCV coinfection. Hepatology. 2006;43:1317–25.

18. World Health Organization. Bench aids for the diagnosis of intestinal parasites. Geneva: WHO; 1994. Available online at: http://apps.who.int/iris/bitstream/10665/37323/1/9789241544764_eng.pdf. Accessed 13 Jan 2018.

19. Allan R, Thoirs K, Phillips M. Accuracy of ultrasound to identify chronic liver disease. World J Gastroenterol. 2010;16:3510–20.

20. Richter J, Hatz C, Campagne G, Bergquist NR, Jenkins JM. Ultrasound in Schistosomiasis. A practical guide to the standardized use of ultrasonography for the assessment of schistosomiasis-related morbidity. Geneva: WHO; 2000. Available online at: http://www.who.int/schistosomiasis/resources/tdr_str_sch_00.1/en/. Accessed 13 Jan 2018.

21. Karita E, Ketter N, Price MA, Kayitenkore K, Kaleebu P, Nanvubya A, et al. CLSI-derived hematology and biochemistry reference intervals for healthy adults in eastern and southern Africa. PLoS One. 2009;4:e4401.

22. Manns MP, Czaja AJ, Gorham JD, Krawitt EL, Mieli-Vergani G, Vergani D, et al. Diagnosis and management of autoimmune hepatitis. Hepatology. 2010;51:2193–213.

23. Chalasani N, Younossi Z, Lavine JE, Diehl AM, Brunt EM, Cusi K, et al. The diagnosis and management of non-alcoholic fatty liver disease: practice guideline by the American Association for the Study of Liver Diseases, American College of Gastroenterology, and the American Gastroenterological Association. Hepatology. 2012;55:2005–23.

24. Mak CM, Lam CW, Tam S. Diagnostic accuracy of serum ceruloplasmin in Wilson disease: determination of sensitivity and specificity by ROC curve analysis among ATP7B-genotyped subjects. Clin Chem. 2008;54:1356–62.

25. Bacon BR, Adams PC, Kowdley KV, Powell LW, Tavill AS, American Association For the study of liver diseases. Diagnosis and management of hemochromatosis: 2011 practice guideline by the American Association for the Study of Liver Diseases. Hepatology. 2011;54:328–43.

26. Rockey DC, Caldwell SH, Goodman ZD, Nelson RC, Smith AD. American Association For the study of liver diseases. Liver biopsy. Hepatology. 2009;49:1017–44.

27. Ishak K, Baptista A, Bianchi L, Callea F, De Groote J, Gudat F, et al. Histological grading and staging of chronic hepatitis. J Hepatol. 1995;22:696–9.

28. Wright M, Goldin R, Fabre A, Lloyd J, Thomas H, Trepo C, et al. Measurement and determinants of the natural history of liver fibrosis in hepatitis C virus infection: a cross sectional and longitudinal study. Gut. 2003;52:574–9.

29. von Elm E, Altman DG, Egger M, Pocock SJ, Gotzsche PC, Vandenbroucke JP, et al. The strengthening the reporting of observational studies in epidemiology (STROBE) statement: guidelines for reporting observational studies. Lancet. 2007;370:1453–7.

30. World Medical Association. World medical association declaration of Helsinki: ethical principles for medical research involving human subjects. JAMA. 2013;310:2191–4.

31. Goldstein NS, Kodali VP, Gordon SC. Histologic spectrum of cryptogenic chronic liver disease and comparison with chronic autoimmune and chronic type C hepatitis. Am J Clin Pathol. 1995;104:567–73.

32. Kodali VP, Gordon SC, Silverman AL, McCray DG. Cryptogenic liver disease in the United States: further evidence for non-a, non-B, and non-C hepatitis. Am J Gastroenterol. 1994;89:1836–9.

33. Czaja AJ. Cryptogenic chronic hepatitis and its changing guise in adults. Dig Dis Sci. 2011;56:3421–38.

34. Mohammed Y, Bekele A. Seroprevalence of transfusion transmitted infection among blood donors at Jijiga blood bank, eastern Ethiopia: retrospective 4 years study. BMC Res Notes. 2016;9:129.

35. World Health Organization. Global Health Observatory data repository: Overweight (body mass index ≥25), age-standardized (%). Estimates by country. Available online at: http://apps.who.int/gho/data/node.main.A897A?lang=en Accessed 13 Jan 2018.

36. Younossi ZM, Koenig AB, Abdelatif D, Fazel Y, Henry L, Wymer M. Global epidemiology of nonalcoholic fatty liver disease-meta-analytic assessment of prevalence, incidence, and outcomes. Hepatology. 2016;64:73–84.

37. Olusanya TO, Lesi OA, Adeyomoye AA, Fasanmade OA. Non alcoholic fatty liver disease in a Nigerian population with type II diabetes mellitus. Pan Afr Med J. 2016;24:20.

38. Chapman MH, Kajihara M, Borges G, O'Beirne J, Patch D, Dhillon AP, et al. Severe, acute liver injury and khat leaves. N Engl J Med. 2010;362:1642–4.

39. Peevers CG, Moorghen M, Collins PL, Gordon FH, McCune CA. Liver disease and cirrhosis because of Khat chewing in UK Somali men: a case series. Liver Int. 2010;30:1242–3.

40. Stuyt RJ, Willems SM, Wagtmans MJ, van Hoek B. Chewing khat and chronic liver disease. Liver Int. 2011;31:434–6.

41. Mahamoud HD, Muse SM, Roberts LR, Fischer PR, Torbenson MS, Khat FT. Chewing and cirrhosis in Somaliland: case series. Afr J Prim Health Care Fam Med. 2016;8:e1–4.

42. Alsalahi A, Abdulla MA, Al-Mamary M, Noordin MI, Abdelwahab SI, Alabsi AM, et al. Toxicological features of Catha Edulis (Khat) on livers and kidneys of male and female Sprague-Dawley rats: a subchronic study. Evid Based Complement Alternat Med. 2012;2012:829401.

43. Brechot C. Pathogenesis of hepatitis B virus-related hepatocellular carcinoma: old and new paradigms. Gastroenterology. 2004;127:S56–61.

44. Makvandi M. Update on occult hepatitis B virus infection. World J Gastroenterol. 2016;22:8720–34.

45. World Health Organization. Global health sector strategy on viral hepatitis. 2016–2021. Geneva: WHO; 2016. Available online at: http://www.who.int/hepatitis/strategy2016-2021/ghss-hep/en/ Accessed 13 Jan 2018.

7

Response of fibroblast growth factor 19 and bile acid synthesis after a body weight-adjusted oral fat tolerance test in overweight and obese NAFLD patients

Dana Friedrich[1]* ⓘ, Hanns-Ulrich Marschall[2] and Frank Lammert[1]

Abstract

Background: Non-alcoholic fatty liver disease (NAFLD) is common both in obese and overweight patients. Fibroblast growth factor 19 (FGF19), an intestinal hormone, could play a role in the complex pathogenesis of NAFLD. The aim of our study was to investigate responses of FGF19 and bile acid (BA) synthesis after a body weight-adjusted oral fat tolerance test (OFTT) in overweight and obese NAFLD patients.

Methods: For this study, we recruited 26 NAFLD patients; 14 overweight (median BMI 28.3 kg/m^2), 12 obese (35.3 kg/m^2) and 16 healthy controls (24.2 kg/m^2). All individuals received 1 g fat (Calogen®) per kg body weight orally. Serum concentrations of FGF19 were determined by ELISA. Concentrations of BAs and BA synthesis marker 7α-hydroxy-4-cholesten-3-one (C4) were measured by gas chromatography-mass spectrometry and high-performance liquid chromatography, respectively; all at 0 (baseline), 2, 4 and 6 h during the OFTT.

Results: BMI correlated negatively with fasting FGF19 concentrations (rho = − 0.439, $p = 0.004$). FGF19 levels of obese NAFLD patients were significantly ($p = 0.01$) lower in the fasting state (median 116.0 vs. 178.5 pg/ml), whereas overweight NAFLD patients had significantly ($p = 0.004$) lower FGF19 concentrations 2 h after the fat load (median 163.0 vs. 244.5 pg/ml), and lowest values at all postprandial time points as compared to controls. Baseline BA concentrations correlated positively with FGF19 values (rho = 0.306, $p = 0.048$). In all groups, we observed BA increases during the OFTT with a peak at 2 h but no change in C4 levels in overweight/obese NAFLD patients.

Conclusions: Reduced basal gastrointestinal FGF19 secretion and decreased postprandial response to oral fat together with blunted effect on BA synthesis indicate alterations in intestinal or hepatic FXR signaling in overweight and obese NAFLD subjects. The precise mechanism of FGF19 signaling after oral fat load needs further evaluation.

Keywords: Bile acids, FGF19, Non-alcoholic fatty liver disease, Oral fat tolerance test

* Correspondence: dana.friedrich@uks.eu
[1]Department of Medicine II, Saarland University Medical Center, Saarland University, 66421 Homburg, Germany
Full list of author information is available at the end of the article

Background

Obesity and fatty liver disease represent increasing medical problems in developed countries. In Germany, the prevalence of obesity increased during the years 1998 to 2011 from 18.9 to 23.3% in men and from 22.5 to 23.9% in women [1]. In the United States, 37% of adults are obese [2]. Obesity is an important risk factor of non-alcoholic fatty liver disease (NAFLD), which has been reported in 30 to 40% of adults [3, 4].

The term NAFLD is used for a wide spectrum of fatty liver diseases that starts with simple steatosis in non-alcoholic fatty liver (NAFL) that may progress to non-alcoholic steatohepatits (NASH), which is complicated by fibrosis, cirrhosis, and eventually hepatocellular carcinoma [5–7]. NAFLD is often associated with the metabolic syndrome and requires exclusion of excessive alcohol consumption as well as viral and autoimmune liver diseases [8]. NAFLD is common in obesity but also in overweight patients [9, 10]. The pathophysiology of NAFLD is complex and still not fully defined [11, 12]. Several metabolic factors have already been identified in the development of NAFLD, including insulin resistance, diabetes mellitus and obesity.

So far there have been only few studies of the importance of gastrointestinal hormones in the pathogenesis of NAFLD [13–15]. The gastrointestinal hormone fibroblast growth factor 19 (FGF19) has emerged as a novel regulator of bile acid, carbohydrate and lipid metabolism. In human metabolic syndrome associated diseases, such as type 2 diabetes mellitus (T2DM) and NAFLD, FGF19 signaling seems to be dysregulated [16]. In animals, FGF19 transgenic mice show resistance to a high-fat diet and decreased liver triglyceride concentrations [17] while the administration of recombinant FGF19 increases the metabolic rate [18]. Accordingly, in humans with NAFLD, reduced fasting FGF19 levels were found [14, 19, 20]. Therefore, the present study focuses on the dietary regulation of FGF19 and its potential role in the pathogenesis of NAFLD.

FGF19 release in the intestine is induced by bile acids (BAs). After a meal, the entry of dietary fat in the duodenum causes gallbladder contraction and BA inflow into the intestinal lumen. The reabsorption of BAs in the terminal ileum activates the canonical BA sensor farnesoid X receptor (FXR), resulting in enhanced transcription and secretion of FGF19 [21, 22]. FGF19 binds on hepatocytes to the FGF receptor 4 (FGFR4) and its cofactor βKlotho [22–24], which triggers a signaling cascade that represses cholesterol 7α-hydroxylase (CYP7A1), the rate-limiting enzyme in BA synthesis from cholesterol [25]. 7α-Hydroxy-4-cholesten-3-one (C4) is an intermediate of BA synthesis, which can be measured in serum [26].

Since the role of FGF19 in the pathogenesis of human NAFLD is unknown, we studied FGF19 and hepatic downstream effects (C4 and BAs) in overweight and obese NAFLD outpatients (and healthy controls) that were subjected to a body weight-adjusted oral fat tolerance test (OFTT). We determined serum concentrations of FGF19, C4 and BAs at baseline and at 2, 4 and 6 h after OFTT. We hypothized that FGF19 levels are lower in obese compared to overweight NAFLD patients.

We aimed to answer the following questions in this study:

1. Do fasting FGF19 serum concentrations differ between normal-weight healthy, overweight and obese NAFLD patients?
2. How does a body weight-adjusted oral fat tolerance test (OFTT) affect serum FGF19 concentrations in these populations?
3. How does a postprandial FGF19 response affect hepatic BA biosynthesis, as assessed by C4?

Methods

Study protocol

The study protocol was approved by the Ethics Committee of the Ärztekammer des Saarlandes, Saarbrücken (ID number 58/09). All subjects (≥ 18 years) were fully informed about the study objectives and methods and gave their written informed consent before participating in this non-randomized controlled pilot trial.

Study subjects

During 2009 and 2010, we recruited overweight and obese NAFLD outpatients in the Department of Internal Medicine II, Saarland University Medical Center, Homburg, as well as healthy controls with normal body weight. Inclusion criteria for NAFLD were ultrasound and/or biopsy findings consistent with fatty liver disease. Exclusion criteria were increased alcohol consumption in medical history and the following acute and chronic liver diseases: cirrhosis, hepatitis A virus (HAV), hepatitis B virus (HBV), hepatitis C virus (HCV), hepatitis D virus (HDV), cytomegalovirus (CMV) and Epstein-Barr Virus (EBV) infections, hemochromatosis, Wilson's disease, α_1-antitrypsin deficiency, and autoimmune hepatitis. Healthy controls included employees of the clinic and medical students with normal BMI and no diseases in history. In controls, no liver and laboratory diagnosis was performed.

Subjects were divided into three groups according to their BMI (healthy controls, normal weight: 19.0–25.4 kg/m^2, overweight NAFLD: 25.5–29.9 kg/m^2, obese NAFLD: ≥ 30.0 kg/m^2) [27, 28].

Liver parameters

In overweight and obese patients ($N = 26$), liver status was assessed by abdominal ultrasound and/or liver biopsy. Ultrasound was performed using the Hitachi EUB-8500 ultrasound scanner (Hitachi Medical Systems, Wiesbaden, Germany). Hepatic steatosis results in abnormal echo patterns on ultrasound scanning; the severity of steatosis was graded as mild (I), moderate (II), or severe (III) [29]. Liver biopsy samples of five patients were examined by an experienced pathologist of Saarland University Medical Center.

Oral fat tolerance test (OFTT)

We used a body weight-adjusted OFTT to investigate postprandial FGF19, BA and C4 responses in our study subjects. For the present study, a standardized test drink Calogen® (Nutricia, Erlangen, Germany) was administered, which is a lipid emulsion based on vegetable fat with 50% long-chain triglycerides [30]. All individuals received 1 g fat per kg body weight orally. The fat load was based on subjects' body weight to adjust the OFTT to hypercaloric (especially high-fat) eating behavior of obese patients [31].

Blood samples

Blood samples were drawn from a peripheral vein at 8:00 AM after an overnight fasting and 2, 4 and 6 h after the oral fat challenge. Samples were centrifuged for 10 min at 3000 g 30 min after blood collection (ROTANTA 46R, Hettich, Tuttlingen, Germany). Subsequently, serum was stored in aliquots at-70 °Cuntil analysis.

Serum FGF19, bile acid and C4 measurements

FGF19 serum concentrations were measured in duplicate by quantitative sandwich enzyme-linked immunosorbent assay, using the FGF19 Quantikine ELISA kit (R&D Systems, Minneapolis, USA). Serum BA concentrations were determined by gas chromatography-mass spectrometry (GCMS) [32]. 7α-hydroxy-4-cholesten-3-one (C4), a valid marker of bile acid biosynthesis [33], was measured by high-performance liquid chromatography (HPLC).

Statistical analysis

Data analysis was performed using SPSS (version 20.0, IBM, Ehningen, Germany). Kruskal-Wallis test was used to analyze quantitative data for differences within the cohort. For the present study with a low number of study subjects ($N < 20$), normal distributions were not expected [34]. Thus, data are expressed as medians and interquartile ranges (IQR 25–75). In addition, Mann-Whitney-U test was used to test differences between two groups. The strength of associations between two parameters was estimated using the non-parametric Spearman correlation test. Spearman's correlation coefficient is presented as rho. For the OFTT, FGF19$_{(0-6h)}$-area under the curve (AUC) and, after correcting for baseline, the incremental AUC (FGF19-IAUC) were computed using GraphPad Prism (version 6.0, GraphPad Software, La Jolla, CA, USA). A p-value < 0.05 denotes statistical significance.

Results
Subject characteristics

Table 1 summarizes the subject characteristics. A total of 42 subjects, 21 women and 21 men, were recruited for our study. Study participants were between 19 and 68 years old (median 47.0 years, IQR 28.8–53.8). Overall, we recruited 14 overweight and 12 obese NAFLD patients as well as 16 healthy controls. Sex and age did not differ between groups. Obese patients had a median BMI of 35.3 kg/m², which corresponds to obesity grade II [28].

NAFLD was diagnosed by ultrasound and/or biopsy. In overweight and obese patients, the steatosis spectrum ranged from grade I, II and III to NASH and fibrosis. In the overweight group ($N = 14$), grade I liver steatosis was

Table 1 Subject characteristics, basal and postprandial FGF19 serum concentrations

Variables	Control	Overweight	Obesity	p-value
N (men/women)	16 (7/9)	14 (8/6)	12 (6/6)	n.s.[a]
Age (years)	29.5 (24.0–53.0)	49.0 (38.8–57.3)	48.0 (37.0–57.3)	0.551[b]
BMI (kg/m²)	24.2 (21.8–26.6)	28.3 (26.3–29.2)	35.3 (32.7–39.0)	< 0.001[b]
FGF19 (pg/ml)				
t = 0 h	178.5 (101.0–257.0)[c]	127.5 (70.0–161.3)	116.0 (51.0–134.3)[c]	0.01[c]
t = 2 h	244.5 (161.5–377.5)[c]	163.0 (78.5–168.3)[c]	181.0 (85.3–393.0)	0.004[c]
t = 4 h	332.5 (202.0–590.8)	207.0 (112.5–365.0)	220.0 (138.8–385.3)	0.445[b]
t = 6 h	211.0 (165.3–296.3)	154.0 (124.0–254.0)	184.5 (110.5–274.3)	0.445[b]

All data are given as median (interquartile range)
[a]Chi-square-test
[b]Kruskal-Wallis-test
[c]Mann-Whitney-U-test

found in six patients (43%), grade II in five patients (36%), and grade III in one patient (7%). NASH was diagnosed in one and fibrosis stage II was documented in one patient. In the obese group ($N = 12$), two patients (17%) displayed liver steatosis grade I, four patients (33%) showed grade II, and three participants (25%) had grade III. In this group, NASH was found in one and fibrosis stage I also in one patient. In one obese study participant, liver status could not be assessed by ultrasound. Additional file 1: Table S1 lists the co-morbidities in overweight and obese NAFLD patients. In overweight patients, hypercholesterolemia and in obese patients, arterial hypertension were the dominant concomitant diseases, respectively. Controls did not take any drugs regularly. Three overweight and eight obese patients were taking medications. These included antidiabetics, antihypertensives, thyroid hormones, analgesics, proton pump inhibitors, antidepressants, non-steroidal antirheumatics, corticoidsteroids and allopurinol, respectively.

Basal and postprandial FGF19 serum concentrations

In the total study group ($N = 42$), fasting FGF19 concentrations ranged from 17.0 to 392.0 pg/ml (median 133.5, IQR 82.8–190.3). Basal FGF19 values were significantly lower in obese NAFLD patients as compared to controls and tended to be lower in overweight NAFLD subjects, too (Table 1, Fig. 1). Basal FGF19 concentrations did not differ between sexes [women, median 126.0 (IQR 80.5–179.0) vs. men, median 138.0 (IQR 93.0–204.0) pg/ml]. Interestingly, fasting FGF19 concentrations were negatively correlated with BMI (Fig. 2).

After the OFTT, FGF19 concentrations increased in controls, overweight and obese patients (Table 1, Fig. 1). Of note, overweight patients displayed lowest FGF19 concentrations at all postprandial time points. Two hours after the OFTT, FGF19 levels ranged from 10.0 to 697.0 pg/ml (median 178.0, IQR 116.5–255.5). At this time, overweight NAFLD patients showed significantly lower FGF19 levels compared with controls (Fig. 1). The FGF19 maximum was found in all three groups after 4 h, with hormone levels ranging from 59.0 to 935.0 pg/ml (median 255.0, IQR 163.3–439.3). At 4 h, FGF19 was highest in controls and twice as high as at baseline. After 6 h, FGF19 values ranged from 48.0 to 802.0 pg/ml (median 189.0, IQR 136.0–269.0) and were still highest in controls.

Both women and men showed the FGF19 maximum at 4 h [women, median 270.0 (IQR 167.5–539.0) vs. men, median 231.0 (IQR 117.5–410.5) pg/ml] but

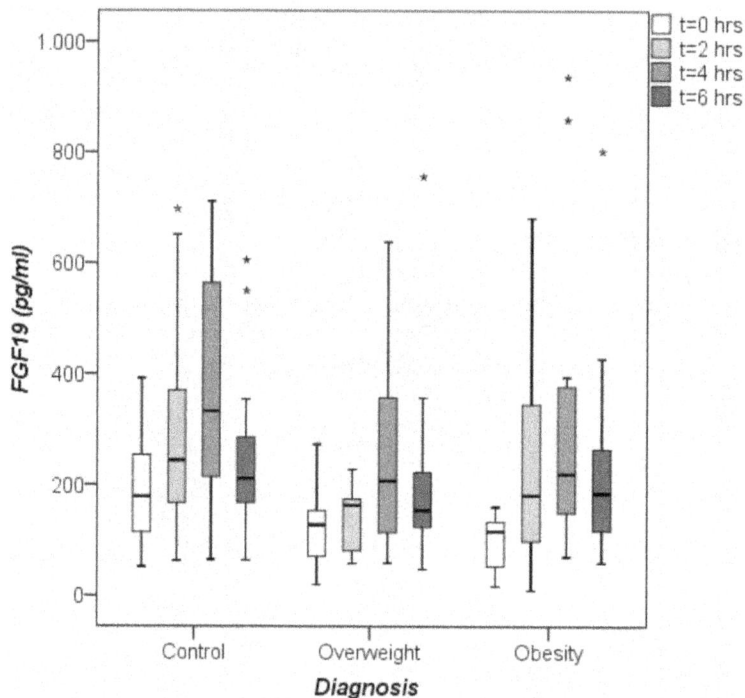

Fig. 1 Fasting and postprandial FGF19 serum concentrations measured by quantitative sandwich enzyme-linked immunosorbent assay (ELISA). Comparison of FGF19 values between healthy controls ($N = 16$), overweight ($N = 14$) and obese ($N = 12$) patients with non-alcoholic fatty liver disease (NAFLD) at baseline (0 h), 2, 4 and 6 h after the oral fat tolerance test (OFTT). Significant difference between basal (0 h) FGF19 concentrations in controls and obese NAFLD patients [controls 178.5 (101.0–257.0) vs. obese 116.0 (51.0–134.3) pg/ml, medians (IQRs), $p = < 0.05$, Mann-Whitney-U-test]. At 2 h, lower FGF19 values in overweight NAFLD patients in comparison to controls [overweight 163.0 (78.5–168.3) vs. controls 244.5 (161.5–377.5) pg/ml, medians (IQRs), $p = 0.004$, Mann-Whitney-U-test], * outlier

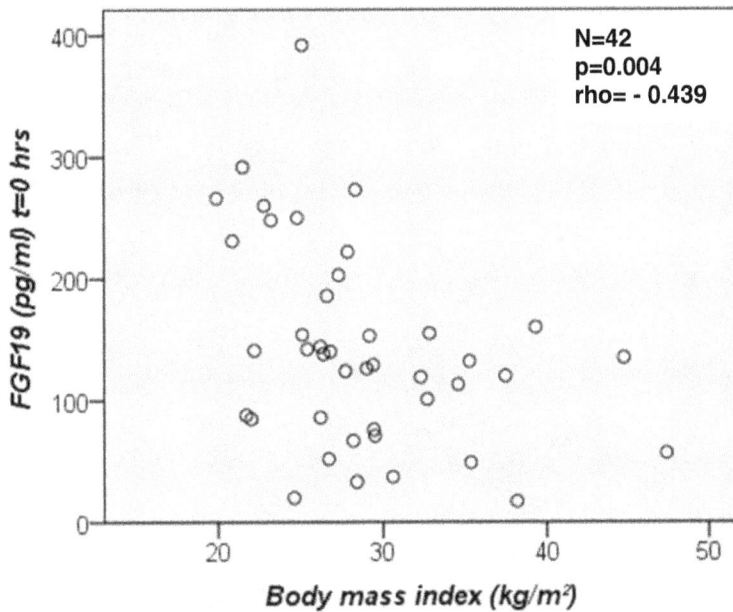

Fig. 2 Fasting FGF19 serum concentrations versus body mass index (BMI) for all study subjects. FGF19 values correlated negatively with BMI. A scattered plot is shown and the Spearman's correlation coefficient was calculated

postprandial levels were higher in women at all time points. Six hours after the oral fat challenge, FGF19 concentrations of both sexes tended to reach a significant difference [women, median 216.0 (IQR 145.0–390.5) vs. men, median 172.0 (IQR124.0–216.5) pg/ml, $p = 0.051$].

Mean FGF19$_{(0-6h)}$-area and mean incremental area under the curve (AUC and IAUC) did not differ significantly between the groups (AUC controls: 1772.8 ± 766.6 vs. overweight: 1130.6 ± 590.0 vs. obese: 1469.3 ± 910.0 pg/ml/6 h; IAUC controls: 699.0 ± 383.7 vs. overweight: 573.3 ± 333.4 vs. obese: 921.5 ± 732.4 pg/ml). FGF19-AUC was highest in controls and lowest in overweight patients ($p = 0.053$); IAUC was higher in obese and lower in overweight patients in comparison

to controls. FGF19-AUC and IAUC did not correlate with body weight-adjusted fat load. In addition, there was no association between FGF19-AUC and BMI; FGF19-IAUC tended to correlate with age (rho = 0.291, $p = 0.062$).

Basal and postprandial BA serum concentrations
Fasting and postprandial bile acid (BA) concentrations did not differ between overweight/obese NAFLD patients and controls. In all three groups, we observed a BA increase after the OFTT with a peak at 2 h (Table 2). Basal FGF19 concentrations correlated positively with basal BA values (Fig. 3).

Table 2 Basal and postprandial BA and C4 serum concentrations

Variables	Control	Overweight	Obesity	p-value
N (men/women)	16 (7/9)	14 (8/6)	12 (6/6)	n.s.[a]
Bile acids (μM)				
t = 0 h	1.1 (0.8–1.7)	1.5 (0.8–2.2)	1.4 (0.9–1.7)	0.343
t = 2 h	1.4 (1.1–4.7)	2.1 (1.2–3.8)	2.4 (1.6–4.1)	0.311
t = 4 h	1.1 (0.7–2.0)	2.0 (1.3–2.5)	2.0 (1.0–2.3)	0.155
t = 6 h	0.7 (0.5–1.6)	1.3 (0.8–2.0)	1.2 (0.8–1.7)	0.087
C4 (nM)				
t = 0 h	41.4 (7.0–69.2)	58.5 (12.8–91.6)	35.1 (1.2–72.3)	0.422
t = 2 h	28.1 (7.1–49.6)	43.1 (10.0–114.0)	35.7 (1.2–118.3)	0.765
t = 4 h	13.0 (6.8–44.7)	40.8 (21.1–99.3)	32.7 (3.3–108.0)	0.343
t = 6 h	11.8 (4.1–34.4)	40.7 (18.1–80.1)	28.6 (3.5–82.4)	0.445

All data are given as median (interquartile range), p-values: Kruskal-Wallis-test,[a]Chi-square-test

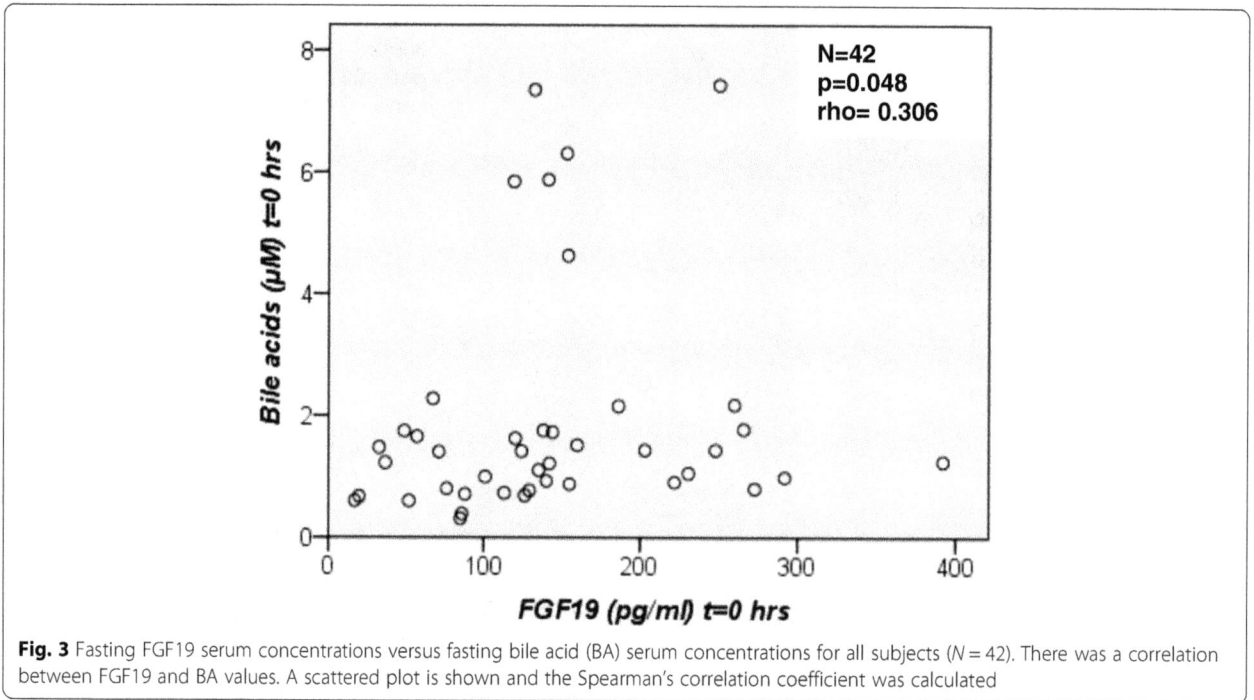

Fig. 3 Fasting FGF19 serum concentrations versus fasting bile acid (BA) serum concentrations for all subjects (*N* = 42). There was a correlation between FGF19 and BA values. A scattered plot is shown and the Spearman's correlation coefficient was calculated

Basal and postprandial C4 serum concentrations

Fasting and postprandial C4 values did not differ significantly between study participants (Table 2, Fig. 4). At all postprandial time points, C4 concentrations were markedly lower in controls in comparison to overweight/ obese NAFLD patients. C4 concentrations in overweight NAFLD patients remained unchanged for 4 h postprandially, despite increasing FGF19 values. In the total study group FGF19 concentrations at 2 h correlated negatively with C4 values at 4 h after the OFTT (Fig. 5). There was

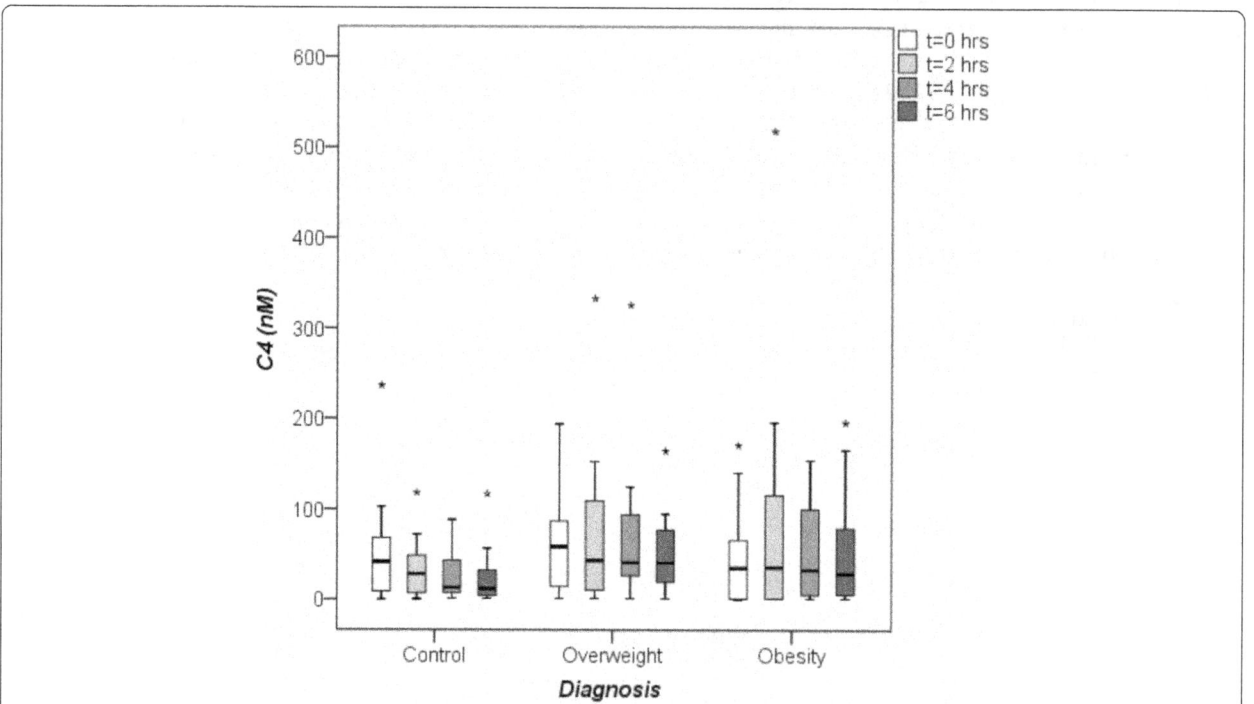

Fig. 4 Fasting and postprandial C4 concentrations. C4, a valid marker of bile acid biosynthesis, was measured by high-performance liquid chromatography (HPLC). Comparison of C4 values between healthy controls (*N* = 16), overweight (*N* = 14) and obese (*N* = 12) patients with non-alcoholic fatty liver disease (NAFLD) at baseline (0 h), 2, 4 and 6 h after the oral fat tolerance test (OFTT). C4 concentrations did not differ between groups (Kruskal-Wallis-test),*outlier

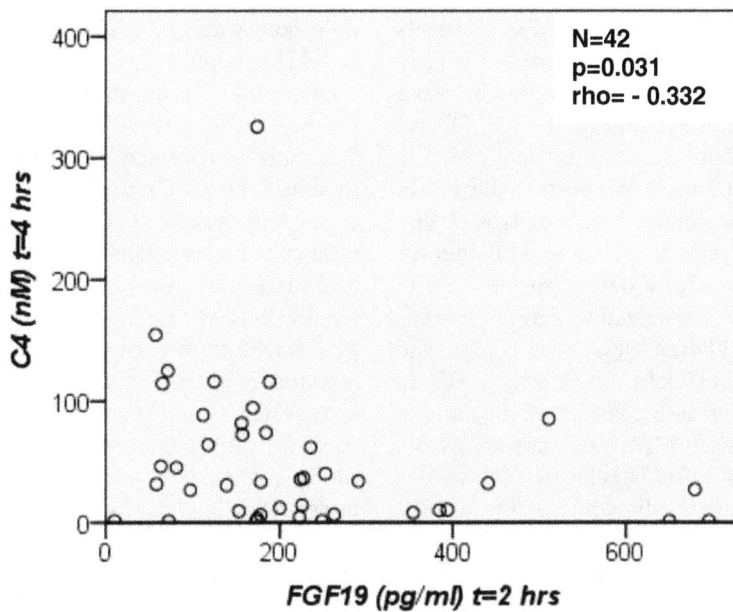

Fig. 5 FGF19 serum concentrations at 2 h versus C4 values at 4 h after the oral fat tolerance test (OFTT) for all subjects ($N = 42$). A scattered plot is shown and the Spearman's correlation coefficient was calculated

also an inverse correlation of FGF19 concentrations at 4 h and C4 values at 6 h after the OFTT in the study group (Fig. 6). These correlations were confirmed for the control group (Additional file 2: Figure S1, Additional file 3: Figure S2). In NAFLD patients, FGF19 concentrations did not correlate with C4 values.

Discussion

The present study investigated serum FGF19, BA, and C4 profiles in overweight and obese NAFLD patients, in comparison to normal-weight healthy controls, after a body weight-adjusted oral fat load. The key findings of our study are (i) fasting FGF19 concentrations were

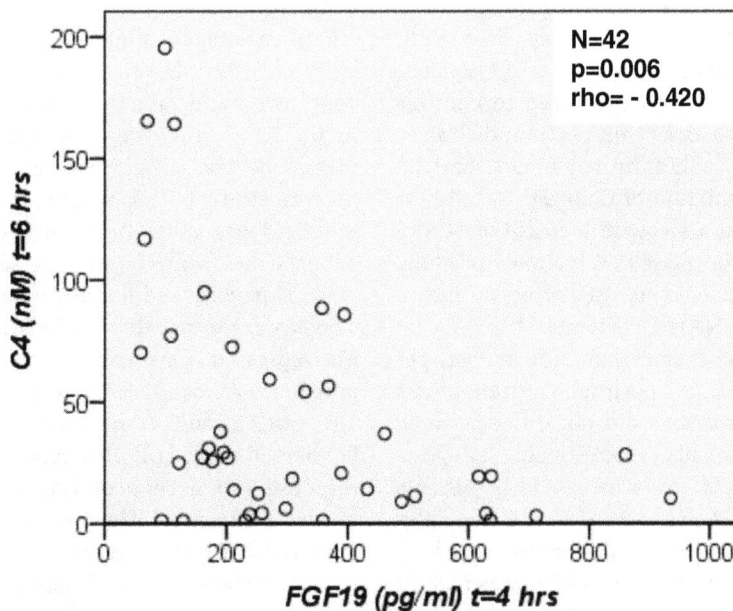

Fig. 6 FGF19 serum concentrations at 4 h versus C4 values at 6 h after the oral fat tolerance test (OFTT) for all subjects ($N = 42$). A scattered plot is shown and the Spearman's correlation coefficient was calculated

significantly lower in obese (grade II) NAFLD patients as compared to controls, (ii) overweight NAFLD patients had significantly lower FGF19 concentrations 2 h after the fat load and lowest values at all postprandial time points and (iii) BAs increased during the OFTT but without changes in C4 levels.

Low FGF19 concentrations have been reported in metabolic syndrome [35], obesity [36] and type 2 diabetes [37, 38]. The findings by Jansen et al. [19] support our results, i.e. the presence of fatty liver disease in obesity is associated with lower fasting FGF19 concentrations. Also in obese children with NAFLD [20] and young obese NASH patients [39] lower fasting FGF19 values were detected whereas Schreuder et al. did not observe differences in fasting FGF19 concentrations between controls and obese NAFLD subjects [13]. In our study, BMI correlated negatively with fasting FGF19 serum concentrations. Our study was too small to correlate FGF19 levels with biopsy-proven severity of NAFLD. In this respect, inverse associations had been found in children [15, 40], but some studies did not find correlations between steatosis grade and FGF19 concentrations [13, 14].

To the best of our knowledge, we are the first group which established a body-weight adjusted oral fat tolerance test (OFTT) to stimulate BA secretion and subsequent FGF19 expression in overweight and obese NAFLD patients. Only a few studies report about postprandial FGF19 concentrations [13, 41, 42]. Similar oral fat load tests have been used for determining postprandial triglyceride concentrations, but to date no standard method is established [43]. Our controls showed the highest FGF19 values during OFTT, suggesting unimpaired intestinal FGF19 release. Remarkably, overweight NAFLD patients had significantly lower FGF19 concentrations 2 h after the fat load as compared to controls and lowest hormone values at all postprandial time points. In another study in healthy volunteers, oral fat load (75 g vegetable fat, mixture of Calogen®, sun flower and olive oil) also showed a stepwise increase of FGF19 between 2 and 4 h and a decrease at 6 h almost reaching fasting levels [41]. Schreuder et al. used whipped cream for their oral fat test in NAFLD patients [13]. The fat challenge was applied with 30 g cream (35% w/v fat) per m^2 of body surface area. Single postprandial time points in plasma FGF19 concentrations did not differ between controls and NAFLD patients. Interestingly, the postprandial FGF19-IAUC was lower in NAFLD patients [13]. In our study, mean AUC and IAUC did not differ significantly, but AUC was highest in controls and lowest in overweight patients; in contrast, IAUC was highest in obese and lower in overweight patients in comparison to controls. In comparison to Schreuder's study [13], our fat challenge was considerably higher, which could have

contributed to differential findings at single postprandial time points and in FGF19-IAUC between controls and NAFLD patients.

Before our study started, we suspected that obese patients would have the highest energy and fat intake. Therefore we decided for a body weight-based fat load to adjust the OFTT to the patient's eating behavior. To check our assumption, we used a 3-day nutritional protocol and calculated energy and macronutrients intake (data not shown). Since there was no significant difference between groups, we suppose under-reporting of food intake in our overweight and obese patients. Most researchers agree that the reported accuracy of food intake decreases with increasing BMI. A systematic review covering studies between 1982 and 2014 showed that a BMI > 30 kg/m^2 is associated with significant under-reporting of food intake. These studies were mostly from Europe and North America [44]. For example, in morbid obese (BMI > 40 kg/m^2) energy intake can reach more than 4000 kcal/day, with high fat intakes of about 40 to 57% of total energy intake [31].

In the present study, higher fat challenge in obese patients could explain their higher FGF19 values in comparison to overweight patients, which indicates that obese can compensate their low fasting FGF19 values by a high fat intake. Sonne and colleagues [42] found that FGF19 concentrations in patients with type 2 diabetes and healthy controls increased with increasing fat and decreasing carbohydrate content in liquid meals (500 kcal, 2.5 vs. 10.0 and 40.0 g fat). FGF19 values tended to be lower in type 2 diabetes patients compared with controls, but were not statistically significant.

Oral fat intake stimulates bile acid (BA) secretion. The entry of dietary fat in the duodenum causes gallbladder contraction and inflow of BA into the intestinal lumen. In the ileum, BA induce secretion of FGF19 that suppresses de novo BA synthesis in the liver [25]. In the present study fasting and postprandial BA concentrations did not differ between overweight/obese NAFLD patients and controls and C4 serum concentrations in NAFLD patients did not decrease as they did in controls. Therefore, the hepatic BA biosynthesis was presumably not repressed. One reason could be that CYP7A1 expression was insufficiently suppressed by FGF19 due to low fasting and postprandial FGF19 concentrations. Schreuder et al. [13] also reported an impaired hepatic response (no decline of C4) in NAFLD patients with insulin resistance. The pathomechanism(s) behind the observed blunted C4 response are unknown. One might speculate about impaired hepatic signaling after binding of FGF19 to the FGF receptor 4/βKlotho heterodimer or other factors within the fatty liver cell that might affect the feedback regulation of BA synthesis.

Our method of bile acid analysis did not yield complete profiles including conjugates with glycine or taurine. Thus, distinct differences in BA profiles between lean controls and NAFLD patients might have affected activation of FXR. This is supported by studies in Chinese children were levels of chenodeoxycholic acid (CDCA) were increased in the moderate/severe stage of NAFLD. The authors report, that decreased circulating level of deoxycholic acid (DCA) in children with mild NAFLD might have a negative effect on the activation of FXR, which subsequently triggers an increasing production of CDCA in patients with moderate to severe NAFLD [45]. In contrast, Jiao and colleagues [39] found increased DCA and decreased CDCA levels in NAFLD patients. In this context, changes in BA composition could also be one reason for altered intestinal FXR signaling, expressed as reduced FGF19 levels, in our overweight and obese NAFLD patients.

Conclusions

Fasting FGF19 serum concentrations were lowest in obese NAFLD patients and highest in normal-weight healthy controls. Our body weight-adjusted oral fat challenge resulted in lowest FGF19 concentrations in overweight NAFLD patients at all postprandial time points. Overweight and obese NAFLD patients showed impaired FGF19 release in fasting and postprandial state. We assume that obese NAFLD patients were able to compensate their low fasting FGF19 values by a high (body weight-adjusted) oral fat intake. Reduced FGF19 values in overweight and obese NAFLD patients might reflect altered intestinal FXR signaling. How the hepatic receptor FGFR4 or its cofactor βKlotho modulate the hepatic response to FGF19 in NAFLD subjects should be examined further in functional studies.

Additional files

Additional file 1: Table S1. Prevalence of comorbidities in overweight ($N = 14$) and obese (12) NAFLD patients. In overweight NAFLD subjects, hypercholesterolemia is the dominant concomitant disease. In obese NAFLD patients, arterial hypertension, hyperlipidemia and hyperuricemia are the most common comorbidities.

Additional file 2: Figure S1. FGF19 serum concentrations at 2 h versus C4 values at 4 h after the oral fat tolerance test (OFTT) in controls ($N = 16$).

Additional file 3: Figure S2. FGF19 serum concentrations at 4 h versus C4 values at 6 h after the oral fat tolerance test (OFTT) in controls ($N = 16$).

Abbreviations

BA: Bile acid; BMI: Body mass index; C4: 7α-hydroxy-4-cholesten-3-one; CDCA: Chenodeoxycholic acid; CYP7A1: Cholesterol 7α-hydroxylase; DCA: Deoxycholic acid; ELISA: Enzyme linked immunosorbent assay; FGF19: Fibroblast growth factor 19; FXR: Farnesoid X receptor; GC MS: Gas chromatography-mass spectrometry; HPLC: High-performance liquid chromatography; hrs: Hours; IQR: Interquartile range; NAFLD: Non-alcoholic fatty liver disease; NASH: Non-alcoholic steatohepatitis; OFTT: Oral fat tolerance test

Acknowledgements
We thank Nutricia GmbH for providing the study test drink Calogen® for our oral fat tolerance test (OFTT).

Authors' contributions
DF developed study design and OFTT, recruited study participants, measured body fat mass, centrifuged and aliquoted blood samples, performed FGF19 ELISA, analyzed the data and wrote the manuscript. FL developed the idea to investigate FGF19 serum levels in NAFLD. HUM measured BA and C4 concentrations. All authors read, edited and approved the final manuscript.

Competing interests
The authors declare that they have no competing interests.

Author details
[1]Department of Medicine II, Saarland University Medical Center, Saarland University, 66421 Homburg, Germany. [2]Department of Molecular and Clinical Medicine, Sahlgrenska Academy, Institute of Medicine, University of Gothenburg, Gothenburg, Sweden.

References
1. Mensink GB, Schienkiewitz A, Haftenberger M, Lampert T, Ziese T, Scheidt-Nave C. Overweight and Obesity in Germany: results of the German health interview and examination survey for adults (DEGS1). Bundesgesundheitsblatt Gesundheitsforschung Gesundheitsschutz. 2013;56:786–94.
2. Ogden CL, Carroll MD, Fryar CD, Flegal KM. Prevalence of obesity among adults and youth: United States, 2011-2014. NCHS Data Brief. 2015;219:1–8.
3. Bellentani S, Scaglioni F, Marino M, Bedogni G. Epidemiology of non-alcoholic fatty liver disease. Dig Dis. 2010;28:155–61.
4. Kirovski G, Schacherer D, Wobser H, Huber H, Niessen C, Beer C, Schölmerich J, Hellerbrand C. Prevalence of ultrasound-diagnosed non-alcoholic fatty liver disease in a hospital cohort and its association with anthropometric, biochemical and sonographic characteristics. Int J ClinExp Med. 2010;3:202–10.
5. Paradis V, Bedossa P. Definition and natural history of metabolic steatosis: histology and cellular aspects. Diabetes Metab. 2008;34:638–42.
6. Cohen JC, Horton JD, Hobbs HH. Human fatty liver disease: old questions and new insights. Sci. 2011;332:1519–23.
7. Weinmann A, Alt Y, Koch S, Nelles C, Düber C, Lang H, Otto G, Zimmermann T, Marquardt JU, Galle PR, Wörns MA, Schattenberg JM. Treatment and survival of non-alcoholic steatohepatitis associated hepatocellular carcinoma. BMC Cancer. 2015;15:210.
8. Roeb E, Steffen HM, Bantel H, Baumann U, Canbay A, Demir M, Drebber U, Geier A, Hampe J, Hellerbrand C, Pathil-Warth A, Schattenberg JM, Schramm C, Seitz HK, Stefan N, Tacke F, Tannapfel A, Lynen Jansen P, Bojunga J. S2k-Leitlinie nicht alkoholische Fettlebererkrankungen. Z Gastroenterol. 2015;53:668–723.
9. Graeter T, Niedermayer PC, Mason RA, Oeztuerk S, Haenle MM, Koenig W, Boehm BO, Kratzer W. Coffee consumption and NAFLD: a community based study on 1223 subjects. BMC Res Notes. 2015;8:640.
10. Hillenbrand A, Kiebler B, Schwab C, Scheja L, Xu P, Henne-Bruns D, Wolf AM, Knippschild U. Prevalence of non-alcoholic fatty liver disease in four different weight related patient groups: association with small bowel length and risk factors. BMC Res Notes. 2015;8:290.
11. Browning JD, Horton JD. Molecular mediators of hepatic steatosis and liver injury. J Clin Invest. 2004;114:147–52.
12. Postic C, Girard J. The role of the lipogenic pathway in the development of hepatic steatosis. Diabetes Metab. 2008;34:643–8.
13. Schreuder TC, Marsman HA, Lenicek M, van Werven JR, Nederveen AJ, Jansen PL, Schaap FG. The hepatic response to FGF19 is impaired in patients with nonalcoholic fatty liver disease and insulin resistance. Am J Physiol Gastrointest Liver Physiol. 2010;298:G440–G5.

14. Eren F, Kurt R, Ermis F, Atug O, Imeryuz N, Yilmaz Y. Preliminary evidence of a reduced serum level of fibroblast growth factor 19 in patients with biopsy-proven nonalcoholic fatty liver disease. Clin Biochem. 2012;45:655–8.

15. Alisi A, Ceccarelli S, Panera N, Prono F, Petrini S, De Stefanis C, Pezzullo M, Tozzi A, Villani A, Bedogni G, Nobili V. Association between serum atypical fibroblast growth factors 21 and 19 and pediatric nonalcoholic fatty liver disease. PLoSOne. 2013;8:e67160.

16. Jahn D, Rau M, Hermanns HM, Geier A. Mechanisms of enterohepatic fibroblast growth factor 15/19 signaling in health and disease. Cytokine Growth Factor Rev. 2015;26:625–35.

17. Tomlinson E, Fu L, John L, Hultgren B, Huang X, Renz M, Stephan JP, Tsai SP, Powell-Braxton L, French D, Stewart TA. Transgenic mice expressing human fibroblast growth factor-19 display increased metabolic rate and decreased adiposity. Endocrinol. 2002;143:1741–7.

18. Fu L, John LM, Adams SH, Yu XX, Tomlinson E, Renz M, Williams PM, Soriano R, Corpuz R, Moffat B, Vandlen R, Simmons L, Foster J, Stephan JP, Tsai SP, Stewart TA. Fibroblast growth factor 19 increases metabolic rate and reverses dietary and leptin-deficient diabetes. Endocrinol. 2004;145: 2594–603.

19. Jansen PL, van Werven J, Aarts E, Berends F, Janssen I, Stoker J, Schaap FG. Alteration of hormonally active fibroblast growth factors after roux-en-Y gastric bypass surgery. Dig Dis. 2011;29:48–51.

20. Wojcik M, Janus D, Dolezal-Oltarzewska K, Kalicka-Kasperczyk A, Poplawska K, Drozdz D, Sztefko K, Starzyk JB. A decrease in fasting FGF19 levels is associated with the development of non-alcoholic fatty liver disease in obese adolescents. J Pediatr Endocrinol Metab. 2012;25:1089–93.

21. Holt JA, Luo G, Billin AN, Bisi J, McNeill YY, Kozarsky KF, Donahee M, Wang DY, Mansfield TA, Kliewer SA, Goodwin B, Jones SA. Definition of novel growth factor-dependent signal cascade for the suppression of bile acid biosynthesis. Genes Dev. 2003;17:1581–91.

22. Kurosu H, Kuro-o M. The klotho gene family as a regulator of endocrine fibroblast growth factors. Mol Cell Endocrinol. 2009;299:72–8.

23. Kharitonenkov A. FGFs and metabolism. Curr Opin Pharmacol. 2009;9:805–10.

24. Inagaki T, Choi M, Moschetta A, Peng L, Cummins CL, McDonald JG, Luo G, Jones SA, Goodwin B, Richardson JA, Gerard RD, Repa JJ, Mangelsdorf DJ, Kliewer SA. Fibroblast growth factor 15 functions as an enterohepatic signal to regulate bile acid homeostasis. Cell Metab. 2005;2:217–25.

25. Chiang JYL. Bile acids: regulation of synthesis. J Lipid Res. 2009;50:1955–66.

26. Kovár J, Lenícek M, Zimolová M, Vítek L, Jirsa M, Pitha J. Regulation of diurnal variation of cholesterol 7alpha-hydroxylase (CYP7A1) activity in healthy subjects. Physiol Res. 2010;59:233–8.

27. Deutsche Gesellschaft für Ernährung (DGE) e.V. Ernährungsbericht. Frankfurt: Deutsche Gesellschaft für Ernährung (DGE) e.V. 1992.

28. WHO. Obesity: preventing and managing the global epidemic. Report of a WHO consultation. World Health Organ Tech Rep Ser. 2000;894(i-xii):1–253.

29. Saverymuttu SH, Joseph AE, Maxwell JD. Ultrasound scanning in the detection of hepatic fibrosis and steatosis. Br Med J (Clin Res Ed). 1986; 292:13–5.

30. Nutricia GmbH. 2012. http://produkte.nutricia.de/de_de/pim/adults/nahrungsmodule/calogen/1300/#. Accessed 06 June 2012.

31. Harbury CM, Verbruggen EE, Callister R, Collins CE. What do individuals with morbid obesity reportas a usual dietary intake? A narrative review of available evidence. Clin Nutr ESPEN. 2016;13:e15-e22.

32. Marschall HU, Wagner M, Zollner G, Fickert P, Diczfalusy U, Gumhold J, Silbert D, Fuchsbichler A, Benthin L, Grundström R, Gustafsson U, Sahlin S, Einarsson C, Trauner M. Complementary stimulation of hepatobiliary transport and detoxification systems by rifampicin and ursodeoxycholic acid in human liver. Gastroenterol. 2005;129:476–85.

33. Axelson M, Bjorkhem I, Reihner E, Einarsson K. The plasma level of 7 alpha-hydroxy-4-cholesten-3-one reflects the activity of hepatic cholesterol 7 alpha-hydroxylase in man. FEBS Lett. 1991;284:216–8.

34. Chan YH. Biostatistics 101: data presentation. Singap Med J. 2003;44:280–5.

35. Stejskal D, Karpísek M, Hanulová Z, Stejskal P. Fibroblast growth factor-19: development, analytical characterization and clinical evaluation of a new ELISA test. Scand J Clin Lab Invest. 2008;68:501–7.

36. Gallego-Escuredo JM, Gómez-Ambrosi J, Catalan V, Domingo P, Giralt M, Frühbeck G, Villarroya F. Opposite alterations in FGF21 and FGF19 levels and disturbed expression of the receptor machinery for endocrine FGFs in obese patients. Int J Obes. 2015;39:121–9.

37. Fang Q, Li H, Song Q, Yang W, Hou X, Ma X, Lu J, Xu A, Jia W. Serum fibroblast growth factor 19 levels are decreased in Chinese subjects with impaired fasting glucose and inversely associated with fasting plasma glucose levels. Diabetes Care. 2013;36:2810–4.

38. Roesch SL, Styer AM, Wood GC, Kosak Z, Seiler J, Benotti P, Petrick AT, Gabrielsen J, Strodel WE, Gerhard GS, Still CD, Argyropoulos G. Perturbations of fibroblast growth factors 19 and 21 in type 2 diabetes. PLoSOne. 2015;10:e0116928.

39. Jiao N, Baker SS, Chapa-Rodriguez A, Liu W, Nugent CA, Tsompana M, Mastrandrea L, Buck MJ, Baker RD, Genco RJ, Zhu R, Zhu L. Suppressed hepatic bile acid signalling despite elevated production of primary and secondary bile acids in NAFLD. Gut. 2017; https://doi.org/10.1136/gutjnl-2017-314307. [Epub ahead of print]

40. Nobili V, Alisi A, Mosca A, Della Corte C, Veraldi S, De Vito R, De Stefanis C, D'Oria V, Jahnel J, Zohrer E, Scorletti E, Byrne CD. Hepatic farnesoid X receptor protein level and circulating fibroblast growth factor 19 concentration in children with NAFLD. Liver Int. 2017; https://doi.org/10.1111/liv.13531. [Epub ahead of print]

41. Schmid A, Leszczak S, Ober I, Karrasch T, Schäffler A. Short-term and divergent regulation of FGF-19 and FGF-21 during oral lipid tolerance test but not oral glucose tolerance test. Exp Clin Endocrinol Diabetes. 2015;123:88–94.

42. Sonne DP, van Nierop FS, Kulik W, Soeters MR, Vilsbøll T, Knop FK. Postprandial plasma concentrations of individual bile acids and FGF-19 in patients with type 2 diabetes. J Clin Endocrinol Metab. 2016;10:3002–9.

43. Mihas C, Kolovou GD, Mikhailidis DP, Kovar J, Lairon D, Nordestgaard BG, Ooi TC, Perez-Martinez P, Bilianou H, Anagnostopoulou K, Panotopoulos G. Diagnostic value of postprandial triglyceride testing in healthy subjects: a meta-analysis. Curr Vasc Pharmacol. 2011;9:271–80.

44. Wehling H, Lusher J. People with a body mass index >30 under-report their dietary intake: a systematic review. J Health Psychol. 2017: 1359105317714318. https://doi.org/10.1177/1359105317714318. [Epub ahead of print]

45. Lu LP, Wan YP, Xun PC, Zhou KJ, Chen C, Cheng SY, Zhang MZ, Wu CH, Lin WW, Jiang Y, Feng HX, Wang JL, He K, Cai W. Serum bile acid level and fatty acid composition in Chinese children with non-alcoholic fatty liver disease. J Dig Dis. 2017;18:461–71.

8

Five-year outcome of conventional and drug-eluting transcatheter arterial chemoembolization in patients with hepatocellular carcinoma

Yi-Sheng Liu, Chia-Ying Lin, Ming-Tsung Chuang, Chia-Ying Lin, Yi-Shan Tsai, Chien-Kuo Wang and Ming-Ching Ou*

Abstract

Background: Currently, no standard of care or therapies have been established for patients with advanced HCC. We evaluated the efficacy and safety of conventional transarterial chemoembolization using gelatin sponges or microspheres plus lipiodol-doxorubicin (cTACE) and TACE with doxorubicin-loaded drug eluting beads (DEB-TACE).

Methods: This retrospective study included 273 patients who received cTACE ($n = 201$) or DEB-TACE. Tumor response, survival, and adverse events were evaluated over a 5-year follow-up period.

Results: During 5-year follow-up, a greater percentage of patients treated with cTACE died than those treated with DEB-TACE (76.1% vs. 66.7%) ($P = 0.045$). At the last evaluation, all surviving patients had disease progression and no differences were seen between treatment groups. However, the time to disease progression differed between groups; median time to disease progression was 11.0 months for cTACE and 16.0 months for DEB-TACE ($P = 0.019$). The median survival time was 37 months in both treatment groups. No significant differences were observed between cTACE and DEB-TACE therapies in subgroups of patients with BCLC stage A or stage B + C either in survival time or time to disease progression (P values > 0.05). No significant differences were observed in survival status or disease progression between cTACE and DEB-TACE in patient subgroups with either tumor number > 5 or with the sum of the diameter of largest five HCC tumors being > 7 cm.

Conclusions: DEB-TACE demonstrates greater long-term benefits than cTACE in treating treatment-naïve patients with HCC. Results of this long-term study support the use of DEB-TACE in treating HCC.

Keywords: Drug-eluting bead transcatheter arterial chemoembolization, DEB-TACE, Hepatocellular carcinoma, Transcatheter arterial chemoembolization, TACE

Background

Hepatocellular carcinoma (HCC) is the third leading cause of cancer-related deaths worldwide and the sixth most common cancer [1, 2]. Due to chronic liver infection resulting from the high incidence of hepatitis C infection and the large number of persons with metabolic syndrome, the incidence of HCC is anticipated to rise [1, 2]. A large percentage of HCC patients are

diagnosed at the intermediate or advanced stage [3, 4]. Currently, no established standard of care or therapeutic possibilities exist for patients with advanced HCC. Only 30 to 40% patients with HCC are candidates for curative treatment such as liver transplant [3, 4]. Hence, most patients can only be treated with locoregional or palliative treatment [5].

Transcatheter arterial chemoembolization (TACE) is used as a palliative local therapeutic option for patients with nonresectable HCC who may be waiting for liver transplant or who are not candidates for liver transplantation. TACE is also used to decrease the tumor burden, allowing for

* Correspondence: emilialiar@yahoo.com.tw
Department of Diagnostic Radiology, National Cheng Kung University Hospital, College of Medicine, National Cheng Kung University, No. 138 Sheng Li Road, Tainan 704, Taiwan, Republic of China

Table 1 Patients' clinical characteristics by cTACE and DEB-TACE groups. ($N = 273$)

Variables	Total ($N = 273$)	cTACE ($n = 201$)	DEB-TACE ($n = 72$)	p-value
Age, years	64.4 ± 10.7	65.3 ± 10.7	61.7 ± 10.3	**0.009**
Sex				
Female	86 (31.5)	63 (31.3)	23 (31.9)	0.925
Male	187 (68.5)	138 (68.7)	49 (68.1)	
Previous treatment				
None	172 (63.0)	126 (62.7)	46 (63.9)	0.166
Operation	53 (19.4)	35 (17.4)	18 (25.0)	
Locoregional treatment	41 (15.0)	33 (16.4)	8 (11.1)	
Operation + locoregional	7 (2.6)	7 (3.5)	0 (0)	
Uni-/Bi-lobar				
Unilobar	136 (49.8)	106 (52.7)	30 (41.7)	0.107
Bilobar	137 (50.2)	95 (47.3)	42 (58.3)	
HBV/HCV				
Non-B or C	22 (8.1)	18 (9.0)	4 (5.6)	0.225
HBV	127 (46.5)	87 (43.3)	40 (55.6)	
HCV	108 (39.6)	82 (40.8)	26 (36.1)	
HBV + HCV	16 (5.9)	14 (7.0)	2 (2.8)	
GOT (IU/L)	70.63 ± 48.72	69.88 ± 50.4	70.63 ± 48.72	0.331
GOT				
Not normal	156 (57.1)	112 (55.7)	44 (61.1)	0.428
Normal	117 (42.9)	89 (44.3)	28 (38.9)	
GPT (IU/L)	72.08 ± 80.27	69.97 ± 81.77	72.08 ± 80.27	0.109
GPT				
Not normal	132 (48.4)	91 (45.3)	41 (56.9)	0.089
Normal	141 (51.6)	110 (54.7)	31 (43.1)	
Bilirubin (mg/dL)	0.76 ± 0.44	0.73 ± 0.42	0.76 ± 0.44	0.087
Bilirubin				
Not normal	22 (8.1)	13 (6.5)	9 (12.5)	0.107
Normal	251 (91.9)	188 (93.5)	63 (87.5)	
AFP (ng/mL)	875.28 ± 4510.43	766.21 ± 4607.3	875.28 ± 4510.43	0.497
AFP				
Negative	224 (82.1)	169 (84.1)	55 (76.4)	0.145
Positive	49 (17.9)	32 (15.9)	17 (23.6)	
Albumin (g/dL)	4 ± 0.49	3.98 ± 0.48	4 ± 0.49	0.312
Albumin				
Not normal	41 (15.0)	29 (14.4)	12 (16.7)	0.648
Normal	232 (85.0)	172 (85.6)	60 (83.3)	
Ascites				
None	257 (94.1)	191 (95.0)	66 (91.7)	0.432
Mild	15 (5.5)	9 (4.5)	6 (8.3)	
Moderate	1 (0.4)	1 (0.5)	0 (0)	

Table 1 Patients' clinical characteristics by cTACE and DEB-TACE groups. (N = 273) (Continued)

Variables	Total (N = 273)	cTACE (n = 201)	DEB-TACE (n = 72)	p-value
Child-Pugh stage				
5	219 (80.2)	161 (80.1)	58 (80.6)	0.883
6	44 (16.1)	33 (16.4)	11 (15.3)	
7	9 (3.3)	6 (3.0)	3 (4.1)	
8	1 (0.4)	1 (0.5)	0 (0)	
ECOG stage				
0	271 (99.3)	199 (99.0)	72 (100)	1.000
1	2 (0.7)	2 (1.0)	0 (0)	
CLIP stage				
0	40 (14.7)	32 (15.9)	8 (11.1)	**0.018**
1	172 (63.0)	132 (65.7)	40 (55.6)	
2	49 (17.9)	29 (14.4)	20 (27.8)	
3	10 (3.7)	8 (4.0)	2 (2.8)	
4	2 (0.7)	0 (0)	2 (2.8)	
Okuda stage				
0	250 (91.6)	185 (92.0)	65 (90.3)	0.471
1	20 (7.3)	13 (6.5)	7 (9.7)	
2	3 (1.1)	3 (1.5)	0 (0)	
BCLC stage				
A	87 (32)	71 (35.7)	16 (22.2)	**0.040**
B + C	184 (67.9)	128 (64.3)	56 (77.8)	
Largest target (cm)	3.64 ± 2.59	3.47 ± 2.32	4.12 ± 3.20	0.175
Tumor numbers	3.5 ± 1.9	3.4 ± 1.9	3.6 ± 2.0	0.690
Tumor numbers ≤5	197 (72.2)	148 (73.6)	49 (68.1)	0.365
Tumor numbers > 5	76 (27.8)	53 (26.4)	23 (31.9)	
Sum of the largest five hepatocellular carcinoma diameter (cm)	6.64 ± 2.33	6.63 ± 2.26	6.66 ± 2.53	0.908

Aspartate aminotransferase (GOT), Alanine aminotransferase (GPT)
Data are summarized as mean ± SD and n (%) for continuous and categorical variables by treatment. Differences between treatments were compared using Mann-Whitney U test for continuous variables and Chi-square test / or Fisher's exact test for categorical variables
Bold p-values indicate statistical significance ($p < 0.05$)

tumor resection [6]. Conventional TACE (cTACE) involves the delivery of embolic material to the tumor plus chemotherapeutic agents such as doxorubicin, either dissolved or emulsified in lipiodol, which is noted for causing both ischemia and strong cytotoxic effects [2, 7]. Lipiodol is a lymphographic agent which is selectively deposited in HCC tumors by arterial infusion and permits the slow release of the chemotherapeutic agent into the tumor [8–10]. In randomized controlled trials, cTACE has demonstrated a survival benefit for HCC patients with non-resectable HCC [11–14] and is recommended as a standard treatment option for patients with Barcelona stage B (BCLC) (intermediate stage) HCC [15, 16]. However, with TACE, the tumor does not always retain the lipiodol, resulting in decreased effectiveness of therapy and risk of liver damage [17, 18].

Drug-eluting beads (DEB) have been introduced into TACE (DEB-TACE) to promote the controlled release of cytotoxic drugs for the treatment of HCC [19, 20]. The drug-eluting microspheres added to TACE result in the delivery of high concentration of chemotherapeutic drugs to the tumor. The use of DEB-TACE is associated with a better safety profile than cTACE; DEB-TACE has been observed to have a lower incidence of adverse events such as abdominal pain, fever, nausea and vomiting [21–24]. A number of clinical studies and meta-analyses have found that DEB-TACE was associated with a significant advantage in tumor response and survival compared with cTACE [21–24]. However, several recent studies failed to demonstrate the superiority of DEB-TACE over cTACE in treatment efficacy, although DEB-TACE was associated with a better safety profile than cTACE [25–28].

Although DEB-TACE has shown benefits relative to TACE in some randomized controlled studies, the method is still controversial in clinical practice. Early results of our study of DEB-TACE and cTACE published in 2015 [29] showed that, at a mean follow-up of 15 months, DEB-TACE was associated with a better safety profile and more patients achieved a complete response and fewer had disease progression than cTACE. The present retrospective study evaluated the long-term benefits of DEB-TACE and cTACE on disease progression and overall survival (OS) during 5-year follow up of patients with HCC.

Methods

This retrospective study recruited consecutive patients with HCC who were treated with TACE at the National Cheng-Kung University Hospital (Tainan, Taiwan) from November 2010 to November 2011. The retrospective analysis was approved by the Ethics Committee of the institutional review board, National Cheng Kung University Hospital (IRB No: A-ER-103-311). The study was performed in accordance with the Declaration of Helsinki and the protocol was reviewed and approved by the Institutional Review Board of the hospital. All patients provided signed informed consent.

Study patients

The study design and protocol were as described previously in Liu et al. [29]. Eligible patients were ≥ 18 years of age with a diagnosis of HCC, had a at least one tumor that had not been treated previously and was > 1 mm in diameter, had Barcelona Clinic Liver Cancer (BCLC) criteria A or B, and had an Eastern Cooperative Oncology Group (ECOG) performance score of 0 or 1. Included patients were also required to have a serum creatinine of < 1.2 mg/dL, aspartate aminotransferase (AST) and alanine aminotransferase (ALT) levels < 100 IU/L, and total bilirubin < 3 mg/dL. Patients were excluded if the tumor had invaded the portal vein, hepatic vein, and/or biliary duct, if the tumor had an extrahepatic arterial supply, or if the patient was diagnosed with atypical HCC such as, for example, infiltrative.

Treatment

A multidisciplinary team determined the treatment for a given patient. All patients were treated with a single cycle of TACE. Study patients either received cTACE with a gelatin sponge or with Embosphere microspheres (Biosphere, Roissy, France), or chemoembolization with doxorubicin-containing DEB (DC Bead, Biocompatibles, Farnham, United Kingdom). Prior to treatment, the attending physician described to the patient the tumor response and complication rates for each treatment method, as determined by the published literature. Subsequently,

the patient decided which method should be used. No other simultaneous or combined treatment was permitted during the cTACE or DEB-TACE treatment period.

On the day of treatment, the patient underwent a complete diagnostic angiographic evaluation of the hepatic artery, superior mesenteric artery, and celiac trunk so as to evaluate the vascular anatomy and portal flow [30]. The segmental and subsegmental arteries feeding the tumor were subsequently catheterized using super-selective angiography with a microcatheter. The right hepatic artery was used in patients whose right hepatic artery came from the superior mesenteric artery. Care was taken to avoid embolization of the cystic and falciform arteries. The phrenic artery was investigated if it was determined to be supplying the tumor.

Patients in the cTACE group were injected with the doxorubicin/lipiodol mixture consisting of 50 mg of doxorubicin mixed with 10 mL of lipiodol. The mixture was injected into a segmental or subsegmental artery, followed by an injection of 500 to 700 μm gelatin sponge (Spongostan standard, Johnson & Johnson, Gargrave, Skipton, United Kingdom), or 100

Table 2 Patients' clinical characteristics after treatment with cTACE and DEB-TACE. (N = 273)

Variables	cTACE (n = 201)	DEB-TACE (n = 72)	p-value
GOT (IU/L)	156.76 ± 176.58	73.31 ± 45.50	**< 0.001**
GOT			
Not normal	153 (76.1)	46 (63.9)	**0.045**
Normal	48 (23.9)	26 (36.1)	
GPT (IU/L)	170.91 ± 266.13	94.17 ± 101.44	**0.014**
GPT			
Not normal	139 (69.2)	47 (65.3)	0.545
Normal	62 (30.8)	25 (34.7)	
Bilirubin (mg/dL)	1.38 ± 0.99	0.98 ± 0.57	**0.002**
Bilirubin			
Not normal	75 (37.3)	14 (19.4)	**0.006**
Normal	126 (62.7)	58 (80.6)	
Albumin (g/dL)	3.81 ± 0.43	3.87 ± 0.42	0.325
Albumin			
Not normal	37 (18.4)	12 (16.7)	0.741
Normal	164 (81.6)	60 (83.3)	
Cholangitis			
No	193 (96)	70 (97.2)	0.641
Yes	8 (4)	2 (2.8)	

Aspartate aminotransferase (GOT), Alanine aminotransferase (GPT)
Data are summarized as mean ± SD and n (%) for continuous and categorical variables by treatment. Differences between treatments were compared using Mann-Whitney U test for continuous variables and Chi-square test / or Fisher's exact test for categorical variables
All serious AE were classified as cholangitis, none as biloma
Bold p-values indicate statistical significance (p < 0.05)

to 300 μm Embosphere microspheres. The amount of lipiodol/doxorubicin injected was determined by the tumor size [31]. The DEB-TACE group was injected with 2 mL of 300 to500 μm DEB combined with 70 mg of doxorubicin [32]. An additional volume(s) of DEB was injected if "near stasis" was not obtained after the first injection until "near stasis" was achieved. The amount of beads injected was based upon the manufacturer's instructions. The study used 300 to 500 μm beads because the 100 to 300 μm beads were not yet approved in Taiwan at the time the study started.

Follow-up and evaluation of treatment response

Tumor status was evaluated every 3 to 4 months according to the modified Response Evaluation Criteria in Solid Tumors (mRECIST) [33]. If the evaluation suggested partial response or stable disease, the patients continued to be followed every 3 to 4 months for up to and over 5 years. Partial response was defined as ≥30% reduction in the sum of the diameter of the visible target lesions compared with baseline. If the assessment indicated progressive disease, patients were treated according to the BCLC guidelines and disease status [34].

Table 3 Survival times and progression times between cTACE and DEB-TACE treatments

Variables	cTACE	DEB-TACE	p-value
Total	(n = 201)	(n = 72)	
Survival status			**0.045**
Died within ≤5 years follow-up	153 (76.1)	48 (66.7)	
Died after more than 5 years follow-up	10 (5.0)	1 (1.4)	
Survived until last follow-up	38 (18.9)	23 (31.9)	
Progression status			0.218
Progression	192 (95.5)	66 (91.7)	
Loss of follow-up/censored	9 (4.5)	6 (8.3)	
Survival time, months	37 (32.2, 41.8)	37 (23.5, 50.5)	0.091
Progression time, months	11.0 (9.6, 12.4)	16.0 (13.1, 18.9)	**0.019**
BCLC stage = A	(n = 73)	(n = 16)	
Survival status			0.083
Died within ≤5 years follow-up	57 (78.1)	9 (56.3)	
Died after more than 5 years follow-up	3 (4.1)	0 (0)	
Survived until last follow-up	13 (17.8)	7 (43.8)	
Progression status			0.219
Progression	70 (95.9)	14 (87.5)	
Loss of follow-up/censored	3 (4.1)	2 (12.5)	
Survival time, months	42 (36.1, 47.9)	45 (0, 90.1)	0.149
Progression time, months	12 (10.5, 13.5)	19 (17.8, 20.2)	0.217
BCLC stage = B + C	(n = 128)	(n = 56)	
Survival status			0.270
Died within ≤5 years follow-up	96 (75)	39 (69.6)	
Died after more than 5 years follow-up	7 (5.5)	1 (1.8)	
Survived until last follow-up	25 (19.5)	16 (28.6)	
Progression status			0.495
Progression	122 (95.3)	52 (92.9)	
Loss of follow-up/censored	6 (4.7)	4 (7.1)	
Survival time, months	33 (27.1, 38.9)	36 (21.3, 50.7)	0.191
Progression time, months	10 (8.1, 11.9)	15 (12.4, 17.7)	**0.032**

Survival and progression status are summarized as n (%) by treatment; Survival time- and progression time-related data are summarized as median (95%CI) by treatment
Differences between treatments were compared using Pearson Chi-square test / or Fisher's exact test for survival and progression status and Log-rank test for survival time or progression time
Bold p-values indicate statistical significance (p < 0.05)

Progressive disease was defined using the mRECIST criteria; i.e., ≥20% increase in the sum of the diameters of the visible target lesions compared with the smallest measurements observed from the start of therapy. Stable disease was defined as cases in which the tumor evaluation did not meet the criteria of partial response or progressive disease [33]. Two experienced radiologists evaluated the images, and any discrepancies were resolved by consensus.

Safety was evaluated throughout the study.

Statistical analysis

Clinical data are summarized as mean ± standard deviation (SD) and n (%) for continuous and categorical variables by treatment. Differences between treatments were compared using Mann-Whitney U test for continuous variables and Chi-square test / or Fisher's exact test for categorical variables and for survival time and progression time. Pearson Chi-square test / or Fisher's exact test were used to evaluate survival and progression status between treatments. The overall survival time and progression time by treatment were graphed using Kaplan-Meier curve and the estimated survival time was presented as median with 95% confidence intervals (95% CI). The log-rank test was applied to compare the difference in OS time between treatments. Results are represented as a P value. All statistical assessments were two-tailed and considered significant at $P < 0.05$. All statistical analyses were carried out using IBM SPSS statistical software version 22 for Windows (IBM Corp. Released 2013. IBM SPSS Statistics for Windows, Version 22.0. Armonk, NY.).

Results

Baseline demographics and disease characteristics

A total of 273 patients (187 males / 86 females) with a mean age of 64.4 years were included in the study (Table 1). Of these, 201 patients were treated with cTACE and 72 with DEB-TACE. The baseline clinical characteristics were similar between treatment groups except for age, CLIP stage, and BCLC stage; patients in the cTACE group were older (65.3 vs. 61.7 years of age; $P = 0.009$), a greater percentage of patients had CLIP stage 0 or 1 cancer (81.6% vs. 66.7%; $P = 0.018$)) and BCLC A stage disease (35.7% vs. 22.2%; $P = 0.040$) than patients in the DEB-TACE group. Across groups, 63% of patients had no prior treatment, about 50% had unilobar disease, and the majority had HCV or HBV infections. About 80% of patients had Child-Pugh stage 5 disease and approximately 99% had an ECOG status of 0. The mean largest tumor size was 3.64 cm and most patients (72.2%) had ≤5 tumors.

Treatment response

Clinical characteristics after treatment differed between cTACE and DEB-TACE patients (Table 2). Mean aspartate aminotransferase (GOT), alanine aminotransferase (GPT) and bilirubin were significantly different between the two groups. DEB-TACE patients had lower mean

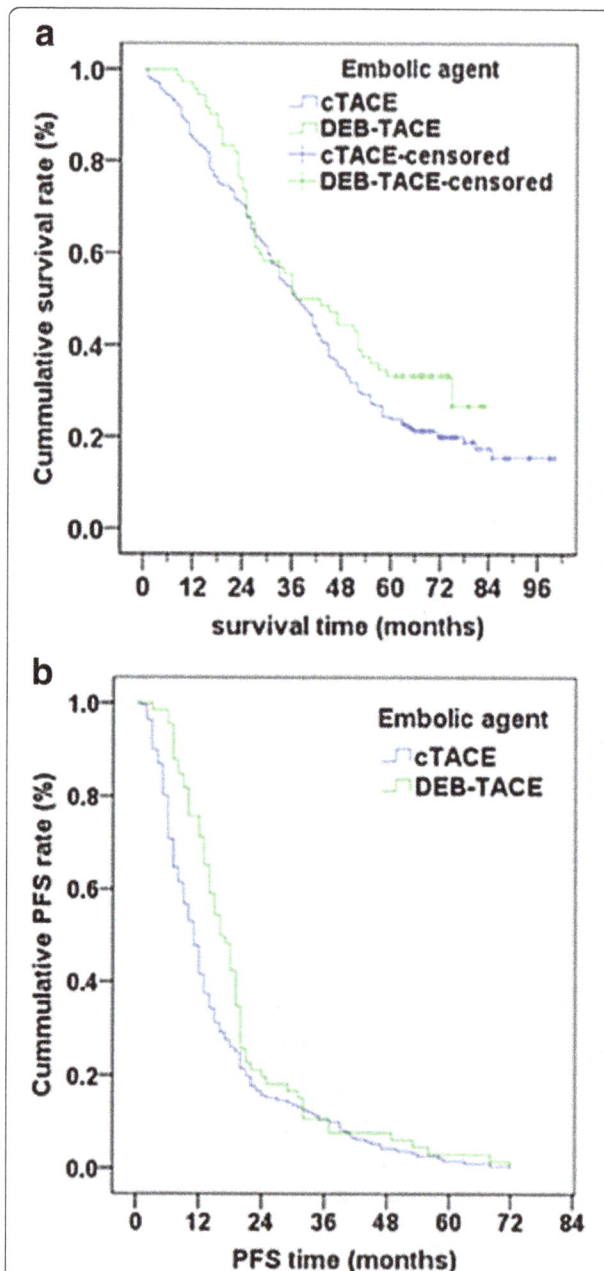

Fig. 1 Kaplan-Meier curve of overall survival time (**a**) and PFS time (**b**) by treatments. **a** The estimated median overall survival time was derived as 37 months (95%CI = 32.2–41.8 months) for cTACE and 37 months (95%CI = 23.5–50.5 months) for DEB-TACE. The log-rank test p-value = 0.091. **b** The estimated median PFS time was derived as 11 months (95%CI = 9.6–12.4 months) for cTACE and 16 months (95%CI = 13.1–18.9 months) for DEB-TACE. The log-rank test p-value = 0.019

GOT (73.31 ± 45.50), and higher percentages had normal GOT values (36.1%). The same was also true for bilirubin levels; DEB-TACE patients had lower mean (0.98 ± 0.57) and higher percentages with normal bilirubin values (80.6%). Compared to cTACE patients, DEB-TACE patients also had significantly lower mean GPT (94.17 ± 101.44), but the percentage of patients with normal values was similar between the two groups. No significant differences were found in the percentage of patients with cholangitis between the cTACE and DEB-TACE groups. (Table 2).

Survival time for the overall population was median 37 months (95% CI = 32.2–41.8 months) for cTACE treatment and a similar median 37 months (95%CI = 23.5–50.5 months) for the DEB-TACE treatment group ($P = 0.091$) (Table 3 and Fig. 1a). Over the 5-year follow-up period, a greater percentage of patients treated with cTACE died than those treated with DEB-TACE (76.1% vs. 66.7%, respectively) ($P = 0.045$). All patients who were still alive at the last evaluation (15 patients died during the 5-year follow-up) had disease progression (Table 3). However, the time to disease progression differed between groups; median time to disease progression was 11.0 months for cTACE and 16.0 months for DEB-TACE ($P = 0.019$). (Table 3 and Fig. 1b).

Survival time and time to disease progression between treatments was also evaluated by BCLC stage, and by patients with > 5 tumors or whose sum of the five largest tumors was > 7 cm in diameter. No significant differences were observed between cTACE and DEB-TACE therapies in the subgroups of patients with BCLC stage A or stage B + C, either in survival time or progression time (P values > 0.05) (Table 3). In addition, no significant differences were observed in survival status or disease progression between cTACE and DEB-TACE in the subgroups of patients with either tumor number > 5 or

the sum of the diameter of the five largest HCC tumors was > 7 cm. (Table 4).

Discussion

This retrospective, observational study compared clinical outcomes of treatment-naive HCC patients who underwent cTACE (conventional TACE) or DEB-TACE (drug-eluting bead TACE). The earlier published findings from the 15-month follow-up of this study population showed that DEB-TACE treatment resulted in a higher percentage of patients with complete response and a lower percentage with disease progression than patients receiving cTACE treatment [29]. In addition, DEB-TACE was associated with a better safety profile than cTACE [29]. The data presented here are those of the same study after 5-years of follow-up. Five-years after treatment, both treatments were associated with a survival time of 37 months. However, over the 5-year follow-up period, a greater percentage of patients treated with cTACE died (76.1%) than those treated with DEB-TACE (66.7%) ($P = 0.045$). After five-years, all surviving patients had disease progression. However, the time to disease progression differed between groups; cTACE was associated with a shorter median time to disease progression (11 months) than DEB-TACE (16.0 months) ($P = 0.019$). Subgroup analysis indicated that survival and disease progression were similar for both treatments in patients with BLCC stage A or stage B + C, and in patients with > 5 tumors, or if the diameter of the patient's five largest tumors was > 7 cm. The findings of the long-term study suggest that DEB-TACE demonstrates long-term benefits in treating treatment-naive HCC patients.

Only a limited number of studies have directly compared the efficacy and safety of DEB-TACE and cTACE in treating HCC. A number of systematic reviews and

Table 4 Survival times and progression times between cTACE and DEB-TACE treatments for patients with tumor number > 5 or sum of the diameter of the largest five HCC tumors was > 7 cm

Variables	cTACE	DEB-TACE	p-value
	(n = 78)	(n = 33)	
Survival status			0.610
Died within ≤5 years follow-up	62 (79.5)	26 (78.8)	
Died after more than 5 years follow-up	3 (3.8)	0 (0)	
Survived until last follow-up	13 (16.7)	7 (21.2)	
Progression status			0.360
Progression	75 (96.2)	30 (90.9)	
Loss of follow-up/censored	3 (3.8)	3 (9.1)	
Survival time, months	31 (26.7, 35.3)	27 (22.3, 31.7)	0.789
Progression time, months	9 (6.7, 11.3)	12 (8.0, 16.0)	0.492

Survival and progression status are summarized as n (%) by treatment; Survival time- and progression time-related data are summarized as median (95%CI) by treatment

Differences between treatments were compared using Pearson Chi-square test / or Fisher's exact test for survival and progression status and Log-rank test for survival time or progression time

meta-analyses have evaluated the effectiveness of cTACE and DEB-TACE in treating HCC [21–24].

Similar to our findings, several of the meta-analyses found DEB-TACE to show treatment benefit and better safety profile compared with cTACE [23, 24]. A systematic review by Martin et al. [21] found DEB-TACE had a significant advantage compared with cTACE in objective response and had greater overall disease control in patients with advanced HCC (P values ≤0.038). Zhou et al. performed a meta-analysis which included nine studies and total of 830 patients [24]. The study found DEB-TACE significantly improved overall survival and increased objective response and disease control rates. Similarly, a meta-analysis performed by Huang et al. [23], which included seven clinical studies with 700 patients, found a significantly better objective response for DEB-TACE than cTACE (P = 0.004), with a relative risk difference of 0.15 (P = 0.0003). Those authors also found that patients with one- and two-year survival were significantly more with DEB-TACE than with cTACE (P values ≤0.007). However, Huang et al. found no difference between treatments for 6-month and 3-year survival (P values ≥0.11). A meta-analysis by Zou et al. [22] found DEB-TACE was associated with higher complete response (Odds ratio [OR], 1.35), overall survival rate (OR, 1.41), and survival time (WMD, 3.03). In contrast to the studies of Huang et al. and Zhou et al., Zou et al. found no difference between treatments for objective response. Those authors also found that the treatments had similar disease control rates. All four meta-analyses found that DEB-TACE was associated with fewer side effects compared with cTACE.

In contrast to the above results, a meta-analysis performed by Facciorusso et al. [25] found that DEB-TACE and cTACE had similar safety and effectiveness. Facciorusso et al. included 12 studies, four of which were randomized controlled trials. The meta-analysis included a total of 1449 patients. The observed 1-, 2- and 3-year survival times were similar between treatment groups (P values ≥0.06). Pooled data of objective response and incidence of adverse events also indicated no differences between the two therapies (P values ≥0.36). However, the study did show a non-significant trend of superiority for DEB-TACE for overall response rate (OR, 1.2), which was confirmed by subgroup and sensitivity analysis.

The difference in findings across the meta-analyses may, in part, reflect the small number of included studies and high heterogeneity in the studies overall. Moreover, the evaluation of response rate across the studies varied, with some of the included studies used EASL criteria and others using mRECIST criteria. In addition, length of follow-up was heterogeneous among the included studies and was found to be one of the main sources of heterogeneity. The present study supports the importance of follow-up in comparing studies. In an earlier phase of the present t study conducted at 15 months post-treatment, DEB-TACE treatment was associated with patients' greater complete response and less disease progression than cTACE. However, at the 5-year follow-up, all surviving patients had disease progression but fewer patients treated with DEB-TACE had died.

The present study has several limitations, including that the study was retrospective in design and only included patients from a single institution. In addition, complete secondary treatment information was not available for the patients and only a small number of patients were treated with DEB-TACE (n = 73).

Conclusions

In conclusion, DEB-TACE shows greater long-term benefit compared with those of cTACE in treating treatment naïve patients with HCC. At 5 years after treatment, HCC patients receiving DEB-TACE have fewer deaths and a longer time to disease progression than patients receiving cTACE. DEB-TACE is also associated with fewer treatment-related adverse events than cTACE. Results of this long-term study support the use of DEB-TACE in treating HCC.

Abbreviations

cTACE: Conventional transarterial chemoembolization; DEB: With doxorubicin-loaded drug eluting beads; ECOG: Eastern cooperative oncology group; HCC: Hepatocellular carcinoma; mRECIST: Modified response evaluation criteria in solid tumors; OS: Overall survival; TACE: Transarterial chemoembolization; TACE: Transarterial chemoembolization; BCLC: Barcelona clinic liver cancer

Acknowledgements

None.

Funding

None.

Authors' contributions

YSL study concepts, study design, literature search, data acquisition, manuscript preparation; CYL study design, literature search, data acquisition, manuscript editing, data analysis, statistical analysis; MTC definition of intellectual content, data analysis, statistical analysis; YST statistical analysis; CKW data acquisition; MCO guarantor of integrity of the entire study, study concepts, study design, definition of intellectual content, manuscript editing, manuscript review. All authors read and approved the manuscript.

Consent for publication

Not applicable.

Competing interests

The authors declare that they have no competing interests.

References

1. Jemal A, Bray F, Center MM, Ferlay J, Ward E, Forman D. Global cancer statistics. CA Cancer J Clin. 2011;61(2):69–90.
2. Thomas MB, Jaffe D, Choti MM, Belghiti J, Curley S, Fong Y, et al. Hepatocellular carcinoma: consensus recommendations of the National Cancer Institute clinical trials planning meeting. J Clin Oncol. 2010;28(25): 3994–4005.
3. Bruix J, Sherman M. American Association for the Study of liver D. Management of hepatocellular carcinoma: an update. Hepatology. 2011; 53(3):1020–2.
4. European Association For The Study Of The L, European Organisation For R, Treatment Of C. EASL-EORTC clinical practice guidelines: management of hepatocellular carcinoma. J Hepatol. 2012;56(4):908–43.
5. Forner A, Llovet JM, Bruix J. Hepatocellular carcinoma. Lancet. 2012; 379(9822):1245–55.
6. Gosalia AJ, Martin P, Jones PD. Advances and future directions in the treatment of hepatocellular carcinoma. Gastroenterol Hepatol. 2017;13(7): 398–410.
7. Ramsey DE, Kernagis LY, Soulen MC, Geschwind JF. Chemoembolization of hepatocellular carcinoma. J Vasc Interv Radiol. 2002;13(9 Pt 2):S211–21.
8. Konno T, Maeda H, Iwai K, Maki S, Tashiro S, Uchida M, et al. Selective targeting of anti-cancer drug and simultaneous image enhancement in solid tumors by arterially administered lipid contrast medium. Cancer. 1984; 54(11):2367–74.
9. Konno T, Maeda H, Iwai K, Tashiro S, Maki S, Morinaga T, et al. Effect of arterial administration of high-molecular-weight anticancer agent SMANCS with lipid lymphographic agent on hepatoma: a preliminary report. Eur J Cancer Clin Oncol. 1983;19(8):1053–65.
10. Jinno K, Moriwaki S, Tanada M, Wada T, Mandai K, Okada Y. Clinicopathological study on combination therapy consisting of arterial infusion of lipiodol-dissolved SMANCS and transcatheter arterial embolization for hepatocellular carcinoma. Cancer Chemother Pharmacol. 1992;31(Suppl):S7–12.
11. Chung GE, Lee JH, Kim HY, Hwang SY, Kim JS, Chung JW, et al. Transarterial chemoembolization can be safely performed in patients with hepatocellular carcinoma invading the main portal vein and may improve the overall survival. Radiology. 2011;258(2):627–34.
12. Lee HS, Kim JS, Choi IJ, Chung JW, Park JH, Kim CY. The safety and efficacy of transcatheter arterial chemoembolization in the treatment of patients with hepatocellular carcinoma and main portal vein obstruction. A prospective controlled study. Cancer. 1997;79(11):2087–94.
13. Luo J, Guo RP, Lai EC, Zhang YJ, Lau WY, Chen MS, et al. Transarterial chemoembolization for unresectable hepatocellular carcinoma with portal vein thrombosis: a prospective comparative study. Ann Surg Oncol. 2011;18(2):413–20.
14. Xue TC, Xie XY, Zhang L, Yin X, Zhang BH, Ren ZG. Transarterial chemoembolization for hepatocellular carcinoma with portal vein tumor thrombus: a meta-analysis. BMC Gastroenterol. 2013;13:60.
15. Llovet JM, Bruix J. Systematic review of randomized trials for unresectable hepatocellular carcinoma: chemoembolization improves survival. Hepatology. 2003;37(2):429–42.
16. Kang JY, Choi MS, Kim SJ, Kil JS, Lee JH, Koh KC, et al. Long-term outcome of preoperative transarterial chemoembolization and hepatic resection in patients with hepatocellular carcinoma. Korean J Hepatol. 2010;16(4):383–8.
17. Poyanli A, Rozanes I, Acunas B, Sencer S. Palliative treatment of hepatocellular carcinoma by chemoembolization. Acta Radiol. 2001;42(6): 602–7.
18. Douhara A, Namisaki T, Moriya K, Kitade M, Kaji K, Kawaratani H, et al. Predisposing factors for hepatocellular carcinoma recurrence following initial remission after transcatheter arterial chemoembolization. Oncol Lett. 2017;14(3):3028–34.
19. Poon RT, Tso WK, Pang RW, Ng KK, Woo R, Tai KS, et al. A phase I/II trial of chemoembolization for hepatocellular carcinoma using a novel intra-arterial drug-eluting bead. Clin Gastroenterol Hepatol. 2007;5(9):1100–8.
20. Nicolini A, Martinetti L, Crespi S, Maggioni M, Sangiovanni A. Transarterial chemoembolization with epirubicin-eluting beads versus transarterial embolization before liver transplantation for hepatocellular carcinoma. J Vasc Interv Radiol. 2010;21(3):327–32.

21. Martin R, Geller D, Espat J, Kooby D, Sellars M, Goldstein R, et al. Safety and efficacy of trans arterial chemoembolization with drug-eluting beads in hepatocellular cancer: a systematic review. Hepato-Gastroenterology. 2012; 59(113):255–60.
22. Zou JH, Zhang L, Ren ZG, Ye SL. Efficacy and safety of cTACE versus DEB-TACE in patients with hepatocellular carcinoma: a meta-analysis. J Dig Dis. 2016;17(8):510–7.
23. Huang K, Zhou Q, Wang R, Cheng D, Ma Y. Doxorubicin-eluting beads versus conventional transarterial chemoembolization for the treatment of hepatocellular carcinoma. J Gastroenterol Hepatol. 2014;29(5):920–5.
24. Zhou X, Tang Z, Wang J, Lin P, Chen Z, Lv L, et al. Doxorubicin-eluting beads versus conventional transarterialchemoembolization for the treatment of hepatocellular carcinoma: a meta-analysis. Int J Clin Exp Med. 2014;7(11):3892–903.
25. Facciorusso A, Di Maso M, Muscatiello N. Drug-eluting beads versus conventional chemoembolization for the treatment of unresectable hepatocellular carcinoma: a meta-analysis. Dig Liver Dis. 2016;48(6):571–7.
26. Lee YK, Jung KS, Kim DY, Choi JY, Kim BK, Kim SU, et al. Conventional versus drug-eluting beads chemoembolization for hepatocellular carcinoma: emphasis on the impact of tumor size. J Gastroenterol Hepatol. 2017;32(2): 487–96.
27. Baur J, Ritter CO, Germer CT, Klein I, Kickuth R, Steger U. Transarterial chemoembolization with drug-eluting beads versus conventional transarterial chemoembolization in locally advanced hepatocellular carcinoma. Hepat Med. 2016;8:69–74.
28. Arabi M, BenMousa A, Bzeizi K, Garad F, Ahmed I, Al-Otaibi M. Doxorubicin-loaded drug-eluting beads versus conventional transarterial chemoembolization for nonresectable hepatocellular carcinoma. Saudi J Gastroenterol. 2015;21(3):175–80.
29. Liu YS, Ou MC, Tsai YS, Lin XZ, Wang CK, Tsai HM, et al. Transarterial chemoembolization using gelatin sponges or microspheres plus lipiodol-doxorubicin versus doxorubicin-loaded beads for the treatment of hepatocellular carcinoma. Korean J Radiol. 2015;16(1):125–32.
30. Covey AM, Brody LA, Maluccio MA, Getrajdman GI, Brown KT. Variant hepatic arterial anatomy revisited: digital subtraction angiography performed in 600 patients. Radiology. 2002;224(2):542–7.
31. Idee JM, Guiu B. Use of Lipiodol as a drug-delivery system for transcatheter arterial chemoembolization of hepatocellular carcinoma: a review. Crit Rev Oncol Hematol. 2013;88(3):530–49.
32. Song MJ, Park CH, Kim JD, Kim HY, Bae SH, Choi JY, et al. Drug-eluting bead loaded with doxorubicin versus conventional Lipiodol-based transarterial chemoembolization in the treatment of hepatocellular carcinoma: a case-control study of Asian patients. Eur J Gastroenterol Hepatol. 2011;23(6):521–7.
33. Lencioni R, Llovet JM. Modified RECIST (mRECIST) assessment for hepatocellular carcinoma. Semin Liver Dis. 2010;30(1):52–60.
34. Graf D, Vallbohmer D, Knoefel WT, Kropil P, Antoch G, Sagir A, et al. Multimodal treatment of hepatocellular carcinoma. Eur J Intern Med. 2014; 25(5):430–7.

9

Dexmedetomidine is safe and reduces the additional dose of midazolam for sedation during endoscopic retrograde cholangiopancreatography in very elderly patients

Osamu Inatomi[1]*(iD), Takayuki Imai[1], Takehide Fujimoto[1], Kenichiro Takahashi[1], Yoshihiro Yokota[1], Noriaki Yamashita[1], Hiroshi Hasegawa[1], Atsushi Nishida[1], Shigeki Bamba[2], Mitsushige Sugimoto[3] and Akira Andoh[1]

Abstract

Background: Endoscopic retrograde cholangiopancreatography (ERCP) often requires deep sedation. Dexmedetomidine, a highly selective α2-adrenoceptor agonist with sedative activity and minimal effects on respiration, has recently been widely used among patients in the intensive care unit. However, its use in endoscopic procedures in very elderly patients is unclear. In this study, we retrospectively investigated the safety and efficacy of dexmedetomidine sedation during ERCP.

Methods: The study included 62 very elderly patients (aged over 80 years) who underwent ERCP from January 2014, with sedation involving dexmedetomidine (i.v. infusion at 3.0 μg/kg/h over 10 min followed by continuous infusion at 0.4 μg/kg/h) along with midazolam. For comparison, the study included 78 patients who underwent ERCP before January 2014, with midazolam alone. We considered additional administration of midazolam as needed to maintain a sedation level of 3–4, according to the Ramsay sedation scale. The outcome measures were amount of midazolam, adverse events associated with sedation, and hemodynamics.

Results: The incidence of decreased SpO_2 and median dose of additional midazolam were significantly lower in the dexmedetomidine group than in the conventional group. The minimum systolic blood pressure and minimum heart rate during and after examination was significantly lower in the dexmedetomidine group than in the conventional group. However, serious acute heart failure or arrhythmia was not noted.

Conclusions: Dexmedetomidine can decrease the incidence of respiratory complications and the total dose of other sedative agents. It can be used as an alternative to conventional methods with midazolam for adequate sedation during ERCP in very elderly patients.

Keywords: Midazolam, Dexmedetomidine, Cholangiopancreatography, Endoscopic

* Correspondence: osam@belle.shiga-med.ac.jp
[1]Division of Gastroenterology, Department of Medicine, Shiga University of Medical Science, Seta Tsukinowa-cho, Otsu, Shiga 520-2192, Japan
Full list of author information is available at the end of the article

Background

Sedation in gastrointestinal endoscopy helps to not only alleviate the discomfort experienced by patients but also to improve the performance of the operator [1–3]. However, sedation can cause serious complications, such as respiratory depression and heart failure. Therefore, it is necessary to consider the safety (frequency of complications) as well as the sedative effects when selecting sedatives. In particular, very elderly patients undergoing endoscopic procedures are generally prone to sedation complications [4, 5].

Currently, benzodiazepines, such as midazolam and propofol, are widely used in endoscopic treatment, and they show an increased dose-dependent frequency of respiratory depression [6–9]. Endoscopic retrograde cholangiopancreatography (ERCP) is more invasive than other endoscopic procedures, and it often requires a comparatively deep sedation [10, 11]. It is known that the combined use of sedatives having different mechanisms of action results in synergistic sedative effects [12, 13]. Thus, the dose of each drug can be decreased, and it is possible to prevent the onset of negative incidents.

Dexmedetomidine (DEX) has low analgesic and sedative effects with low respiratory depression, and its usefulness for sedation in intensive care and local anesthesia treatment has been reported in recent years [14–16]. As it is associated with low respiratory suppression, its usefulness has been reported for sedation in endoscopic treatment [17–19]; however, its effectiveness and safety are unclear in very elderly patients undergoing ERCP. In this study, we retrospectively analyzed the influence of the combined use of DEX and midazolam for sedation during ERCP in very elderly patients.

Methods

Patients

Between January 2014 and June 2016, 62 consecutive patients aged over 80 years received DEX for sedation during ERCP at our hospital, and they were included in the DEX group. Between April 2012 and December 2013, 78 consecutive patients received midazolam alone, and they were included in the conventional group. The patients that the baseline percutaneous arterial blood oxygen saturation (SpO_2) was less than 90, the systolic blood pressure was 60 mmHg or less, or the heart rate was 40 beats/min or less were excluded from analysis. All patients provided informed written consent prior to undergoing ERCP. The study was conducted in agreement with the Declaration of Helsinki and received approval from the ethics committee of Shiga University of Medical Sciences and conformed to its guidelines.

Sedation procedure

Endoscopic examination was performed by three expert gastrointestinal endoscopists. In all patients, the sedative was administered by a sedative physician (non-anesthesiologist) who was familiar with the use of sedatives. The JF-260 V system (Olympus Medical Systems, Tokyo, Japan) was used. Oxygen (2 L/min) was administered at the start of the examination. During the examination, blood pressure, heart rate, and SpO_2 were continuously monitored, and an electrocardiogram was continuously obtained.

In the DEX group, the initial dose of DEX (Presedex, Pfizer, Tokyo, Japan) was set at 3 µg/kg/h, and after loading for 10 min, the dose was reduced to 0.4 µg/kg/h with the range described in previous reports [18, 20].Continuous infusion was carried out with the maintenance dose until the end of the examination. Additionally, 2.5 mg of midazolam (Astellas Pharma, Tokyo, Japan) was intravenously injected at the start of the examination. A single intravenous injection of 2 mg of midazolam was repeated to maintain the sedation level at 3–4, according to the Ramsay sedation scale (RSS) [21].

In the conventional group, 2.5 mg of midazolam was intravenously injected at the start of the examination. A single intravenous injection of 2 mg of midazolam was repeated to maintain the sedation level at 4 according to the RSS, as in the DEX group (Fig. 1).

In both groups, catecholamine was administered when the systolic blood pressure was 60 mmHg or less, and atropine was administered when the heart rate was 40 beats/min or less for more than 10 s.

Endpoints and evaluation

The main endpoint of effectiveness was the amount of midazolam. The secondary endpoint was the frequency of respiratory depression associated with sedation, the frequency of occurrence of acute heart failure and brady-arrhythmia, and time-dependent changes in blood pressure and heart rate and the frequency of administration of catecholamine and atropine. Blood pressure and heart rate were continuously measured from the start of sedation until the end of the examination, and the pre-examination values (at the time of entering the examination room), the lowest values during examination (minimum blood pressure/minimum heart rate), and the post-examination values (10 min after examination) were evaluated. Respiratory depression was defined as $SpO_2 < 90$ during the examination. Procedure time was defined as the time from endoscope insertion to end of the examination.

Statistical analysis

Measurement results are shown as median and quartile range for variables with non-normal distribution (amount

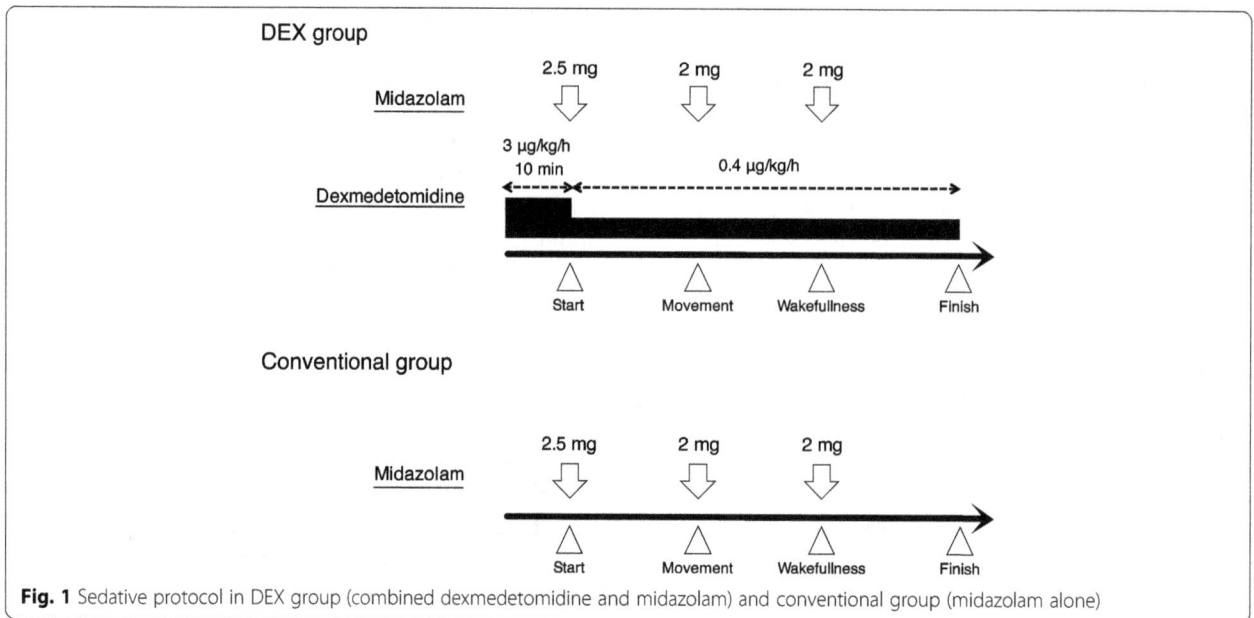

Fig. 1 Sedative protocol in DEX group (combined dexmedetomidine and midazolam) and conventional group (midazolam alone)

of drug used) and mean ± standard deviation for variables with normal distribution (blood pressure, heart rate, and oxygen dose). Drug use was analyzed using the Mann–Whitney U test; background factors and complication frequency were analyzed using the chi-square test, and circulatory dynamics over time were analyzed using repeated measures analysis of variance (ANOVA). A P-value < 0.05 was considered to indicate a significant difference.

Results

Patient background

There was no significant difference between the DEX group and conventional group with regard to age, sex, body mass index (BMI), medical history, NYHA classification, reason for examination, content of enforcement treatment, and mean examination time (Table 1).

Comparison of total dose of midazolam

The median dose of midazolam was significantly lower in the DEX group (10.0 mg) than in the conventional group (18.0 mg) ($p < 0.001$) (Fig. 2).

The frequency of respiratory depression

The frequency of respiratory depression was significantly lower in the DEX group (0%) than in the conventional group (6.9%) ($p = 0.04$). In the two patients of the conventional group we could not continue the examination due to respiratory insufficiency.

Sedation-related complications

Issues related to circulatory dynamics, including heart failure, sick sinus syndrome, and advanced atrioventricular block, were not observed in both groups. Atropine

Table 1 Patient background

	DEX group ($n = 62$)	Conventional group ($n = 87$)	P-value
Age	85.2 (81–94)	85.4 (80–99)	0.30
Sex (M/F)	39/23	30/57	0.13
BMI (kg/m^2)	21.1	19.7	0.08
Comorbidity			
Ischemic heart disease	15	23	0.85
Chronic heart failure	28	34	0.50
Arrhythmia	22	23	0.28
NYHA classification			
No cardiovascular disease	34	53	0.50
Class I	25	32	0.73
≥ Class II	3	2	0.65
Diagnosis			
Biliary stone	40	44	0.10
Biliary cancer	20	38	0.18
Others	2	5	1.0
Procedure			
EST	21	23	0.37
EPBD	12	8	0.43
ENBD	10	14	1.0
Biliary stent	24	42	0.31
Procedure time (min, mean ± SD)	45.0 ± 30.1	48.5 ± 31.2	0.94

EST endoscopic sphincterotomy, *EPBD* endoscopic papillary balloon dilatation, *ENBD* endoscopic nasobiliary drainage

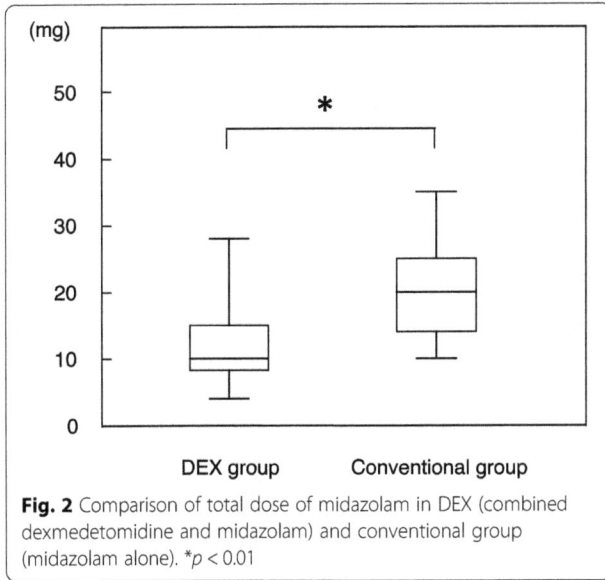

Fig. 2 Comparison of total dose of midazolam in DEX (combined dexmedetomidine and midazolam) and conventional group (midazolam alone). *$p < 0.01$

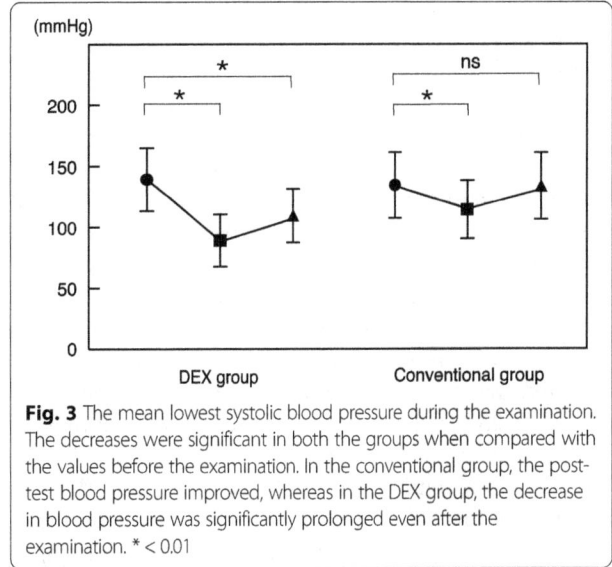

Fig. 3 The mean lowest systolic blood pressure during the examination. The decreases were significant in both the groups when compared with the values before the examination. In the conventional group, the post-test blood pressure improved, whereas in the DEX group, the decrease in blood pressure was significantly prolonged even after the examination. * < 0.01

(0.5 mg, iv) was administered in 2 patients from the DEX group (3.2%) due to bradycardia, and in no patient from the conventional group ($p = 0.34$). Dopamine (3 µg/kg/min for 3 min) was administered because of hypotension in 1 patient from the DEX group (1.6%) and in no patient from the conventional group ($p = 0.17$) (Table 2). The three patients who had received atropine or catecholamine recovered promptly after discontinuing the administration of DEX and received all the procedure, and there was no serious respiratory or circulatory failure that would cause clinical problems during the recovery period.

Time-dependent changes in circulatory dynamics
The mean lowest systolic blood pressure during the examination was 89.1 mmHg in the DEX group and 114.3 mmHg in the conventional group, and the decreases were significant ($p < 0.001$) in both the groups when compared with the values before the examination. In the conventional group, the post-test blood pressure improved, whereas in the DEX group, the decrease in blood pressure was significantly prolonged even after the examination (Fig. 3).

In the DEX group, the mean lowest heart rate during the examination was 62.1 beats/min, and the value was significantly lower than that before the examination ($p < 0.001$).

In the conventional group, the mean heart rate was 75.4 beats/min, and the value was similar to that before the examination. In addition, in the DEX group, the decrease in heart rate was significantly prolonged even after the examination (mean 67.2 beats/min), whereas in the conventional group, the heart rate after the examination improved (mean 79.9 beats/min) (Fig. 4).

Discussion
In this study, the combined use of DEX was found to significantly reduce the amount of midazolam, resulting in a decrease in the frequency of respiratory suppression events in very elderly patients undergoing ERCP. Although DEX tended to lower the minimum blood pressure and heart rate during examination, complications related to serious circulatory dynamics did not occur.

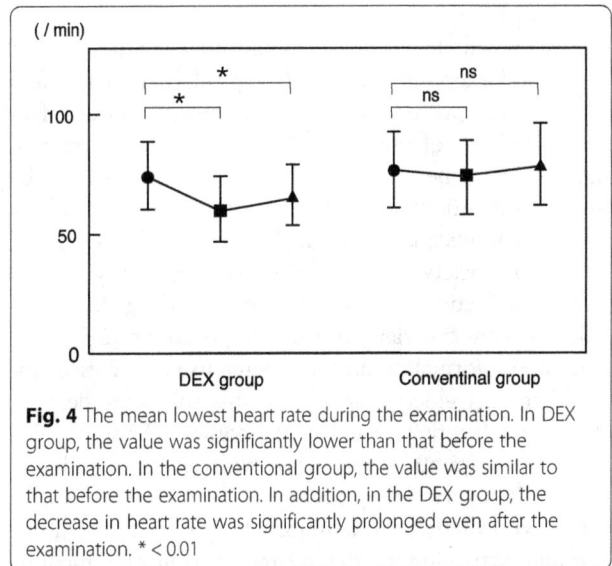

Fig. 4 The mean lowest heart rate during the examination. In DEX group, the value was significantly lower than that before the examination. In the conventional group, the value was similar to that before the examination. In addition, in the DEX group, the decrease in heart rate was significantly prolonged even after the examination. * < 0.01

Table 2 Sedation-related complications

	DEX group (n = 62)	Conventional group (n = 87)	P-value
Respiratory depression	0 (0%)	6 (6.9%)	0.04
Use atropine for bradycardia	2 (3.2%)	0 (0%)	0.34
Use vasopressor for hypotension	1 (1.6%)	0 (0%)	0.17

DEX acts on the locus ceruleus located in the pons, and it activates the α2-receptor present in noradrenaline neurons and induces sedation by suppressing upper neuron activity through negative feedback. In contrast to many other sedatives, it is characterized by limited affinity for gamma-aminobutyric acid (GABA) receptors, and therefore, there is almost no respiratory depression [21].

Although sedation by DEX has been reported for its usefulness in other endoscopic procedures, such as upper and lower endoscopy for screening purposes and endoscopic submucosal dissection (ESD), its effectiveness in ERCP is controversial. Muller et al. and Mazanikov et al. reported that it was not sufficiently effective when used alone [22, 23], while Lee et al. reported the effectiveness of the combined use of midazolam and pethidine hydrochloride in randomized trials [24]. The reason for this discrepancy is that ERCP is a more invasive procedure than other endoscopic procedures, and it is known that injection of contrast medium into the pancreatic duct and bile duct or mechanical expansion of the papilla, including endoscopic papillary balloon dilation, is painful, while mucosal resection in ESD is usually painless. DEX is considered to be somewhat weaker as a sedative than benzodiazepine and other sedative drugs [15], and a single use does not provide sufficient sedative effect for ERCP.

Conventional sedation agents, such as benzodiazepines and propofol, have been widely used for sedation in endoscopic procedures in recent years, and they have many advantages, such as good strength of the sedation effect; however, they are likely to cause side effects in a dose-dependent manner, especially the suppression of respiration [25]. Respiratory depression tends to occur in ERCP. In a prospective study using midazolam and pethidine hydrochloride, the frequency of deep sedation accompanied by respiratory depression was 86% in ERCP compared to only 26% in upper gastrointestinal endoscopy [11].

It is known that various complications tend to occur in the endoscopic treatment of very elderly patients, and it has been reported that one of the most important factors is the use of sedatives [4]. In very elderly patients, the actions of benzodiazepines and propofol tend to be excessive [5, 10, 26], and respiratory depression can be a critical complication. Although the guidelines of the American Society of Gastrointestinal Endoscopy recommend a reduction in the dose of sedative drugs in elderly patients from the viewpoint of complications [27], there is limited information on the specific use of sedatives for ERCP in very elderly patients. In this study, we demonstrated for the first time that the combined use of DEX with low respiratory depression was effective and safe for ERCP in very elderly patients.

It is known that DEX inhibits the sympathetic nerve through activation of the α2-receptor in the medulla

oblongata and affects circulatory dynamics [28, 29]. In this study, the minimum systolic blood pressure and heart rate during and after the examination decreased significantly with DEX when compared to that with conventional sedation. Although catecholamine and atropine were used in some patients, we judged it was clinically acceptable as blood pressure and heart rate recovered promptly after discontinuing the administration of DEX, and there was no serious circulatory problem such as acute heart failure or severe atrioventricular block failure during the recovery period in the all patients. However, comparative study with other sedative such as propofol may be needed for more safe sedation in circulation dynamics.

In addition, DEX may not be suitable for ERCP in the case of emergency as protocol with DEX include loading time for about 10 min before the start of ERCP procedure. Improvement of the protocol with shorter loading time might solve this problem.

The present study has some limitations. This was a retrospective study performed at a single center, and it did not involve blinding. However, information bias was minimal as we used DEX in consecutive cases and adjusted the dose by setting certain criteria for reducing/adding sedatives. A prospective, randomized study is needed to clarify the appropriate sedative protocol for ERCP in very elderly patients.

Conclusion
Dexmedetomidine can decrease the incidence of respiratory complications and the total dose of other sedative agents. Combined protocol using sedative agents with different pharmacokinetics may minimize the side effects of each. Dexmedetomidine can be used as an alternative to conventional methods with midazolam for adequate sedation during ERCP in very elderly patients.

Abbreviations
ANOVA: Analysis of variance; DEX: Dexmedetomidine; ERCP: Endoscopic retrograde cholangiopancreatography; ESD: Endoscopic submucosal dissection; GABA: Gamma-aminobutyric acid; RSS: Ramsay sedation scale; SpO$_2$: Percutaneous arterial blood oxygen saturation

Acknowledgements
There are no further sources of funding for the study, authors, or preparation of the manuscript.

Funding
All authors disclosed no financial relationships relevant to this study.

Authors' contributions
OI was involved in analyzing the results and writing the manuscript. TI, YY, and NY participated in the design of the study and performed the statistical analysis. TF, KT and HH helped procedure for ERCP. SB, MS and AA conceived of the study, and participated in its design and coordination and helped to draft the manuscript. All authors read and approved the final manuscript.

Consent for publication
Not applicable

Competing interests
The authors declare that they have no competing interests.

Author details
[1]Division of Gastroenterology, Department of Medicine, Shiga University of Medical Science, Seta Tsukinowa-cho, Otsu, Shiga 520-2192, Japan. [2]Division of Clinical Nutrition, Department of Medicine, Shiga University of Medical Science, Otsu, Japan. [3]Division of Digestive Endoscopy, Shiga University of Medical Science Hospital, Otsu, Japan.

References

1. Cohen LB, Wecsler JS, Gaetano JN, Benson AA, Miller KM, Durkalski V, et al. Endoscopic sedation in the United States: results from a nationwide survey. Am J Gastroenterol. 2006;101:967–74.
2. Cohen LB, Delegge MH, Aisenberg J, Brill JV, Inadomi JM, Kochman ML, et al. AGA Institute review of endoscopic sedation. Gastroenterology. 2007;133:675–701.
3. McQuaid KR, Laine L. A systematic review and meta-analysis of randomized, controlled trials of moderate sedation for routine endoscopic procedures. Gastrointest Endosc. 2008;67:910–23.
4. Travis AC, Pievsky D, Saltzman JR. Endoscopy in the elderly. Am J Gastroenterol. 2012;107:1495–501.
5. Clarke GA, Jacobson BC, Hammett RJ, Carr-Locke DL. The indications, utilization and safety of gastrointestinal endoscopy in an extremely elderly patient cohort. Endoscopy. 2001;33:580–4.
6. Ross WA. Premedication for upper gastrointestinal endoscopy. Gastrointest Endosc. 1989;35:120–6.
7. Freeman ML. Sedation and monitoring for gastrointestinal endoscopy. Gastrointest Endosc Clin N Am. 1994;4:475–99.
8. Faigel DO, Baron TH, Goldstein JL, Hirota WK, Jacobson BC, Johanson JF, et al. Guidelines for the use of deep sedation and anesthesia for GI endoscopy. Gastrointest Endosc. 2002;56:613–7.
9. Perel A. Non-anaesthesiologists should not be allowed to administer propofol for procedural sedation: a consensus statement of 21 European National Societies of Anaesthesia. Eur J Anaesthesiol. 2011;28:580–4.
10. Riphaus A, Stergiou N, Wehrmann T. Sedation with propofol for routine ERCP in high-risk octogenarians: a randomized, controlled study. Am J Gastroenterol. 2005;100:1957–63.
11. Patel S, Vargo JJ, Khandwala F, Lopez R, Trolli P, Dumot JA, et al. Deep sedation occurs frequently during elective endoscopy with meperidine and midazolam. Am J Gastroenterol. 2005;100:2689–95.
12. Salonen M, Onaivi ES, Maze M. Dexmedetomidine synergism with midazolam in the elevated plus-maze test in rats. Psychopharmacology. 1992;108:229–34.
13. Bergese SD, Patrick Bender S, McSweeney TD, Fernandez S, Dzwonczyk R, Sage K. A comparative study of dexmedetomidine with midazolam and midazolam alone for sedation during elective awake fiberoptic intubation. J Clin Anesth. 2010;22:35–40.
14. Bradley C. Dexmedetomidine--a novel sedative for postoperative sedation. Intensive Crit Care Nurs. 2000;16:328–9.
15. Hall JE, Uhrich TD, Barney JA, Arain SR, Ebert TJ. Sedative, amnestic, and analgesic properties of small-dose dexmedetomidine infusions. Anesth Analg. 2000;90:699–705.
16. Riker RR, Shehabi Y, Bokesch PM, Ceraso D, Wisemandle W, Koura F, et al. Dexmedetomidine vs midazolam for sedation of critically ill patients: a randomized trial. JAMA. 2009;301:489–99.
17. Demiraran Y, Korkut E, Tamer A, Yorulmaz I, Kocaman B, Sezen G, et al. The comparison of dexmedetomidine and midazolam used for sedation of patients during upper endoscopy: a prospective, randomized study. Can J Gastroenterol. 2007;21:25–9.
18. Takimoto K, Ueda T, Shimamoto F, Kojima Y, Fujinaga Y, Kashiwa A, et al. Sedation with dexmedetomidine hydrochloride during endoscopic submucosal dissection of gastric cancer. Dig Endosc. 2011;23:176–81.
19. Nishizawa T, Suzuki H, Sagara S, Kanai T, Yahagi N. Dexmedetomidine versus midazolam for gastrointestinal endoscopy: A meta-analysis. Dig Endosc. 2015;27:8–15.
20. Nonaka T, Inamori M, Miyashita T, Harada S, Inoh Y, Kanoshima K, et al. Feasibility of deep sedation with a combination of propofol and dexmedetomidine hydrochloride for esophageal endoscopic submucosal dissection. Dig Endosc. 2015;28:145–51.
21. Hayashi Y, Sumikawa K, Maze M, Yamatodani A, Kamibayashi T, Kuro M, et al. Dexmedetomidine prevents epinephrine-induced arrhythmias through stimulation of central α2 adrenoceptors in halothane-anesthetized dogs. Anesthesiology. 1991;75:113–7.
22. Muller S, Borowics SM, Fortis EAF, Stefani LC, Soares G, Maguilnik I, et al. Clinical efficacy of dexmedetomidine alone is less than propofol for conscious sedation during ERCP. Gastrointest Endosc. 2008;67:651–9.
23. Mazanikov M, Udd M, Kylänpää L, Mustonen H, Lindström O, Halttunen J, et al. Dexmedetomidine impairs success of patient-controlled sedation in alcoholics during ERCP: a randomized, double-blind, placebo-controlled study. Surg Endosc. 2013;27:2163–8.
24. Lee BS, Ryu J, Lee SH, Lee MG, Jang SE, Hwang J-H, et al. Midazolam with meperidine and dexmedetomidine vs. midazolam with meperidine for sedation during ERCP: prospective, randomized, double-blinded trial. Endoscopy. 2014;46:291–8.
25. Kim EH, Park JC, Shin SK, Lee YC, Lee SK. Effect of the midazolam added with propofol-based sedation in esophagogastroduodenoscopy: a randomized trial. J Gastroenterol Hepatol. 2018;33:894–9.
26. Salminen P, Grönroos JM. Anesthesiologist assistance in endoscopic retrograde cholangiopancreatography procedures in the elderly: is it worthwhile? J Laparoendosc Adv Surg Tech A. 2011;21:517–9.
27. Qureshi WA, Zuckerman MJ, Adler DG, Davila RE, Egan JV, Gan SI, et al. ASGE guideline: modifications in endoscopic practice for the elderly. Gastrointest Endosc. 2006;63:566–9.
28. Venn RM, Grounds RM. Comparison between dexmedetomidine and propofol for sedation in the intensive care unit: patient and clinician perceptions. Br J Anaesth. 2001;87:684–90.
29. Herr DL, Sum-Ping STJ, England M. ICU sedation after coronary artery bypass graft surgery: dexmedetomidine-based versus propofol-based sedation regimens. J Cardiothorac Vasc Anesth. 2003;17:576–84.

10

First clinical experience in 14 patients treated with ADVOS: a study on feasibility, safety and efficacy of a new type of albumin dialysis

Wolfgang Huber[1*†], Benedikt Henschel[2†], Roland Schmid[1] and Ahmed Al-Chalabi[3]

Abstract

Background: Liver failure (LF) is associated with prolonged hospital stay, increased cost and substantial mortality. Due to the limited number of donor organs, extracorporeal liver support is suggested as an appealing concept to "bridge to transplant" or to avoid transplant in case of recovery. ADVanced Organ Support (ADVOS) is a new type of albumin dialysis, that provides rapid regeneration of toxin-binding albumin by two purification circuits altering the binding capacities of albumin by biochemical (changing of pH) and physical (changing of temperature) modulation of the dialysate.

It was the aim of this study to evaluate feasibility, efficacy and safety of ADVOS in the first 14 patients ever treated with this procedure.

Methods: Patients included suffered from acute on chronic LF ($n = 9$) or "secondary" LF ($n = 5$) which resulted from non-hepatic diseases such as sepsis. The primary endpoint was the change of serum bilirubin, creatinine and serum BUN levels before and after the first treatment with ADVOS. The Wilcoxon Signed Rank test for paired samples was used to analyze the data.

Results: A total of 239 treatments (1 up to 101 per patient) were performed in 14 patients (6 female, 8 male). Mean age 54 ± 13; MELD-score 34 ± 7; CLIF-SOFA 15 ± 3. Serum bilirubin levels were significantly decreased by 32% during the first session (26.0 ± 15.4 vs. 17.7 ± 10.5 mg/dl; $p = 0.001$). Similarly, serum creatinine (2.2 ± 0.8 vs. 1.6 ± 0.7 mg/dl; $p = 0.005$) and serum BUN (49.4 ± 23.3 vs. 31.1 ± 19.7 mg/dl; $p = 0.003$), were significantly lowered by 27% and 37%, respectively. None of the treatment sessions had to be interrupted due to side effects related to the procedure.

Conclusion: ADVOS efficiently eliminates water- and protein-bound toxins in humans with LF. ADVOS is feasible in patients with advanced LF which is emphasized by a total number of more than 100 treatment sessions in one single patient.

Keywords: Chronic liver failure, Acute-on-chronic-liver failure, Acute liver failure, Extracorporeal liver support, Liver transplantation, Single pass albumin dialysis, Molecular Adsorbent Recirculating System, Fractionated plasma separation and adsorption, CLIF-SOFA, MELD

* Correspondence: Wolfgang.Huber@lrz.tum.de
†Equal contributors
[1]II. Medizinische Klinik und Poliklinik, Klinikum rechts der Isar, Technische Universität München, Ismaninger Straße 22, D-81675 Munich, Germany
Full list of author information is available at the end of the article

Background

Based on its course, liver failure (LF) is classified as acute (ALF), chronic (CLF) or acute-on-chronic (ACLF) [1–3]. In addition to the primary hepatic origin of LF, "secondary" LF may result from non-hepatic diseases such as sepsis [4]. All entities of LF are associated with prolonged hospital stay, increased costs and substantial mortality. LF of any origin frequently results in secondary organ dysfunction, most commonly leading to renal, circulatory and cerebral failure. Particularly in ACLF the number of organ failures is associated with poor short-term outcome approaching a 28-days- mortality of about 80% in ACLF if three or more organs fail [5]. In critically ill patients, "secondary" LF contributes more to mortality than any other organ failure, as demonstrated by a large prospective multi-centric cohort study [4]. Furthermore, any LF can progress to an irreversible state which requires liver transplantation (LTX). Because of the limited number of donor organs and contraindications to transplantation in a substantial number of patients, extracorporeal liver support (ELS) is considered an appealing concept to avoid transplant in case of reversible LF or as a "bridge to transplant". This is further emphasized by a strong pathophysiological rationale to remove toxic mediators which frequently result in secondary failure of other organs. Several concepts including single pass albumin dialysis SPAD [6, 7], Molecular Adsorbent Recirculating System (MARS;[7–16]), plasma exchange [17, 18], fractionated plasma separation and adsorption [19] and bio-artificial devices [20, 21] have been investigated. For most of these procedures, improvement in secondary endpoints has been demonstrated in pre-clinical trials and clinical case series [6, 22, 23]. However, benefits regarding mortality or other strong endpoints have not been proven in a randomized controlled trial. With regard to multiple confounders and modifiers of outcome in this particular group of patients, a large number of patients would be required for an appropriately powered randomized controlled trial (RCT) using the currently available devices. These large numbers of patients for such a RCT are unlikely to be achieved due to treatment costs and organizational expenses. Therefore, optimization of ELS to increase its effect size and safety as well as offering additional features for advanced multi-organ support to enhance applicability might help to validate the clinical usefulness of advanced ELS.

The ADVanced Organ Support (ADVOS) procedure is a newly introduced ELS (ADVOS multi, manufactured by Hepa Wash GmbH Munich, Germany), which potentially offers multi-organ support facilities. Rapid detoxification and continuous regeneration of toxin-binding albumin is provided by tertiary circuits, which alter the binding capacities of albumin by biochemical (changing of pH) and physical (change of temperature) modulation of the effluent dialysate (Fig. 1; see Materials and Methods). Feasibility and effective detoxification have been shown in an animal study [24]. However, so far there were no reports on ADVOS treatment in humans.

Therefore, it was the aim of our study to investigate the efficacy of the elimination of bilirubin, creatinine and BUN in the first 14 patients ever treated with the ADVOS procedure.

Methods

Patients

The initial concept to evaluate the ADVOS procedure comprised two separate randomized trials including patients with ACLF (HEPATICUS-1/Trial-Registration:

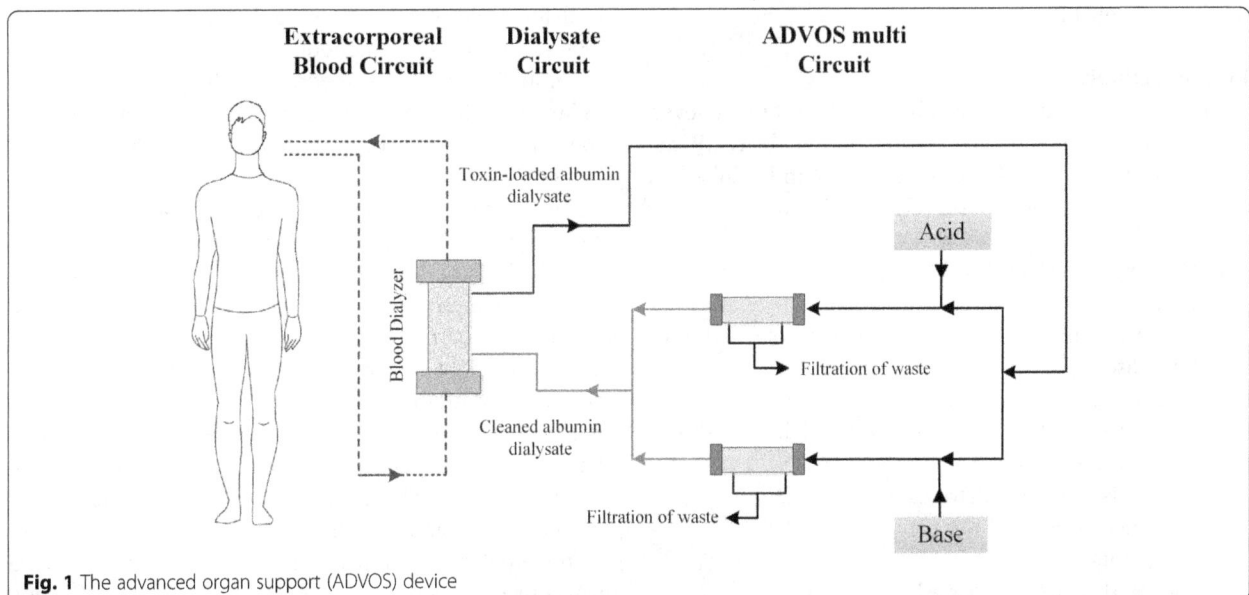

Fig. 1 The advanced organ support (ADVOS) device

NCT01079091) and with "secondary" LF due to sepsis, multi-organ failure or acute LF without cirrhosis (HEPATICUS-2/Trial-Registration: NCT01079104). A "run-in" phase with up to five patients per study was part of the concept. These patients were not randomized, but were treated according to the protocols for the treatment groups of HEPATICUS-1 and –2. This approach was approved by the local Ethics Committee ("Ethikkommission der Fakultät für Medizin der Technischen Universität München", reference number 2695/10; 2696/10). After the run-in phase, the studies HEPATICUS-1 and HEPATICUS-2 have not been continued due to lack of feasibility of the trial-concept. This decision was also based on the results of recently published randomized trials on MARS and fractionated plasma separation and adsorption. Consequently, the power calculation for HEPATICUS-1 and –2 was reanalyzed. Using a more "conservative" – i.e. pessimistic - estimation of the effect-size also including the experiences from HELIOS and RELIEF suggested that up to more than 700 patients might be needed for each trial.

The local Ethics Committee agreed on the evaluation of the seven patients treated in the run-in-phase of these studies and of another seven patients who were treated after the ADVOS procedure had received the CE-certificate in July 2013 (Ethikkommission der Fakultät für Medizin der Technischen Universität München", reference number 18/15). The need for informed consent was waived for the patients after CE certification due to the retrospective design of the study regarding those seven patients. Informed consent was obtained from the seven patients included in the HEPATICUS-trials or their legal representatives.

The study was conducted in an eight-bed general intensive care unit of a German university hospital. Patients for the HEPATICUS-trials were included between October 2012 and August 2012.

Inclusion criteria

Three patients of the run-in phase and six out of seven patients included after CE-certification had ACLF according to the CANONIC criteria [3, 25] and fulfilled all mandatory criteria of the HEPATICUS-1 trial:

1. Documented clinical or histological evidence of cirrhosis AND
2. Acute decompensation in previously stable cirrhotic liver disease AND
3. Bilirubin ≥2 mg/dl AND
4. SOFA score ≥9 [26] calculated after 12 h of optimal medical therapy AND
5. Patient is in the intensive care unit AND
6. Informed consent of the patient or the legal representative AND
7. Age of 18 years or older AND

8. Enrollment of patients within 96 h of fulfilling inclusion criteria 1–5

The inclusion criteria 6 and 8 were not mandatory for the seven post-CE certification patients.

Five patients suffered from "secondary" liver failure defined as acute liver failure of non-hepatic (e.g. sepsis, shock) or hepatic (e.g. ASH) origin in patients without evidence of chronic liver impairment. These patients fulfilled all mandatory criteria of the HEPATICUS-2-trial:

1. Patient is in the intensive care unit AND
2. Bilirubin ≥2 mg/dl AND
3. SOFA score ≥9 calculated 12 h after initial resuscitation measures AND
4. Signed informed consent of the patient or the legal representative AND
5. Age of 18 years or older AND
6. Enrollment of patients within 96 h of fulfilling inclusion criteria [1–5].

Criteria 4 and 6 were not mandatory for the post-CE certification patients

For exclusion criteria see Table 1

The ADVOS procedure

The ADVOS multi device designed for extracorporeal liver and kidney support was used for all treatments. The device is composed of three circuits: A *blood circuit* to perfuse a commercially available dialyzer (FX 80; Fresenius Medical Care; D-61352 Bad Homburg; Germany) was established using a conventional double-lumen dialysis catheter (Gambro Gam Cath Dolphin; Gambro Hospal GmbH, Gröbenzell, Germany). Catheters with a length of 250 mm and a diameter of 13 F were used for femoral access and catheters with a length of 150–175 mm and a diameter of 13 F were used for internal jugular access, respectively. The primary and secondary circuits were established using a commercially available CRRT device (CF 200, Infomed SA, Geneva, Switzerland).

The *second circuit* was perfused by the albumin dialysate running on the dialysate side of the dialyzer *in parallel* with the blood flow. According to the information of the manufacturer several ex-vivo experiments had shown that for the elimination of *protein*-bound toxins concurrent flow is not inferior to countercurrent flow. The recycled albumin containing dialysate has a volume of approximately 2 liters. The composition of albumin dialysate was similar to a conventional hemodialysis dialysate with the only exception of addition of human albumin with an end-concentration of 2–4%.

The *third circuit* represents the proprietary ADVOS procedure and aims at regeneration and detoxification

Table 1 Exclusion criteria of HEPATICUS-1 and of HEPATICUS-2 trial

Exclusion criteria for both HEPATICUS-1 and HEPATICUS-2	
Patients, whose mortality approaches 100%, or who are not likely to benefit from treatment (intervention with ADVOS is likely to be futile)	
Patients, whose current medical condition does not allow treatment with any extracorporeal procedure	
Potential conflict with good clinical practice (GCP) or with the declaration of Helsinki	
$P_aO_2/F_iO_2 \leq 100$ mmHg (respiratory SOFA score of 4)	
Patient testament excludes the use of life-prolonging measures	
Post-operative patients whose liver failure is related to liver surgery	
Participation in another clinical study	
Patients diagnosed with Creutzfeldt-Jakob disease	
Pregnancy	
Weight ≥ 120 kg	
Uncontrolled seizures	
Mean arterial pressure ≤ 50 mmHg despite conventional medical treatment	
Active or uncontrolled bleeding	
Untreatable extrahepatic cholestasis	
Patients with MELD-score of 40	
Exclusion criteria specific for HEPATICUS-1	Exclusion criteria specific for HEPATICUS-2
Patients with creatinine >5 mg/dl or urine output <200 ml/day (renal SOFA-score of 4)	Patient with known history of chronic liver disease
Patients who receive a vasopressor support of Dopamine >15 µg/kg/min or epinephrine >0.1 µg/kg/min or norepinephrine >0.1 µg/kg/min (cardiovascular SOFA-score of 4)	

of toxin-loaded albumin. In this ADVOS circuit, the toxin-loaded albumin effluent from the dialyzer is branched into two parts. Each part undergoes a change of pH by adding acid or base before passing through the dialyzers resulting in a release of albumin-bound toxins in the dialysate. The unbound toxins are removed by a tertiary filtration process. Finally, the acidified and the alkalinized albumin dialysates converge so that an albumin dialysate with physiological pH (range 6.9–7.6) is generated again. In addition to biochemical modulation of the binding capacities of albumin, the ADVOS procedure also provides physical altering of albumin binding by heating and cooling of the dialysate. The primary temperature modulation can be performed by cooling of the dialysate to 28°. To keep this modulation "regional" the re-transfused blood is re-warmed to the pre-treatment body-temperature. Irrespective of our study – in which no systemic modulations of blood temperature were performed – this feature also allows for modulation of the body temperature (heating or cooling of the patient), if this is considered useful within the multi-organ support facilities of the ADVOS device.

Finally, the de-toxified dialysate containing unloaded albumin re-circles to the affluent connector of the dialysate compartment of the dialyzers.

Anticoagulation

Anticoagulation was performed as required for conventional dialysis and modified for the patients' individual coagulation state at the discretion of the treating physician.

Pre- and post-dilution

No pre- or post-dilution was used during any treatment session.

Length of treatment session

For ethical reasons and to optimize the individual therapeutic effect, there was no strictly pre-defined treatment period. Regarding the available experience with other devices for liver support the protocol aimed at treatment periods of 6–12 h which were achieved in the majority of first treatment sessions (see Table 3). Taking into consideration the disease severity of most of the patients, the treatment periods were modified according to other diagnostic or therapeutic requirements and according to the individual condition of the patient.

During ADVOS therapy no additional renal replacement therapy (serial or in parallel) was performed.

Endpoints

With regard to efficacy and "proof of concept", a comparison of pre- and post-treatment values of bilirubin, creatinine and blood urea nitrogen (BUN) was chosen as the primary endpoint. These blood analyses were performed immediately before connection and after disconnection to the ADVOS procedure. Due to the markedly different number of treatment sessions (1–101), analyses regarding the primary endpoint was restricted to the first treatment session in each patient.

Statistics

The Wilcoxon-Test for paired samples was used to detect significant treatment effects. Spearman correlation was calculated to analyze the association of absolute and relative decreases in bilirubin, creatinine and BUN. P-values <0.05 were considered as statistically significant. All statistical tests were performed using IBM SPSS Statistics 23 (SPSS Inc., Chicago, IL, USA).

Results
Patients' characteristics

The patients' characteristics are shown in Table 2.

All patients were critically ill with a high predicted mortality according to different scores of HF and general prognostic scores for critically ill patients: All but one patient with ACLF had the highest score of the CANONIC-ACLF staging (stage C) [3]. The MELD-score [27] in these patients was 34 ± 7 points. The mean CLIF-SOFA [3] was 15 ± 3 points. Only two patients were listed for liver transplant. None of the patients underwent liver transplantation due to unavailable organ or acute contraindications for transplantations.

The most frequent precipitating event of ACLF was acute alcoholic hepatitis in four of nine cases. Two more cases of ACLF were related to infectious complications. Another two patients without ACLF suffered from first episodes of alcoholic steatohepatitis without evidence of cirrhosis which precludes listing for liver transplantation for six months according to German allocation laws. The other three cases of secondary LF were induced by sepsis. Among those patients were two patients with malignancies.

All 14 patients suffered from acute renal failure according to the AKIN criteria. Seven of 14 patients had undergone renal replacement therapy before the first ADVOS treatment.

Primary endpoint: treatment efficacy

The 14 first treatment sessions were performed for a mean of 575 ± 193 min without interruption or need for disconnection due to technical reasons or adverse events related to the procedure. The serum levels of both protein-bound and water-soluble toxins were significantly decreased during treatment with the ADVOS procedure: Se5rum bilirubin levels were significantly decreased by 32% after a single ADVOS procedure (17.7 ± 10.5 mg/dl vs. 26.0 mg/dl ± 15.4 mg/dl; $p = 0.001$). Similarly, serum creatinine (1.6 ± 0.7 mg/dl vs. 2.2 ± 0.8 mg/dl; $p = 0.005$) and BUN (31.1 ± 20.29 mg/dl vs. 49.4 ± 23.3 mg/dl; $p = 0.003$) were significantly lowered by a mean of 27% and 37% by a single ADVOS treatment, respectively (Table 3; Figs. 2, 3 and 4).

Treatment efficacy at different starting values

There was a significant correlation between the baseline serum levels of bilirubin, creatinine and BUN with their absolute reduction induced by the first ADVOS treatment ($r = 0.911$, $p < 0.001$; $r = 0.756$, $p = 0.002$; $r = 0.644$, $p = 0.013$), respectively (see also Table 3). By contrast, the relative changes in serum bilirubin, creatinine and BUN were not associated to their baseline levels ($r = 0.383$ $p = 0.177$; $r = 0.236$ $p = 0.417$; $r = 0.247$ $p = 0.395$).

Safety and outcome

In summary, the ADVOS treatment was hemodynamically well tolerated during a mean of 9.7 ± 3.5 h of therapy. Overall, 239 treatments were carried out (17 ± 26; 1–101 treatments per patient). None of the treatment sessions had to be interrupted due to complications that were likely related to the ADVOS procedure. The 28-days survival rate was 5/15 (36%). Finally, two patients (14%) were discharged home.

Discussion

At present, there are three procedures of extracorporeal liver support based on albumin-dialysis used in clinical practice. Albumin-dialysis aims at the elimination of albumin-bound endogenous toxins such as bile-acids that accumulate in case of LF via a semipermeable membrane. For this purpose, albumin has to be added to the dialysate in a final concentration between 2% and 20% [6, 7, 10, 11, 28]. In SPAD, dialysate flow rates range between 0.5 L/h and 2 L/h. SPAD is easily available, can be performed with standard renal replacement therapy (RRT) devices and has the advantage of "naïve" albumin in the dialysate which provides maximum detoxification capacities of the dialysate [6]. However, with repeated treatment sessions up to 24 h and a market price of commercially available 20% human albumin solutions up to 150€ per 100 mL, a total albumin cost of approximately 1500€ per session has been estimated [6]. Therefore, attempts have been made to recirculate albumin after regeneration (cleansing). MARS, the second type of albumin-dialysis, helps to save albumin resources. Its efficacy in elimination of albumin bound toxins has been demonstrated in several case-series and studies

Table 2 Patients' baseline characteristics

Patient	Study	Type of Liver failure (LF)	Aetiology	Precipitating event	Age [years]	Gender	CANONIC [ACLF-grade]	Child-Pugh [points]	MELD [points]	CLIF-SOFA [points]	Acute renal failure
P1	Post-CE	acute-on-chronic LF	alcoholic	SBP	59	female	3	12 (C)	40	12	+
P2	Post-CE	acute-on-chronic LF	alcoholic	ASH	52	female	2	12 (C)	26	14	+
P3	Post-CE	acute-on-chronic LF	alcoholic	ASH	53	male	3	13 (C)	37	15	+
P4	Post-CE	acute-on-chronic LF	alcoholic	Infection	61	male	3	11 (C)	35	15	+
P5	Post-CE	acute-on-chronic LF	alcoholic	Ischemia	68	female	3	12 (C)	24	18	+
P6	Post-CE	acute-on-chronic LF	alcoholic	ASH, sepsis	48	female	3	12 (C)	44	13	+
P7	HEPATICUS-1	acute-on-chronic LF	alcoholic	GI-bleeding	54	male	3	14 (C)	29	14	+
P8	HEPATICUS-1	acute-on-chronic LF	alcoholic	GI-bleeding	38	male	3	13 (C)	32	17	+
P9	HEPATICUS-1	acute-on-chronic LF	alcoholic	ASH	28	male	3	11 (C)	34	13	+
P10	HEPATICUS-2	"Secondary" LF	Sepsis	n.a.	66	female	n.a.	n.a.	19	18	+
P11	HEPATICUS-2	"Secondary" LF	ASH	n.a.	39	male	n.a.	n.a.	39	9	+
P12	HEPATICUS-2	"Secondary" LF	Drug-induced	n.a.	73	male	n.a.	n.a.	38	15	+
P13	HEPATICUS-2	"Secondary" LF	ASH	n.a.	56	female	n.a.	n.a.	35	14	+
P14	Post-CE	"Secondary" LF	Sepsis	n.a.	67	male	n.a.	n.a.	40	18	+
Mean ± SD or number [%]					54 ± 13	8 male; 6 female	2.9 ± 0.3	12 ± 1	34 ± 7	15 ± 3	100%

ASH alcoholic steatohepatitis, *SBP* spontaneous bacterial peritonitis, *MELD* model of end-stage liver disease
CLIF-SOFA chronic liver-failure sequential organ failure assessment, *CANONIC* CLIF acute-on-chronic liver failure in cirrhosis
n.a not applicable

Table 3 Treatment data and outcome

Patient	Treat-ment time [min] [19]	Serum bilirubin [mg/dl]				Serum creatinine [mg/dl]				Serum BUN [mg/dl]				No. of treatments	28d survival
		Day before ADVOS	Before start of ADVOS	After ADVOS	Delta [mg/dl]	Day before ADVOS	Before start of ADVOS	After ADVOS	Delta [mg/dl]	Day before ADVOS	Before start of ADVOS	After ADVOS	Delta [mg/dl]		
P1	745	37.4	41.1	25.4	-15.7	0.7	0.8	0.5	-0.3	59	76	28	-48	19	-
P2	800	22.8	24.0	12.8	-11.2	1.0	1.0	0.9	-0.1	26	25	14	-11	10	-
P3	730	20.8	22.3	14.1	-8.2	1.8	1.6	1.5	-0.1	21	20	18	-2	7	-
P4	770	16.3	15.9	13.2	-2.7	2.4	1.9	1.5	-0.4	27	20	18	-2	29	-
P5	800	n.d.	11.6	9.2	-2.4	n.d.	2.8	1.2	-1.6	n.d.	45	13	-32	3	-
P6	600	43.5	41.6	34.2	-7.4	3.9	3.3	2.2	-1.1	91	97	63	-34	22	+
P7	720	3.1	5.3	3.9	-1.4	1.7	3.0	2.1	-0.9	19	33	22	-11	17	+
P8	420	21.6	20.7	17.8	-2.9	1.3	2.0	2.8	+0.8	44	69	82	+13	9	-
P9	570	26.4	26.2	20.3	-5.9	1.9	2.3	1.7	-0.6	43	51	35	-16	6	+
P10	300	1.9	2.0	1.5	-0.5	1.7	1.3	0.7	-0.6	54	31	16	-15	1	-
P11	240	40.4	41.6	29.0	-12.6	3.0	3.2	2.0	-01.2	35	40	27	-13	101	+
P12	510	18.3	17.5	10.9	-6.6	1.4	2.9	2.1	-0.8	40	49	27	-22	3	-
P13	360	38.2	42.1	19.9	-22.2	3.0	2.3	1.2	-1.1	79	68	33	-35	11	+
P14	480	49.3	51.8	35.7	-16.1	3.0	3.0	2.2	-0.8	54	67	39	-28	1	-
Mean ± SD Number [%]	575± 193	26.2± 14.9	26.0± 15.4	17.7± 10.5	-8.3± 6.5	2.0± 0.9	2.2± 0.8	1.6± 0.7	-0.6± 0.6	46± 22	49± 23	31± 20	-18± 16	17± 26 [1-101]	5/14 [36%]

ADVOS advanced organ support

BUN blood urea nitrogen

n.d. not done

Delta absolute changes when comparing values immediately before and after the first ADVOS session

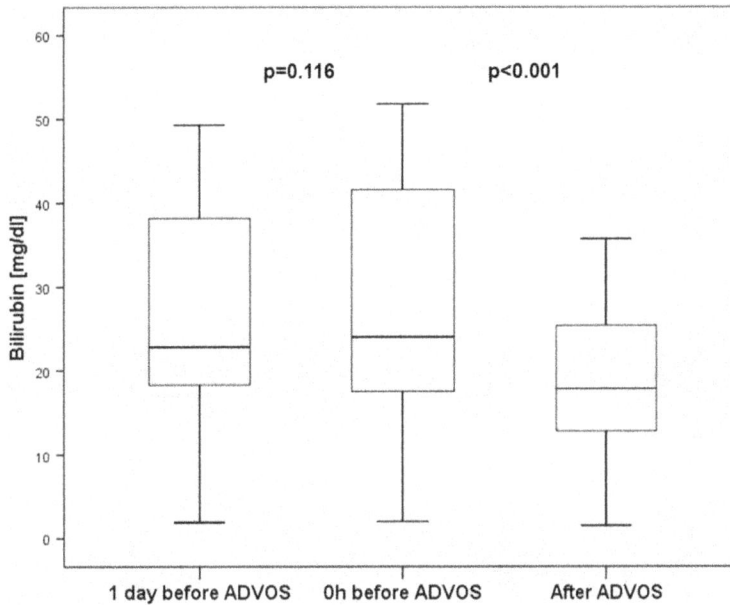

Fig. 2 Boxplots depicting the time course of serum bilirubin

[7, 10, 11, 28]. While MARS uses a charcoal column and an anion exchange resin column to unload albumin-bound toxins and to regenerate albumin, the recently introduced ADVOS procedure continuously unloads and regenerates albumin by intermittent alteration of its binding capacities [7, 10, 11, 24, 28]. This is achieved by biochemical (changing of pH) and physical (change of temperature) modulation of the effluent dialysate. In addition to its features as ELS, ADVOS – at least from a theoretical viewpoint - offers the advantage of multi-organ support by providing the potential to modulate the acid–base-balance and the body temperature of the patient. While MARS is usually performed with 600 mL of 20% albumin, this amount is further reduced in the ADVOS procedure to 200 mL [24].

Nevertheless, similar to MARS, regeneration of albumin carries the potential for its denaturation and loss of efficacy.

Our study in 14 patients primarily analyzed the efficacy of elimination of protein-bound and water-soluble

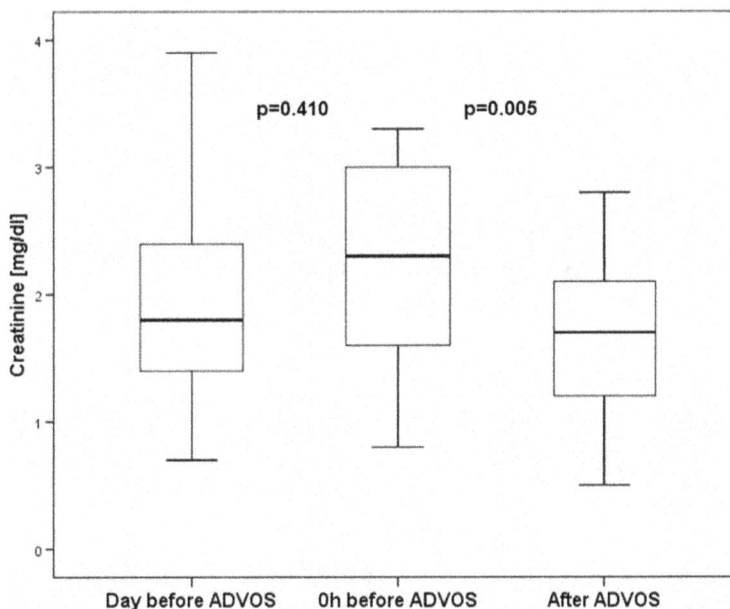

Fig. 3 Boxplots depicting the time course of serum creatinine

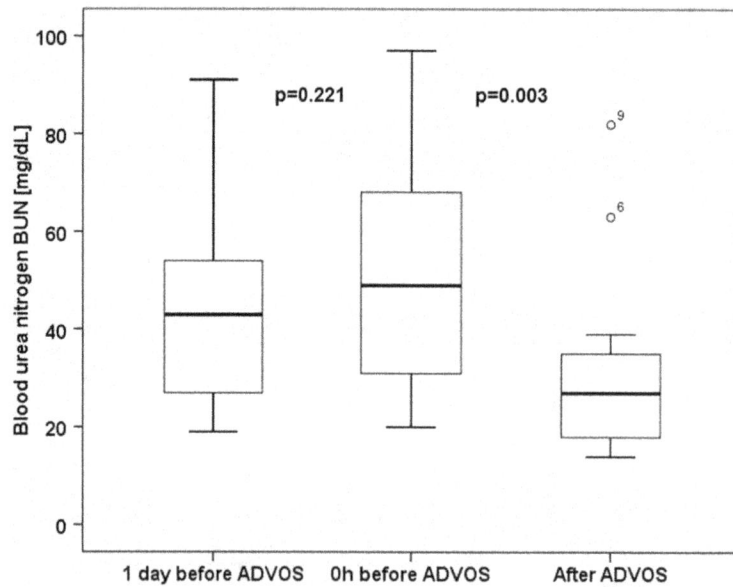

Fig. 4 Boxplots depicting the time course of serum BUN

toxins by the ADVOS procedure. As demonstrated in Table 2 and Table 4, ADVOS significantly reduced serum bilirubin, creatinine and BUN by 32%, 27% and 37%, respectively. Although cross-comparison with data from other recent studies with different inclusion criteria and populations has to be performed with caution, our data suggest at least comparable elimination capacities of ADVOS to those reported for MARS, fractionized plasma separation and adsorption (Prometheus) and SPAD in the most recent studies (Table 4). Furthermore,

Table 4 Comparison of patients' characteristics and elimination efficacy

Trial/Reference	Banares [10]	Kribben [19]	Sponholz MARS [7]	Sponholz SPAD [7]	Own study
Device	MARS	Prometheus	MARS	SPAD	ADVOS
Patients' characteristics					
Clinical setting	19 ICUs	10 ICUs	Surgical ICU		Medical ICU
Type of LF					
- ACLF	100%	100%	56%		64%
- ALF	-	-	28%		-
- "secondary" LF	-	-	-		36%
- Graft failure	-	-	16%		-
(CLIF)-SOFA	8 ± 3	10 ± 3	13 ± 4		15 ± 3
MELD	26 ± 8	28 ± 10			34 ± 7
Child-Pugh	11 ± 2	12 ± 1			12 ± 1
Efficacy analysis					
No. of treatments for efficacy analysis	4	8 (mean)	2.2 (mean)	2.2 (mean)	1
Delta-Bilirubin relative	−26% (day 4)	−23% (day 28)	−23%	−23%	−32%
Delta-Bilirubin absolute [mg/dL]	−8.7 (day 4)	−6 (day 28)	−4.3	−4.2	−8.3
Delta-creatinine relative	−20% (day 4)	−13% (day 28)	−18%	+5%	−27%
Delta-creatinine absolute [mg/dL]	−0.3 (day 4)	−0.2 (day 28)	−0.4	+0.1	−0.6
Delta-BUN relative	n.d.	n.d.	−9%	+5%	−37%
Delta-BUN absolute [mg/dL]	n.d	n.d.	−12	+8	−18
Maximum number of treatments	10	11	4	4	101

it has to be kept in mind that these elimination rates were achieved by a single ADVOS treatment compared to repeated (two up to eight) sessions performed in the reference studies with the other devices. Treatment periods between seven and ten hours were comparable for all methods.

Similarly, the interpretation of feasibility and safety data is limited due to the small number of patients treated and due to the lack of a direct control group. However, our conclusions are supported by the high number of total treatment sessions that was done reaching up to 101 sessions in one single patient.

Although we have to clearly admit that this study was not powered for mortality analysis and lacked a control group, the final outcome of the patients is worth mentioning. Due to the lack of direct controls, the outcome of our patients has to be compared to the data available from large scoring databases (e.g. CLIF-SOFA). These databases provide validated outcome estimates for patients comparable those in our study. At first glance, survival was poor with 28-days and in-hospital mortality rates of 65% and 86%, respectively. This might be related to several reasons: As supported by all scoring systems investigated, the patients were more severely ill compared to the randomized trials summarized in Table 4. All but one patient with ACLF had Grade 3 according to the CANONIC criteria, which has been associated in a recent study with 28-days- and 3-months-mortality rates of 83.6% and 87.3%, respectively [5]. For the mean CLIF-SOFA score of 15 points in our patients, the same study predicts a high 28-days-mortality approaching 90%. Furthermore, two of our patients suffered from malignancies, and in at least five patients active alcoholism was suggested by the presence of ASH. Ongoing alcoholism - precluding LTX according to German allocation rules – was also evident in three patients with ACLF. Two patients suffered from "secondary" (see above) liver failure due to severe sepsis and was classified as nontransplantable. This may explain why only two patients were listed for liver transplantation. None of these patients underwent LTX during the observation period. These individual medical histories emphasize that extracorporeal liver support was initiated in most of our patients as a rescue treatment, since LTX was not feasible.

Strengths and limitations of the study

This study demonstrated feasibility and efficacy of a new approach to ELS. To the best of our knowledge a total number of 101 treatment sessions in one single patient has not been reported for any other procedure of ELS. Elimination rates for surrogate markers were among the highest ever reported (Table 4) suggesting a high efficacy during the first treatment. The patients included are heterogenous regarding the aetiology of liver failure and

also regarding the number of treatment sessions. This heterogeneity could be considered as a methodological limitation. On the other hand, this heterogeneity might give first hints on potential indications and general applicability of the procedure in different groups of patients with severe liver failure. Furthermore, any reporting bias could be avoided, since we reported on all patients who have ever been treated with ADVOS in our ICU. Despite feasibility, safety and efficacy of the intervention, the overall outcome was poor, which might be related to the use of ADVOS as a rescue therapy in this study which predominantly included patients without the option to undergo LTX. Another limitation is the low number of patients included that precludes more robust conclusions regarding the outcome. Conclusions regarding the outcome are further limited by the lack of a randomized control group or matched controls. Finally, even in case of randomized controls the statistical power would be low due to the restricted number of comparisons.

Conclusion

ADVOS efficiently eliminates water- and protein-bound toxins in humans with LF. ADVOS is feasible in patients with advanced LF which is emphasized by a total number of more than 100 treatment sessions in one single patient.

Abbreviations
ACLF: Acute-on-chronic liver failure; ADVOS: Advanced organ support; BUN: Blood urea nitrogen; CANONIC: CLIF acute-on-chronic liver failure in cirrhosis; CLIF: Chronic liver failure; ELS: Extracorporeal liver support; FPSA: Fractionated plasma separation and adsorption; LF: Liver failure; LTX: Liver transplantation; MARS: Molecular adsorbents recirculating system; MELD: Model for end-stage liver disease; RRT: Renal replacement therapy; SPAD: Single pass albumin dialysis

Acknowledgements
We express our gratitude to the physicians and to the nursing staff of the intensive care unit 2/11 (II. Medizinische Klinik; Klinikum rechts der Isar; Technische Universität München) for their support to perform this study.

Funding
The trials HEPATICUS-1 and HEPATICUS-2 were financed by the Hepa Wash GmbH, Munich, Germany.

Authors' contributions
AA, WH and RS designed the study. WH and BH collected the data, performed statistical analysis and drafted the manuscript. AA also collected data and helped to draft the manuscript. RS also participated in analysis of the data and drafting the manuscript. All authors read and approved the final manuscript.

Competing interests
The authors declare that they have no competing interests.

Consent for publication
Not applicable.

Ethics approval and consent to participate
The initial concept to evaluate the ADVOS procedure comprised two separate randomized trials including patients with ACLF (HEPATICUS-1/Trial-Registration: NCT01079091) and with "secondary" LF due to sepsis, multi-organ failure or acute LF without cirrhosis (HEPATICUS-2/Trial-Registration: NCT01079104). A "run-in" phase with up to five patients per study was part of the concept. These patients were not randomized, but were treated according to the protocols for the treatment groups of HEPATICUS-1 and –2. This approach was approved by the local Ethics Committee ("Ethikkommission der Fakultät für Medizin der Technischen Universität München", reference number 2695/10; 2696/10). After the run-in phase, the studies HEPATICUS-1 and HEPATICUS-2 have not been continued due to lack of feasibility of the trial-concept.
The local Ethics Committee agreed on the evaluation of the seven patients treated in the run-in-phase of these studies and of another seven patients who were treated after the ADVOS procedure had received the CE-certificate in July 2013 (Ethikkommission der Fakultät für Medizin der Technischen Universität München", reference number 18/15). The need for informed consent was waived for the patients after CE certification due to the retrospective design of the study regarding those seven patients. Informed consent was obtained from the seven patients included in the HEPATICUS-trials or their legal representatives.

Author details
[1]II. Medizinische Klinik und Poliklinik, Klinikum rechts der Isar, Technische Universität München, Ismaninger Straße 22, D-81675 Munich, Germany. [2]Klinik für Anaesthesiologie der Universität München, Campus Großhadern, Marchioninistraße, 15 81377 Munich, Germany. [3]Jamaica Hospital Medical Center, 8900 Van Wyck Expy, Jamaica, NY 11418, USA.

References
1. Jalan R, Gines P, Olson JC, Mookerjee RP, Moreau R, Garcia-Tsao G, et al. Acute-on chronic liver failure. J Hepatol. 2012;57(6):1336–48. Epub 2012/07/04.
2. Moreau R, Arroyo V. Acute-on-chronic liver failure: a new clinical entity. Clin Gastroenterol Hepatol. 2015;13(5):836–41. Epub 2014/03/04.
3. Moreau R, Jalan R, Gines P, Pavesi M, Angeli P, Cordoba J, et al. Acute-on-chronic liver failure is a distinct syndrome that develops in patients with acute decompensation of cirrhosis. Gastroenterology. 2013;144(7):1426–37. 37 e1-9. Epub 2013/03/12.
4. Kramer L, Jordan B, Druml W, Bauer P, Metnitz PG. Incidence and prognosis of early hepatic dysfunction in critically ill patients–a prospective multicenter study. Crit Care Med. 2007;35(4):1099–104. Epub 2007/03/06.
5. Lee M, Lee JH, Oh S, Jang Y, Lee W, Lee HJ, et al. CLIF-SOFA scoring system accurately predicts short-term mortality in acutely decompensated patients with alcoholic cirrhosis: a retrospective analysis. Liver Int. 2015;35(1):46–57. Epub 2014/09/10.
6. Kreymann B, Seige M, Schweigart U, Kopp KF, Classen M. Albumin dialysis: effective removal of copper in a patient with fulminant Wilson disease and successful bridging to liver transplantation: a new possibility for the elimination of protein-bound toxins. J Hepatol. 1999;31(6):1080–5. Epub 1999/12/22.
7. Sponholz C, Matthes K, Rupp D, Backaus W, Klammt S, Karailieva D, et al. Molecular adsorbent recirculating system and single-pass albumin dialysis in liver failure - a prospective, randomised crossover study. Crit Care. 2016;20(1):2. Epub 2016/01/06.
8. Hassanein TI, Schade RR, Hepburn IS. Acute-on-chronic liver failure: extracorporeal liver assist devices. Curr Opin Crit Care. 2011;17(2):195–203. Epub 2011/02/25.
9. Laleman W, Wilmer A, Evenepoel P, Elst IV, Zeegers M, Zaman Z, et al. Effect of the molecular adsorbent recirculating system and Prometheus devices on systemic haemodynamics and vasoactive agents in patients with acute-on-chronic alcoholic liver failure. Crit Care. 2006;10(4):R108. Epub 2006/07/25.
10. Banares R, Nevens F, Larsen FS, Jalan R, Albillos A, Dollinger M, et al. Extracorporeal albumin dialysis with the molecular adsorbent recirculating system in acute-on-chronic liver failure: the RELIEF trial. Hepatology. 2013;57(3):1153–62. Epub 2012/12/06.
11. Heemann U, Treichel U, Loock J, Philipp T, Gerken G, Malago M, et al. Albumin dialysis in cirrhosis with superimposed acute liver injury: a prospective, controlled study. Hepatology. 2002;36(4 Pt 1):949–58. Epub 2002/09/26.
12. Kortgen A, Rauchfuss F, Gotz M, Settmacher U, Bauer M, Sponholz C. Albumin dialysis in liver failure: comparison of molecular adsorbent recirculating system and single pass albumin dialysis–a retrospective analysis. Ther Apher Dial. 2009;13(5):419–25. Epub 2009/10/01.
13. Sen S, Davies NA, Mookerjee RP, Cheshire LM, Hodges SJ, Williams R, et al. Pathophysiological effects of albumin dialysis in acute-on-chronic liver failure: a randomized controlled study. Liver Transpl. 2004;10(9):1109–19. Epub 2004/09/07.
14. Saliba F, Camus C, Durand F, Mathurin P, Letierce A, Delafosse B, et al. Albumin dialysis with a noncell artificial liver support device in patients with acute liver failure: a randomized, controlled trial. Ann Intern Med. 2013;159(8):522–31. Epub 2013/10/16.
15. Schmidt LE, Wang LP, Hansen BA, Larsen FS. Systemic hemodynamic effects of treatment with the molecular adsorbents recirculating system in patients with hyperacute liver failure: a prospective controlled trial. Liver Transpl. 2003;9(3):290–7. Epub 2003/03/06.
16. Hessel FP, Bramlage P, Wasem J, Mitzner SR. Cost-effectiveness of the artificial liver support system MARS in patients with acute-on-chronic liver failure. Eur J Gastroenterol Hepatol. 2010;22(2):213–20. Epub 2009/09/24.
17. Qin G, Shao JG, Wang B, Shen Y, Zheng J, Liu XJ, et al. Artificial liver support system improves short- and long-term outcomes of patients with HBV-associated acute-on-chronic liver failure: a single-center experience. Medicine. 2014;93(28):e338. Epub 2014/12/20.
18. Xu X, Liu X, Ling Q, Wei Q, Liu Z, Zhou L, et al. Artificial liver support system combined with liver transplantation in the treatment of patients with acute-on-chronic liver failure. PLoS One. 2013;8(3):e58738. Epub 2013/03/22.
19. Kribben A, Gerken G, Haag S, Herget-Rosenthal S, Treichel U, Betz C, et al. Effects of fractionated plasma separation and adsorption on survival in patients with acute-on-chronic liver failure. Gastroenterology. 2012;142(4):782–9. e3. Epub 2012/01/18.
20. Figaro S, Pereira U, Rada H, Semenzato N, Pouchoulin D, Legallais C. Development and validation of a bioartificial liver device with fluidized bed bioreactors hosting alginate-encapsulated hepatocyte spheroids. Conf Proc IEEE Eng Med Biol Soc. 2015;2015:1335–8. Epub 2016/01/07.
21. Nastos C, Kalimeris K, Papoutsidakis N, Defterevos G, Pafiti A, Kalogeropoulou E, et al. Bioartificial liver attenuates intestinal mucosa injury and gut barrier dysfunction after major hepatectomy: Study in a porcine model. Surgery. 2016. Epub 2016/02/06.
22. Hassanein TI, Tofteng F, Brown Jr RS, McGuire B, Lynch P, Mehta R, et al. Randomized controlled study of extracorporeal albumin dialysis for hepatic encephalopathy in advanced cirrhosis. Hepatology. 2007;46(6):1853–62. Epub 2007/11/03.
23. Seige M, Kreymann B, Jeschke B, Schweigart U, Kopp KF, Classen M. Long-term treatment of patients with acute exacerbation of chronic liver failure by albumin dialysis. Transplant Proc. 1999;31(1–2):1371–5. Epub 1999/03/20.
24. Al-Chalabi A, Matevossian E, AK VT, Luppa P, Neiss A, Schuster T, et al. Evaluation of the Hepa Wash(R) treatment in pigs with acute liver failure. BMC Gastroenterol. 2013;13:83. Epub 2013/05/15.
25. Arroyo V, Moreau R, Jalan R, Gines P. Acute-on-chronic liver failure: A new syndrome that will re-classify cirrhosis. J Hepatol. 2015;62(1 Suppl):S131–43. Epub 2015/04/29.
26. Vincent JL, Moreno R, Takala J, Willatts S, De Mendonca A, Bruining H, et al. The SOFA (Sepsis-related Organ Failure Assessment) score to describe organ dysfunction/failure. On behalf of the Working Group on Sepsis-Related Problems of the European Society of Intensive Care Medicine. Intensive Care Med. 1996;22(7):707–10. Epub 1996/07/01.
27. Wiesner RH, McDiarmid SV, Kamath PS, Edwards EB, Malinchoc M, Kremers WK, et al. MELD and PELD: application of survival models to liver allocation. Liver Transpl. 2001;7(7):567–80. Epub 2001/07/19.
28. Mitzner SR. Extracorporeal liver support-albumin dialysis with the Molecular Adsorbent Recirculating System (MARS). Ann Hepatol. 2011;10 Suppl 1:S21–8. Epub 2011/05/20.

11

Health-related quality of Life in patients with chronic hepatitis C receiving Sofosbuvir-based treatment, with and without Interferon

Naglaa F. A. Youssef[1], Mohamed El Kassas[2], Amany Farag[1] and Ashley Shepherd[3*] (iD)

Abstract

Background: The Egyptian government introduced the first directly acting antivirals (DAAs) into Egypt through the government funded National Treatment Program. As yet, there has been no investigation into the effects of these new DAAs therapies on patient reported outcomes (PROs). This study aimed to (1) assess the PROs (health-related quality of life (HRQoL), mental health and perceived social support) of HCV patients receiving DAAs therapy prior, during and at the end of therapy; (2) evaluate PROs of Interferon-free (dual) users versus Interferon-containing (triple) users cross the three different time periods; and (3) identify the predictors of HRQoL of DAAs therapy users cross the three different time periods.

Methods: A prospective observational design was used. Patients with chronic HCV undergoing treatment following the Egyptian National Guidelines at one of the national treatment centers were approached. Data collection occurred in the period from February to October 2015. Data was collected at three time points: (1) baseline (time 0: T0), before initiating therapy); (2) 5/6 weeks after initiation of therapy (time 1 of therapy: T1) and at the end of the therapy (Time 2: T2). Four PROs questionnaires were utilized for data collection: (1) Multidimensional Scale of Perceived Social Support (MSPSS), (2) The Depression Anxiety Stress Scales (DASS-21), (3) the Liver Disease Symptom Index-2.0 (LDSI-2.0) for testing disease specific HRQoL and (4) the Center for Adherence Support Evaluation (CASE) Index, alongside the background data sheet.

Results: Sixty-two patients participated. There was a change in HRQoL, symptom experience and mental health across the three different time periods. HRQoL was impaired more after starting the course of therapy (T1) than at baseline (T0) and end of therapy (T2), $z \geq -2.04$, $p \leq .04$. Also, symptom experience deteriorated more during the treatment period than at the baseline, $Z \geq -1.97$, $p \leq .04$. Anxiety and stress were significantly higher during the treatment period than at the end of treatment. Perceived social support was significantly higher during the treatment period than at baseline and end of therapy, $Z \geq -2.27$, $p \leq .023$. During the course of therapy, triple users were more likely to report poorer HRQoL and anxiety than dual users ($p \leq .04$). By the end of therapy, the two arms of therapy had no significant differences in any of the PROs.

At baseline, the predictor model significantly ($p = .000$) explained 37.5% of the variation in the HRQoL prior to

(Continued on next page)

* Correspondence: ashley.shepherd@stir.ac.uk
[3]Faculty of Health Sciences and Sport, University of Stirling, Stirling FK9 4LA, Scotland, UK
Full list of author information is available at the end of the article

(Continued from previous page)

therapy. Depression was the main variable that contributed to (41.3%) predicting change in HRQoL prior to therapy. During therapy, the model significantly ($p = .000$) explained 76% of the variation in the HRQoL-T1. Stress-T1, body mass index (BMI)-T1 and HRQoL-T0 significantly and respectively predicted 44.4, 46.5 and 31.1% of the variation in HRQoL-T1. At the end of therapy, the model significantly ($p = .000$) predicted 80.5% of the variation in the HRQoL-T2. HRQoL-T1 and anxiety-T2 significantly predicted 72.3 and 61.6% of the variation in HRQoL-T2.

Conclusions: Baseline HRQoL, depression and BMI should be systematically assessed before starting the antiviral therapy for early detection and the improvement of the impairment before the initiation of therapy. Anxiety should be frequently assessed and followed up through the course of antiviral therapy. The triple group required more nursing and practitioner attention due to increased anxiety levels and impaired HRQoL during the treatment therapy.

Keywords: Directly acting antivirals-DAAs, Health related quality of life, Social support, Patient reported outcomes (PROs), Hepatitis C Virus antiviral therapy

Background

Worldwide, the prevalence of the hepatitis C virus (HCV) is 2.8%, causing a considerable global burden of morbidity and mortality [1, 2]. According to a nationally representative survey carried out in 2008 [3], Egypt has the highest HCV prevalence in the world; with 14.7% sero prevalence. Hepatitis C has been associated with substantial resource utilization as a result of its effect on the liver as well as other organ systems (the extrahepatic manifestations of HCV) [4, 5]. It has been widely reported to have a profound negative impact on patient's health-related quality of life (HRQoL) because of the associated complications of advanced liver disease (i.e. encephalopathy, variceal hemorrhage, ascites) [6]. Also, employees being treated for hepatitis C had high rates of absenteeism and impairment of their work productivity [7]. HCV affects HRQoL through other avenues, such as fatigue, persistent flu-like symptoms, joint pain, itching, sleep disturbances, appetite changes, nausea, and depression [8, 9].

Patient reported outcomes (PROs) have become increasingly important data in clinical research, since they can provide the most complete assessment of the impact of chronic hepatitis C and its treatment on patients' health status [10]. PROs have been defined as measurements that are based on reports that come directly from the patients about their health status without any amendment or interpretation by healthcare providers [11]. There are a number of important PROs that provide insight into patients' experiences such as HRQoL. HRQoL has been defined as the patients' subjective perception of the impact of their disease and/or its treatment on their daily life, and their physical, psychological and social functioning. These definitions clearly acknowledge that HRQoL is a multidimensional concept. Therefore, it has been considered the gold standard to measure patients' experiences with their disease and treatment [12].

A number of antiviral therapies have been developed. Antiviral therapies can eradicate the virus resulting in improvements in liver histology, which prevents liver-related mortality [13] and enhances HRQoL because of symptoms' alleviation and an increase in associated economic and social benefits. For example, work force participation and removal of social stigma can follow after successful treatment [13–15]. However, the toxicity associated with antiviral treatments can negatively affect HRQoL by way of diminished physical, emotional and social functioning [7, 16].

A pegylated interferon (peg-IFN)-based regimen has long been the standard treatment for patients with HCV [17]. Treatment with a peg-IFN-containing regimen has been shown to severely impair all PROs including work productivity, leading to negative patient experiences and lower adherence to the treatment regimen [7, 16].

The arrival of direct acting antivirals (DAAs), such as boceprevir and telaprevir, in triple combination with peg-IFN and ribavirin, increased HCV clearance rates but might cause adverse effects that can further decrease HRQoL [18, 19]. Over the past few years, the treatment landscape for HCV has been changing rapidly, leading to the introduction of newer and improved, DAAs. Even in patients who were considered difficult to treat; these agents have reduced toxicity, increased barriers to resistance and led to reduced side effects [20–23] such as fatigue and neuropsychiatric problems [24]. The interferon-free treatment (dual) can potentially provide a number of important advantages; including higher efficacy, lower side effects and shorter duration of treatment, which can substantially increase adherence level and improve PROs [25].

The Egyptian government introduced sofosbuvir as the first DAAs into Egypt through the government funded National Treatment Program [26]. The first DAAs regimen used in the country was sofosbuvir, which was administered either as a triple therapy in combination with peg-IFN and ribavirin or as a dual therapy combined only with ribavirin (for interferon non-eligible patients). As of July 2015, other treatment options, including an all DAAs therapy with simepravir and sofosbuvir were introduced, with many more DAAs containing therapies soon to be approved [26].

To date, there have been no investigations into how Egyptian HCV patients receiving the new DAAs perceive their HRQoL. Therefore, this study is the first to evaluate a number of PROs, including health-related quality of life (HRQoL), mental health status (i.e. depression, anxiety and stress), and perceived social support among HCV patients, while receiving DAAs therapy; either an interferon-free or interferon-containing *regimen*.

Specifically this study aimed to:

1) Assess the PROs (i.e. health-related quality of life, mental health and perceived social support) of HCV patients receiving direct acting antivirals (DAAs) therapy prior, during and at the end of therapy.
2) Evaluate PROs of Interferon-free (dual) users versus Interferon-containing (triple) users prior, during and at the end of treatment.
3) Identify the predictors of HRQoL of DAAs therapy users prior, during and at the end of therapy.

Methods
Study design
A prospective observational design was used to conduct this study. Patients with chronic HCV being treated, using the Egyptian National Guidelines at one of the national treatment centres, were approached to participate. According to the most updated treatment protocol, patients undergo therapy for a relatively short period (3 to 6 months).

Study population
A total of 80 patients were invited to participate in the study in the period from February to October 2015. Patients were randomly selected from HCV patients visiting the HCV specialized clinic. Patients were eligible to participate in the study if they met the following criteria:

- Had no significant psychiatric illnesses (diagnosed by psychiatrist),
- Aged 18 years or older,
- Eligible for starting DAAs therapy and
- Gave written consent to participate.

Data collection
This study was conducted at the Outpatients clinic of the National Hepatology and Tropical Medicine Research Institute (NHTMRI), Cairo, Egypt. This institute is one of 42 specialized national treatment centres for treatment of viral hepatitis distributed throughout the country; and it is the largest of all these centres. This institute serves patients from different regions in Egypt and of various socioeconomic status. All the centres follow the same set of national guidelines for the treatment of patients with chronic HCV and are supervised by the National Committee for Control of Viral Hepatitis.

Data was collected at three points in time: (1) baseline [time 0 (T0), before initiating therapy]; (2) 5th or 6th week after initiation of therapy [time 1 (T1) of therapy] and (3) at the final week of therapy [time 2 (T2)]. At time 0, the patients were first interviewed following an appointment with the consultant in the outpatients' clinic, where it was confirmed that they were eligible to start the HCV therapy.

Protocol of therapy
According to the 2014 Egyptian HCV national patient treatment guidelines, antiviral therapy was administered either as Interferon-free (dual) or Interferon-containing (triple) therapies. The recommended regimen for patients who were not eligible to receive peg-IFN (dual group) was daily Sofosbuvir (400 mg) plus weight-based RBV (1000 mg [<75 kg] to 1200 mg [>75 kg]) for 24 weeks. Inclusion criteria for treatment of patients who would be treated with Interferon free regimen was defined with the presence of any or all the following;

a) Child score up to 8
b) Total bilirubin ≤ 5
c) Albumin ≥ 2.5
d) Platelet count ≥ 30,000
e) Prtothrombin concentration ≥ 50%
f) Hemoglobin concentration ≥ 10 mg

Patients who were eligible to receive Interferon (triple group) would be treated with daily Sofosbuvir (400 mg) and weight-based RBV (1000 mg [<75 kg] to 1200 mg [>75 kg]) plus weekly Peg-INF for 12 weeks.

Collection data procedure
Questionnaires and data collection
Four instruments were utilized for data collection alongside the background data sheet. Participants were interviewed face to face for around 30–40 min each, based on the patient co-operation and literacy level, to complete all the questionnaires.

The Multidimensional Scale of Perceived Social Support (MSPSS) [27] is a commonly used instrument for measuring the perceived adequacy of social support from three specific sources: family, friends and significant others [26]. Each subscale has four items that are rated on a seven point scale in the English version or on a three point scale in the Arabic version. The MSPSS can be computed to give the total and subscale scores for each of the three sources of support. The total score and subscale scores are calculated by adding up the participant's responses. An increasing score represents increasing perceived adequacy of social support. This is the most appropriate tool for measuring perceived social support among patients waiting for OHS for many reasons. (1) It is the shortest and simplest tool available (12 items); (2) An Arabic version of MSPSS is available [27] and has been widely used among Arabic speaking people [26]. It has a high construct validity and internal consistency reliability with Cronbach's alpha for total MSPSS = 0.74 [27].

The Depression Anxiety Stress Scale (DASS-21) [28] was used to assess mental health. The DASS-21 questionnaire includes 21 questions that measure anxiety, stress and depression separately, where each scale has seven questions. Each question is scored on a 4-point combined severity/frequency scale over the past week. The score ranges from 0 (did not apply to me at all) to 3 (applied to me very much, or most of the time). The overall score ranges from 0 to 21. Scores 0–4, 0–3 and 0–7 show normal levels of depression, anxiety and stress respectively; scores 5–7, 4–5 and 8–9 show low levels of depression, anxiety and stress respectively; scores of 8–11, 5–7 and 10–13 show moderate levels of depression, anxiety and stress respectively; scores 12–15, 8–9 and 14–17 show severe levels of depression, anxiety and stress respectively; and scores of 25+, 10+ and 18+ show extreme severe levels of depression, anxiety and stress respectively. Scores for depression, anxiety and stress are calculated by adding the scores for the relevant items. The Arabic version of this tool has been psychometrically validated.

The Liver Disease Symptom Index (LDSI)-2.0 is a short and psychometrically tested disease specific HRQoL questionnaire, which has been widely used with patients at different stages of a chronic infection with HCV [29, 30]. It is available in Arabic [29]. The LDSI-2.0 has two subscales that are used to assess symptom severity, and the impact of these symptoms on patients' daily activities (symptom hindrance). The participants were asked if a symptom was experienced during the past week. If yes, the participants were asked to what extent it was affecting their daily lives and social contacts on a five-point Likert scale, with 0 = not at all, and 4 = to a high extent. Possible scores for each subscale ranged from 0 to 60 for the severity dimension and 0–36 for hindrance dimension. A higher score on the severity dimension represents a higher perception of the symptoms' severity, and a higher score on the hindrance dimension represents a higher perception of the limitations of daily activities because of these symptoms. It also provides an overall total score that represents a disease specific HRQoL [29, 30].

The Center for Adherence Support Evaluation (CASE) Index [31] is a valid, reliable, simple and easy to administer instrument that measures self-reported antiretroviral therapy adherence. It is composed of three questions: Question 1: Self-reported frequency of 'difficulty taking HCV medications on time', with responses being: never, rarely, most of the time or all of the time. Question 2: Self-reported 'average number of days per week at least one dose of HCV medications was missed', with responses being: every day, 4–6 days per week, 2–3 days per week, once a week, less than once a week or never. Question 3: Self-reported 'last time missed at least one dose of HCV medications', with responses being: within the past week, 1–2 weeks ago, 3–4 weeks ago, between 1 and 3 months ago, more than 3 months ago or never. The total index score (INDEXSCORE) > 10 indicates good adherence, while < 10 indicates poor adherence.

Socio-demographic and medical data sheets were designed by the researchers and divided into two parts: (i) the socio-demographic sheet was used to collect data related to the participants' characteristics; such as age, gender, employment status, occupation, education level, marital status and medical history, and (ii) the medical data sheet was used to record the diagnosis, disease duration, type of antiviral therapy, comorbidity (i.e. diabetes, hypertension), and other factors. The Body Mass Index (BMI) was calculated using the standard formula: BMI = kg/m^2.

Statistical methods

The Statistical Package for the Social Sciences 20 (IBM SPSS, Armonk, New York, United States) was used for the data analysis. Descriptive statistics were computed to summarize data. Individual variables were examined by percentages, means, and SDs. A non-parametric statistical technique, such as chi-square for independence, was used to compare the frequencies of nominal variables. Differences among the two arms of therapy were examined by independent t test. Friedman test was used to examine the change in HRQoL, mental health and social support at the three time points. Wilcoxon Signed Rank Test (Post-hoc pairwise) with Bonferroni correction was performed for HRQoL, mental health and social support across the three time points. A multiple linear regression analysis using "stepwise forward method" was used to investigate the factors associated with HRQoL. Since this was an exploratory study, there was no prior decision regarding the order of entering the variables in the model [32]. The multiple regression assumptions were investigated and there was no violation of normality, linearity, and multicollinearity. All statistical analyses were two tailed with $p < .05$ as the significance level.

Results

Characteristics of the participants

Sixty-two patients in total participated in this study at T0 and T1; and 36 participated at T2 (Fig. 1). The baseline demographic and medical characteristics revealed that the mean age of the sample ($n = 62$) was 54.06 ± [standard deviation (SD) 10.41 years] (Table 1). The sample contained an almost equal number of males (48.4%) and females (51.6%). Most of the sample were married (72.6%), and employed (64.3%). There was an equal distribution between cirrhotic and non-cirrhotic participants, with disease discovery duration ranging from 3 to 216 months. Half of the participants had a medical comorbidity, with diabetes (30.6%) and hypertension (24.2%) the most commonly reported comorbidities (Table 1). About 87.1% of the patients were treatment naïve which meant they had never received HCV antiviral therapy before this study. Experienced patients had previously received HCV antiviral therapy (peg-IFN).

Comparison between males and females

A comparison between males ($n = 30$) and females ($n = 32$) demographic and medical data at baseline and their PROs through the three time points was conducted. Only significant results are presented in Table 2. As has been observed, females were more likely to be older and obese than males. Prior to therapy, females had a poorer HRQoL, higher levels of symptoms' severity, hindrance of symptoms in their daily life, and a higher level of

depression, than males. During the course of therapy, depression remained higher among females than males. At the end of therapy, there was no significant difference between males' and females' PROs.

Objective 1: PROs (health-related quality of life, mental health and perceived social support) of HCV patients receiving DAAs therapy prior, during and at the end of therapy

Friedman test for repeated measures was computed, among the patients who participated at the three different time points ($n = 36$), to compare HRQoL [LDSI-2.0 total score], symptom experience [two subscales of LDSI-2.0: severity and hindrance], mental health [depression, anxiety and stress], and perceived social support across the three different time points (Table 3).

There was a significant effect for time on HRQoL, $X^2 = 8.35$, $p = .015$. A Wilcoxon Signed Rank Test with Bonferroni correction was performed between each of the time points with r indicating the effect size based on the Cohen criteria. A Wilcoxon Signed Rank Test revealed there was a statistically significant impairment of HRQoL after starting the course of therapy (T1) than at baseline (T0) and end of therapy (T2), $z \geq -2.04$, $p \leq .04$, with a medium effect size ($r \geq -.26$) (Table 3).

Also, there was a significant effect for time (T0 vs. T1) on symptom experience (severity & hindrance) and mental health (depression & anxiety), ($X^2 = 5.41$, 9.89, 8.79, 6.82 respectively, $p < .05$). A Wilcoxon Signed Rank Test revealed there was a statistically significant impairment of symptom experience and mental health during the treatment period (T1, 5/6 weeks) than at the baseline, $Z \geq -1.97$, $p \leq .04$, with a medium effect size ($r \geq -.25$). Additionally, anxiety and stress were significantly higher during the treatment period than at the end of treatment. Perceived social support was also significantly higher during the treatment period than at baseline (T0) and end of therapy (T2), $Z \geq -2.27$, $p \leq .023$, with a medium effect size ($r \geq -.29$) (Table 3).

Comparison of basic demographic and medical data between dual and triple users

For the purpose of comparing dual and triple therapy users, the baseline demographic and medical characteristics of the two groups of participants were initially compared using the nonparametric statistical tests (i.e. Chi-square test and independent-samples Mann-Whitney U Test). Dual participants were more likely to live in urban areas (Pearson Chi-Square = 7.123, $p = .02$) and more cirrhotic (Pearson Chi-Square = 7.806, $p = .01$) than triple therapy participants. However, the rates of baseline factors that could potentially impact HRQoL-T1 (i.e. age, gender, employment status, depression-T0, anxiety-T0, stress-T0, disease duration, PCR-T0, BMI-

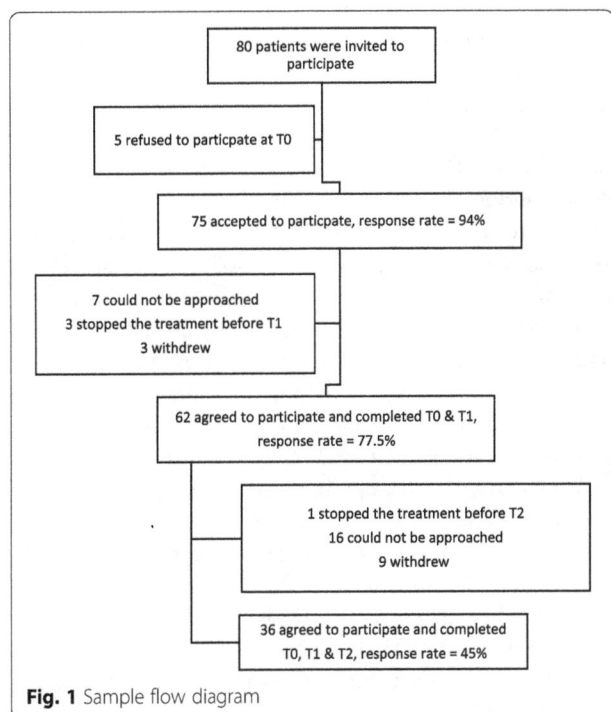

Fig. 1 Sample flow diagram

Table 1 Baseline demographic and clinical characteristics of the participants

	Number (total 62)	Percent
Age	54.06 ± 10.41*	
Gender		
• Males	30	48.40
• Females	32	51.60
Education		
• Uneducated	24	38.70
• Can read and write or preparatory	12	29.00
• Secondary	12	19.40
• University	8	12.90
Marital status		
• Unmarried	17	27.40
• Married	45	72.60
Employment status		
• Unemployed	17	27.40
• Employed	17	27.40
• Housewife	28	45.20
Residence area		
• Rural	15	24.20
• Urban	47	75.80
Diseases stage		
• Non cirrhotic	31	50
• Cirrhotic	31	50
Number of comorbidities		
• 0	31	50
• 1	17	27.4
• 2	11	17.7
• 3	3	4.8
Type of comorbidity		
• Hypertension	15	24.20
• Diabetes	19	30.60
• Others (renal disease, disc, heart disease, asthma, peptic ulcer)	11	17.70
Disease duration (Range from 3 to 216 months)	71.10 ± 57.72*	
Type of treatment		
• Dual	31	50
• Triple	31	50
Treatment experience		
• Naive	54	87.10
• Experienced	8	12.90
Treatment paying method		
• Self	6	9.70
• Governmental	56	90.30

Table 1 Baseline demographic and clinical characteristics of the participants (Continued)

BMI		
T0	30.6 ± 4.24*	
T1	30.4 ± 4.53*	
PCR at T1 (50 cases)		
• Negative	32	64
• Positive	18	36

BMI body mass index, PCR Polymerase Chain Reaction, T0 Time 0, T1 time 1
*Mean ± SD
*P value: * ≤ .05 at two tailed

T0, symptom severity-T0, symptom hindrance-T1 and HRQoL-T0) were similar between the two arms of therapy (all $P \geq .05$) (Table 4).

Comparison of HRQoL, mental health and symptom experience between dual and triple users

Table 4 presents the comparison of PROs (i.e. HRQoL, mental health and symptom experience) between the dual and triple therapy users at the three points in time. During the course of therapy (after 5/6 weeks), triple users ($n = 31$) were more likely to report poorer HRQoL and anxiety than dual users ($n = 31$) ($p \leq .04$). Using Pearson correlation showed that there is a high significant association between anxiety and HRQoL during the treatment period (r - = .78, $p = .000$). Anxiety during the time period was significantly correlated with baseline HRQoL (r = .51. $p = .000$). By the end of therapy, the two arms of therapy had no significant differences in any of the PROs (Table 5). A post hoc power calculation for the Mann Whitney U test of differences in HRQoL between the dual and triple therapy group during treatment is estimated power of 0.33.

Objective 2: PROs of dual users versus triple users prior, during and at the end of treatment

The pattern of change in PROs among triple ($n = 26$) and dual ($n = 10$) therapy users prior, during and at the end of therapy was considered using Friedman test (Table 6). Results revealed that the triple therapy group had significantly poorer HRQoL, symptom severity, symptom hindrance and depression, and more increase in perceived social support score at T1 than at baseline, (Chi-Square ≥ 6.653, $p \leq .036$). In contrast, dual users had no significant change in their HRQoL, symptom experience and mental health (Chi-Square ≤ 5.706, $p \geq .058$), while their perceived social support was significantly increased during T1 in comparing to T0 and T2 ($p = .037$) like triple users (Table 6). A post hoc power calculation for the Friedman test of change in HRQoL in the dual group over time is estimated power between 0.21 and 0.41.

Table 2 Comparison between males and females

	Mean ± Std. Deviation	t
Age		
• Male	49.48 ± 12.19	-3.68**
• Female	58.34 ± 5.92	
PCR-T0		
• Male = 28	890248.43 ± 1049454.60	2.22*
• Female = 28	411320.44 ± 451668.92	
BMI-T0		
• Male	29.10 ± 3.86	-2.83**
• Female	31.99 ± 4.15	
MBI-T1		
• Male	28.88 ± 3.83	-2.74**
• Female	31.88 ± 4.71	
HRQoL-T0		
• Male	23.73 ± 15.89	-3.43**
• Female	39.06 ± 19.66	
Symptom Severity-T0		
• Male	18.53 ± 10.30	-3.12**
• Female	27.43 ± 12.28	
Symptom Hindrance-T0		
• Male	5.20 ± 6.66	-3.27**
• Female	11.62 ± 8.57	
Depression-T0		
• Male	5.56 ± 5.88	-3.52**
• Female	11.47 ± 7.19	
Depression-T1		
• Male	7.20 ± 6.46	-2.32*
• Female	11.28 ± 7.69	

Note: only significant results are presented, sample of male = 30 & female = 32
PCR-T0 Polymerase Chain Reaction time0, *BMI-T0* body mass index time 0, *BMI-T1* body mass index time 1, *HRQoL-T0* health-related quality of life time 0
*P value: * ≤ .05, ** ≤ .001, *** ≤ .0001 at two tailed

Objective 3: Predictors of HRQoL of DAAs therapy users prior, during and at the end of therapy

At baseline, the developed model could significantly (P = .000) predict 37.5% (R^2 = 39.8, AdjR^2 = 37.5) the variance in the HRQoL prior to therapy. Depression and anxiety were significant variables that contributed to predict the change in HRQoL prior to therapy (41.3 & 29.1% respectively) (Table 7). All the other variables were excluded from the model as they could not significantly predict the HRQoL-T1: age, gender, PCR-T0, BMI-T0, MSPSS-T0 and stressT0.

After 5/6 weeks of therapy (T1), the model significantly (P = .000) explained 76% (R^2 = 78.2, AdjR^2 = 76) the variance in the HRQoL. Out of 15 independent factors that entered the model, only HRQoLT0 & BMIT0 prior to therapy; and StressT1, Anxiety-T1 & BMI-T1

during therapy significantly explained the variation in HRQoL during the course of therapy. The five variables could significantly and prospectively predict 31.1, 35, 44.4, 24.4 & 46.5% of the variations in HRQoL during therapy (Table 7). All the other variables could not significantly predict the HRQoL during therapy: age, gender, PCR-T0, MSPSS-T0, MSPS-T1, depression-T0, anxiety-T0, stress-T0 and depressionT1, NDEXSCORE-T1, type of therapy.

At the end of therapy (T2), the model significantly (P = .000) predicted 80.5% (R^2 = 83, AdjR^2 = 80.5) of the variance in the HRQoL-T2. Out of 22 independent variables, four variables (HRQoL-T1, Anxiety-T1, Anxiety-T2, MSPSS-T2,) could significantly predict the variation in HRQoL. HRQoL & anxiety during the course of therapy and perceived support & anxiety at the end of therapy significantly and respectively predict 72.3, 33.1, 25.3 & 61.6% of the variations in HRQoL-T2 at the end of therapy (Table 7). All the other variables could not significantly predict the HRQoL-T2: depression-T2, stress-T2, HRQoL-T0, MSPSS-T0, MSPSS-T1, depression-T0, anxiety-T0, stress-T0, depression-T1, stress-T1, INDEXSCORE-T1, T1INDEXSCORE-T2, age, gender, disease duration, PCR-T1, BM-IT0 and MBI-T1.

The key finding of this study is that anxiety was always the constant variable that could significantly predict change in HRQoL during the three different time periods.

Discussion

Healthcare consumers, whether patients or policy makers, are increasingly interested in how medical intervention impacts PROs, such as patient's HRQoL [33–36]. Therefore, several studies examined the HRQoL among HCV on antiviral therapy; and agreed that Peg-IFN and ribavirin therapy of chronic HCV remains problematic, as it causes unpleasant side effects that could affect the patients' HRQoL [34, 35]. Therefore, a new DAAs therapy has been developed and has been found to be a well-tolerated therapy with low adverse side effects [10, 13]. Although the benefits of DAAs therapy are well established; its effects on HRQoL are less certain [10, 37]. Therefore, this prospective observational study is the first study to evaluate a number of PROs, including HRQoL, mental health status (i.e. depression, anxiety and stress), and perceived social support among Egyptian HCV patients, while receiving DAAs therapy; either a dual or triple therapy. Consequently, this section provides an interpretation of the study's results based on the stated three aims, implications for nursing practice and suggested recommendations for future research and limitations of the study.

This study recruited 62 patients with HCV who were treated with DAAs. Our study provides several new and important lines of evidence about these patients'

Table 3 PROs of HCV patients receiving DAAs therapy prior, during and at the end of therapy

Variables/Time	N	Mean + SD	Friedman test		Wilcoxon test		
			Chi-Square	P-value	T	Z	P value (r)
HRQoL							
T0	36	31.02 ± 15.30	8.35	.01	T0 - T1 = 436	-2.37	.01 (-.30)
T1	36	39.63 ± 21.11					
T2	36	34.50 ± 19.96			T1 –T2 = 178.50	-2.04	.04(-.26)
Symptom experience							
Symptom severity							
T0	36	23.19 ± 10.21	5.41	.06	T0 - T1 = 458	-1.97	.04(-.25)
T1	36	27.36 ± 13.07					
T2	36	24.25 ± 12.75					
Symptom hindrance							
T0	36	7.83 ± 6.40	9.89	.007	T0 - T1 = 358	-2.58	.01(-.33)
T1	36	12.27 ± 9.00					
T2	36	10.25 ± 7.89					
Mental Health							
Depression							
T0	36	8.91 ± 7.25	8.79	.01	T0 - T1 = 385	-2.28	.02(-.29)
T1	36	10.77 ± 7.18					
T2	36	8.97 ± 6.57					
Anxiety							
T0	36	7.33 ± 5.80	6.82	.03	T0 - T1 = 379	-2.57	.01(-.33)
T1	36	8.88 ± 5.87					
T2	36	6.86 ± 6.05			T1 - T2 = 80	-2.63	.009(-.34)
Stress							
T0	36	10.94 ± 7.35	4.86	.08	T1 - T2 = 103.50	-2.47	.01(-.32)
T1	36	12.05 ± 6.83					
T2	36	9.75 ± 6.80					
MSPSS							
T0	36	2.41 ± .47	11.35	.003	T0 - T1 = 212	-2.27	.02(-.29)
T1	36	2.51 ± .37					
T2	36	2.41 ± .39			T1 - T2 = 146	-2.77	.006(-.36)

HRQoL Health-related quality of life time 0, *T0* time 0, *T1* time 1, *T2* time 2
P value significant at two tailed

HRQoL, symptom experience, mental health and perceived social support of patients receiving DAAs (Dual and triple therapy) that will enhance health care providers' insight about these patients' needs during the course of therapy.

Objective 1: PROs of HCV patients receiving DAAs therapy prior, during and at the end of therapy

Our study clearly documented the effect of time on HRQoL, symptom experience, mental health and perceived social support. There was a significant effect for time on HRQoL; it was significantly poorer after 5/ 6 weeks (peak point of impairment) of therapy than at the baseline and at the end of therapy. It is interesting that the HRQoL score significantly increased from T0 to T1, indicting impairment of HRQoL and then backed to baseline score. This finding is very important as it confirms the need for follow up and tracking of the HRQoL among patients on antiviral therapy. Previously, it was ascertained that in addition to the baseline impairment of HRQoL in patients with chronic HCV, treatment regimens can impose additional PROs burdens [38]. This impairment is further amplified by the antiviral (peg-IFN and RBV) side effects, particularly anemia and depression. Similarly, non cirrhotic patients who received triple

Table 4 Comparison of basic demographic and medical data between dual and triple users

Variables	Type of therapy		P value Sig. (2-tailed)
	Dual (n = 31)	Triple (n = 31)	
Gender			
• Male	12	18	.20
• Female	19	13	
Education			
• Uneducated	17	7	.02
• Educated	14	24	
Employment			
• Employed	6	11	.24
• Unemployed	8	9	
• Housewives	17	11	
Martial status			
• Single	8	9	.50
• Married	23	22	
Area of residence			
• Rural	3	12	.02
• Urban	28	19	
Treatment experience			
• Naïve	30	24	.05
• Experience	1	7	
Diagnosis			
• Non-cirrhotic	10	21	.01
• Cirrhotic	21	10	
Mean ± SD			
Age	56.47 ± 9.32	51.65 ± 11.03	.07
Disease duration (months)	81.71 ± 62.86	60.48 ± 50.94	.15
PCR-T0	655845.81 ± 997681.03	645348.15 ± 638028.61	.96
PCR-T1 (50 cases)			
• Negative 32 (51.6%)			
• Positive 18 (29.0%)			

PCR-T0 Polymerase Chain Reaction time 0, PCR-T1 Polymerase Chain Reaction time 1
P value significant at two tailed

therapy had significant impairments in HRQoL using Short Form (SF)-36. Dual therapy was also associated with moderate HRQoL and work productivity impairment regardless of the stage of fibrosis for role physical and role emotional of SF-36, but this impairment was significantly lower when compared to triple therapy [10]. Younossi et al [10]. showed that at week 4 of active treatment with

DAAs therapy (Ledipasvir and Sofosbuvir), a significant decline in some domains of HRQoL was observed in patients without and with mild fibrosis, including physical and social functioning, role physical and emotional, and vitality of SF-36, physical and functional well-being and fatigue, and activity/energy domain of Chronic Liver Disease Questionnaire-HCV (CLDQ-HCV).

However, our study showed that by the end of therapy the scores of HRQoL, mental health and symptom experience were almost back to baseline score. A previous study on other hand showed that by the end of treatment, a more substantial deterioration was observed in most of the HRQoL domains including role physical and role emotional of SF-36 regardless of patients' fibrosis status [10]. Furthermore, at the end of treatment, perceived general health, emotional well-being, and worry domains significantly improved in both fibrosis cohorts. At follow-up, all HRQL domains and work productivity returned to their baseline levels or moderately improved as early as post-treatment week 4 [10].

Time also significantly impacted on symptom experience (severity & hindrance) and mental health (depression & anxiety). Symptom hindrance and mental health were significantly poorer at T1 (5/6 weeks of therapy) than at baseline (T0). Additionally, anxiety and stress were significantly higher during the treatment period (T1) than at the end of treatment (T2). Interestingly, anxiety at baseline, after 5/6 weeks and at the end of therapy, was significantly associated with severity and hindrance of symptoms and HRQoL at different points in time ($p < 0.02$, r ranged from 0.38 to 0.79). Previously, it was ascertained that in addition to the baseline impairment of mental health of patients with chronic HCV, treatment regimens can impose additional mental health impairment [25]. Therefore, it was unsurprising to find perceived social support significantly higher during the treatment period than at baseline (T0) and end of therapy (T2). For that reason, more healthcare support is required during the course of therapy, particularly to improve HRQoL, symptom experience and mental health, which have been found to significantly worsen during the course of therapy.

Comparison of basic demographic and medical data between dual and triple users

For the purpose of comparing the dual vs. the triple therapy users, the baseline demographic and medical characteristics of the two groups of participants were initially compared. We found that the dual participants were less educated, more likely to live in urban areas and more cirrhotic than triple users. At the time of data collection in Egypt, two treatment regimens were delivered according to the guideline protocol of the National Committee of Control HCV (NCCVH) for patients with

Table 5 PROs prior, during and at the end of treatment among dual and triple users

	Type of therapy		Independent-samples Mann-Whitney U Test
	Dual N =31	Triple N = 31	P value Sig. (2-tailed)
Baseline	X ± SD		
BMI-T0	31.26 ± 4.16	29.92 ± 4.26	.31
HRQoL-T0	32.54 ± 21.23	30.74 ± 17.67	.85
Symptom Severity-T0	23.32 ± 13.14	22.93 ± 11.24	.97
Symptom Hindrance-T0	9.22 ± 9.09	7.80 ± 7.50	.64
MSPSS-T0	2.22 ± .57	2.49 ± .39	.05
Depression-T0	9.12 ± 7.51	8.09 ± 6.92	.59
Anxiety-T0	6.41 ± 5.83	7.51 ± 6.03	.53
Stress-T0	8.64 ± 6.61	10.80 ± 7.63	.29
After 5/6 weeks	X ± SD		
BM-IT1	31.24 ± 4.47	29.60 ± 4.50	.16
HRQoL-T1	31.06 ± 24.06	41.54 ± 21.62	.04
Symptom Severity-T1	21.77 ± 15.09	28.51 ± 12.72	.05
Symptom Hindrance-T1	9.29 ± 9.64	13.03 ± 9.67	.09
MSPSS-T1	2.34 ± .55	2.54 ± .38	.23
Depression-T1	9.12 ± 7.67	9.48 ± 7.15	.72
Anxiety-T1	5.64 ± 5.77	9.19 ± 6.16	.01
Stress-T1	9.00 ± 7.46	11.87 ± 7.09	.11
INDEXSCORE-T1	15.74 ± .77	15.45 ± 1.45	.87
At the end of therapy	X ± SD		
HRQoL-T2	26.60 ± 17.01	37.53 ± 20.47	.15
Symptom Severity-T2	18.20 ± 12.50	26.57 ± 12.29	.06
Symptom Hindrance-T2	8.40 ± 5.10	10.96 ± 8.72	.52
MSPSS-T2	2.40 ± .40	2.41 ± .40	.84
Depression-T2	6.20 ± 6.49	10.03 ± 6.40	.10
Anxiety-T2	4.50 ± 3.53	7.76 ± 6.61	.27
Stress-T2	6.40 ± 5.16	11.03 ± 6.99	.08
INDEXSCORE-T2	15.90 ± .31	15.30 ± 1.46	.41

BMI-T0 body mass index time 0, HRQoL-T0 health-related quality of life time 0, MSPSS-T0 Multidimensional Scale of Perceived Social Support time 0, BMI-T1 body mass index time 1, HRQoL-T1 health-related quality of life time 1, MSPSS-T1 Multidimensional Scale of Perceived Social Support time 1, INDEXSCORE-T1 The total index score of the Center for Adherence Support Evaluation (CASE) Index time 1, HRQoL-T2 health-related quality of life time 2, MSPSS-T2 Multidimensional Scale of Perceived Social Support time 2, INDEXSCORE-T2 The total index score of the Center for Adherence Support Evaluation (CASE) Index time 2
P value significant at two tailed

HCV. According to this guideline, patients with more advanced liver disease were always ineligible for peg-IFN treatment and thus dual therapy was presented to them. This could help explain our findings, which also confirm that our sample was representative of HCV patients who received DAAs therapy at that time.

Comparison of HRQoL, mental health and symptom experience between dual and triple users

Similar to an earlier study [36], we found that prior to therapy HRQoL was not significantly different between dual and triple users. Also, mental health status, symptom experience and perceived support were similar. However the triple users were more likely to experience more deterioration in their HRQoL and higher levels of anxiety during the course of therapy. These findings might be due to the fact that the effect of Peg-IFN on patients' HRQoL and anxiety was found to be higher than the effect of a Peg-IFN-free regimen. However, the adherence score was high and similar in dual and triple users, indicating the effect of treatment on HRQoL and anxiety. It is well established that HCV infection is associated with poorer HRQoL and a part of impaired health of these patients is related to comorbid psychiatric disorders and interferon treatment. Interferon treatment is an

Table 6 Pattern of change in PROs among dual and triple users prior, during and at the end of treatment

Variables/Time	Triple therapy $N = 26$			Dual therapy $N = 10$		
	Mean + SD	Chi-Square	P-value	Mean + SD	Chi-Square	P-value
HRQoL						
T0	29.81 ± 15.87	10.26	.006	34.20 ± 13.98	.47	.79
T1	43.35 ± 21.15			30.00 ± 18.63		
T2	37.54 ± 20.47			26.60 ± 17.02		
Symptom experience						
Symptom severity						
T0	22.69 ± 10.29	8.00	.01	24.50 ± 10.46	.68	.71
T1	29.77 ± 12.31			21.10 ± 13.54		
T2	26.58 ± 12.29			18.20 ± 12.51		
Symptom hindrance						
T0	7.12 ± 6.67	13.01	.001	9.70 ± 5.54	.15	.92
T1	13.58 ± 9.66			8.90 ± 6.23		
T2	10.96 ± 8.72			8.40 ± 5.10		
Mental Health						
Depression						
T0	8.58 ± 6.65	11.40	.003	9.80 ± 8.99	5.70	.05
T1	10.62 ± 6.93			11.20 ± 8.18		
T2	10.04 ± 6.40			6.20 ± 6.49		
Anxiety						
T0	7.69 ± 6.04	4.95	.08	6.40 ± 5.29	2.10	.34
T1	9.62 ± 5.97			7.00 ± 5.46		
T2	7.77 ± 6.62			4.50 ± 3.54		
Stress						
T0	11.54 ± 7.27	4.93	.08	9.40 ± 7.72	.70	.70
T1	12.92 ± 6.63			9.80 ± 7.19		
T2	11.04 ± 6.99			6.40 ± 5.17		
MSPSS						
T0	2.45 ± .40	6.65	.03	2.31 ± .64	6.58	.03
T1	2.54 ± .35			2.43 ± .44		
T2	2.42 ± .40			2.41 ± .41		

HRQoL health-related quality of life, T0 time 0, T1 time 1, T2 time 2, MSPSS Multidimensional Scale of Perceived Social Support
P value significant at two tailed

important cause of depression and anxiety in HCV patients and is sometimes associated with irritability, manic episodes, or acute confusional state [39]. Interferon is associated significantly with increased somatic but not cognitive affective symptoms of depression and with increased anxiety and fatigue during treatment [40].

At the end of therapy, the perceived support was not significantly different among dual and triple users. However, there was a significant effect of time on changing the score of perceived social support, where dual and triple users reported higher perceived support during the course of therapy than in baseline and end of therapy. This finding was similar to previous studies that reported that with increasing disease severity there is increased family support [29, 41].

By the end of therapy, it was observed that the mean score of HRQoL, symptom severity and hindrance, depression, anxiety and stress, had improved in the two arms of therapy, with no significant difference between them. On the other hand, in the only recent large identified study, fatigue, HRQoL using a disease specific CLDQ-HCV and generic SF-36 and work productivity were examined between patients receiving the triple therapy and patients receiving dual therapy [25]. It was found that patients receiving the triple therapy ($n = 327$)

Table 7 Predictors of HRQoL of DAAs therapy users prior, during and at the end of therapy

Model		Summary of the model			Unstandardized Coefficients	Standardized Coefficients			95.0% Confidence Interval for B		Collinearity Statistics	
		R	R^2	AdjR^2	B	Beta	t	Sig.	Lower Bound	Upper Bound	Tolerance	VIF
T0	(Constant)	.63	.39	.38	15.79		4.46	.000	8.69	22.89		
	Depression-T0				1.11	.41	3.13	.003	.39	1.83	.65	1.53
	Anxiety-T0				.98	.29	2.21	.032	.09	1.87	.65	1.53
T1	(Constant)	.88	.78	.76	18.13		1.45	.153	-6.95	43.21		
	Stress-T1				1.39	.44	4.04	.000	.70	2.09	.36	2.76
	HRQoL-T0				.37	.31	3.54	.001	.16	.58	.56	1.77
	Anxiety-T1				.91	.24	2.27	.028	.10	1.72	.37	2.66
	BMI-T1				-2.39	-.47	-2.82	.007	-4.11	-.69	.16	6.25
	BMI-T0				1.91	.35	2.12	.040	.09	3.730	.15	6.32
T2	(Constant)	.91	.83	.81	34.92		3.42	.002	13.97	55.87		
	HRQoL-T1				.68	.72	5.52	.000	.43	.93	.36	2.72
	Anxiety-T2				2.11	.66	5.27	.000	1.29	2.93	.46	2.17
	MSPSS-T2				-12.81	-.25	-3.09	.005	-21.33	-4.29	.93	1.06
	Anxiety-T1				-1.14	-.33	-2.11	.044	-2.25	-.03	.25	3.91

HRQoL-T0 health-related quality of life time 0, BMI-T1 body mass index time 1, BMI-T0 body mass index time 0, HRQoL-T1 health-related quality of life time 1, MSPSS-T2 Multidimensional Scale of Perceived Social Support time 2
P value significant at two tailed

experienced poorer HRQoL and work productivity than patients receiving the dual therapy ($n = 201$) ($p \leq 0.01$) at the end of treatment [25]. Interferon in general has a negative impact on patients' HRQoL during the course of therapy and the potential low adherence to the treatment regimen was confirmed [42, 43]. Otherwise, our study found no significant difference between the two regimens, although the dual therapy had a minimal negative impact on patients' HRQoL compared to the triple therapy. Our explanation is that the shorter duration of the treatment course (24/12 weeks according to the regimen type) may have been related to the lower treatment-related PROs burden of these patients and therefore enhancing their adherence level to medication would be expected [25]. However, it may also be due to the difference in methodology used between our study and Younossi's study [25] in terms of questionnaires used and time point measurements. Also, the sample size was smaller than previous studies, which might not be helpful in finding a significant difference at the end of therapy between the two groups of therapy.

Objective 2: PROs of dual users versus triple users prior, during and at the end of treatment

A comparison of the pattern of change in PROs among triple and dual therapy users through the three time periods revealed that triple therapy users were significantly more likely to report poorer HRQoL, symptom severity, symptom hindrance and depression, and increase in

perceived social support score at T1 than at baseline. In contrast, dual users had no significant change in their HRQoL, symptom experience and mental health, while their perceived social support was significantly increased during T1 in comparing to T0 and T2 like triple therapy users. This finding indicates that whatever the type of therapy, patients reported a high perceived support from their spouse, family and friends. Culturally this finding is unsurprising as social support increases during illness. Previously, interferon-free regimens have a modest negative effect on PROs whatever the disease stage [44].

Objective 3: Predictors of HRQoL of DAAs therapy users prior, during and at the end of therapy

A number of multivariate analyses were run to identify the independent predictors of HRQoL at the three different points in time. At baseline, the eight factors in the model significantly explained 37.5% of the variance in overall HRQoL prior to therapy. However, only anxiety and depression were significant variables, which appear to be the key determinants for HRQoL prior to therapy. Similar to a previous study [25], our study showed that pre-treatment depression and anxiety are the major factors associated with impaired HRQoL among patients with HCV before initiation of treatment. The high prevalence of depression, stress and anxiety in patients with HCV before the initiation of treatment has previously been reported [36]. Using the backwards multivariate linear regression, Bonkovsky et al [33] found that depression and anxiety [using the Beck Depression Inventory (BDI)] were significantly associated with impaired HRQoL summary scores (using the SF-36). It was also reported that the severity of depressive symptoms was highly correlated with fatigue severity, functional disability and somatization [45]. Baseline depression, anxiety, treatment-related adverse events and cirrhosis have been found to be the most consistent independent predictors of disease specific quality of life using the CLDQ-HCV at all points in time [25, 36]. In patients with cirrhosis who were treated with dual or triple therapy, the multivariate analysis at baseline showed that, being female, baseline depression, anxiety, insomnia, fatigue, a history of unsuccessful treatment, and having cirrhosis were associated with more impairment in PROs (i.e. Functional Assessment of Chronic Illness Therapy-Fatigue, CLDQ-HCV, Work Productivity and Activity Impairment Questionnaire: Specific Health Problem [WPAI-SHP]) scores. Furthermore, during treatment, receiving an IFN-containing regimen was another independent predictor of PROs impairment, whereas having cirrhosis was no longer associated with any of the PROs impairment during treatment [44].

Accordingly, whatever the liver disease stage and the instruments that were used to examine the association between mental health status and HRQoL, it has been found that depression and anxiety were significantly associated with HRQoL of patients with HCV. Therefore, the high prevalence of depression and anxiety symptoms among HCV patients not receiving antiviral therapy have justified the importance of regular psychosocial screening and support for them independent of antiviral therapy [45]. It is important to keep in mind that, prior to the initiation of treatment, patients with HCV appeared to experience impairment of their HRQoL [38]. In a cross-sectional study of 81 HCV-infected patients who were not receiving antiviral therapy, anxiety, depression, psychopathological symptoms, social support and resilience were assessed [41]. It was found that depression and anxiety scores were significantly higher among HCV patients than in a healthy control group [41] as 62.9% of HCV patients had a major depressive disorder diagnosis, and 42.3% had significant depressive symptoms, according to the BDI-II [46].

After 5 to 6 weeks of therapy (T1), the model significantly explained 76% of the variance in the HRQoL. HRQoL T0 & BMI T0 prior to therapy; and Stress T1, Anxiety T1 & BMI T1 during therapy significantly explained the variation in HRQoL during the course of therapy. These findings give support to the important role that these factors play in HRQoL of HCV patients during therapy. These results were previously unknown; therefore, it was difficult to compare our study's findings with previous studies. In patients with cirrhosis who

were treated with dual or triple therapy, the multivariate analysis during treatment (4 weeks after starting therapy) showed that being female, baseline depression, anxiety, insomnia, fatigue, and having a history of unsuccessful treatment, and receiving an IFN-containing regimen were the predictors of PROs impairment [Functional Assessment of Chronic Illness Therapy-Fatigue, CLDQ-HCV, WPAI-SHP]), whereas having cirrhosis was not associated with any of the PROs impairment during treatment [44].

Based on our study's findings, we recommend that baseline HRQoL and BMI should be systematically assessed before starting the antiviral therapy for early detection and the improvement of the impairment before the initiation of therapy. Also, the patients' anxiety, stress and BMI should be frequently assessed and followed up through the course of antiviral therapy. Additionally, HRQoL & anxiety during the course of therapy and perceived support & anxiety at the end of therapy significantly and respectively predict the variations in HRQoL T2 at the end of therapy. A pervious study found that a history of pre-treatment anxiety, depression, fatigue, female gender, and presence of cirrhosis were major predictors of disease specific quality of life impairment [25].

Additionally, our results confirmed previously reported data that anxiety is one of the major constant predictors of HRQoL impairment (at different time points) [25]. Therefore, health care providers should develop a supportive care program to help decrease anxiety levels that might later impact on these patients HRQoL. Studying this relationship in these patients is highly recommended. Also, a comprehensive care plan including all these associated factors is urgently needed to avoid the deterioration of patients' HRQoL during the course of therapy. Also, an exploration of the causes of increased anxiety among HCV patients at baseline and during the course of antiviral therapy is required.

Comparison between males and females

We found that females had a higher depression level and an increased impaired HRQoL than males prior to treatment even after controlling for age, PCR T0, BMI T0 and duration of disease in months. A comparison between male and female patients revealed that our findings were similar to a previous study [36]. Bonkovsky et al. [33], using a multivariate model, found that female gender, greater BMI, older age, current cigarette smoking, a higher depression score, and use of antidepressant or anxiolytic medications at baseline were significant predictors of poor HRQoL, particularly of the physical summary score among HCV patients [33]. However, at the end of treatment, our study did not agree with the findings of a previous study [36] which found that females had poorer PRQs than males at the end of treatment.

Interestingly, although females had a significantly lower PCR (viral load) than males prior to therapy, they experienced poorer HRQoL, higher depression, higher symptom severity and hindrance of symptoms. Similarly, Younossi et al (2014) [36] found that females, without considering the viral load, showed more impairment in PROs than males; including physical components of SF-36, physical well-being, fatigue, systematic domains of CLDQ-HCV and activity impairment. Clearly, further research is required to investigate this further.

Nurses and healthcare providers should therefore care for these female patients, particularly their mental health status and depression symptoms, by developing intervention programs that aim to improve their mental health status, which will be reflected on their HRQoL and their overall life. Due to the reduced sample size at time points two and three (T1 & T2), there is an urgent need to repeat this study, but using a larger balanced sample of male and female patients in Egypt and elsewhere.

Recommendations

Anxiety has been found to be high in patients receiving HCV antiviral therapy, particularly those following triple therapy. Consequently, we highly recommend that anxiety among these patients be systematically researched and analysed and a nursing intervention plan be developed to support these individuals. The patient's perspective in terms of PROs (i.e. HRQoL, mental health and perceived social support) must be considered by nurses and healthcare providers regularly in the plan of care to improve treatment experience by decreasing the treatment burden.

A symptom management program should be developed and delivered by highly qualified and well trained nurses to HCV-patients who attend regular consultations during the antiviral therapy. Also, a phone number should be available for delivering symptom management advice at any time and at any place according to the patient's needs and without interrupting the health care providers' work. Designing simple illustrated educational materials as guidance would be helpful to answer some of these patients' questions and explain the treatments adverse effects as well as how to overcome them during the course of therapy.

Although this study used a quantitative approach, some patients gave qualitative comments to "explain" their answer, which increased the understanding of patients' suffering as well as their needs. Therefore, a qualitative approach is recommended to explore psychosocial needs and to suggest self-care approaches that can help

these patients to overcome the medications adverse effects as well as symptom hindrance.

Face to face interviews were used to complete the instruments, as most of the patients were uneducated. This approach was time consuming to the researcher as well as to the participants. Thus, it was appropriate to use only a disease specific HRQoL questionnaire (i.e. LDSI-2.0) alongside the other instruments. Using a disease specific HRQoL questionnaire was helpful in identifying the unique symptoms experienced by patients on antiviral therapy. Subsequently, we recommend that future studies demonstrate both generic and disease specific HRQoL measurements to gain more insights into patterns of change in various domains of HRQoL among these patients, and which domains are more likely to be affected during the course of therapy.

Health-related quality of life is a complex concept with numerous dimensions. It should be an important outcome measure for all persons with HCV generally, and on antiviral therapy specifically, to ensure that the healthcare resources and medical treatment, as well as nursing interventions offered to this population are providing an improvement in patient's daily activities and well-being. Ascertaining HRQoL requires engaging the patients in their plan of treatment and intervention, as this cannot be ascertained independently by a clinician or the nurse.

Potential limitations

The fact that patients know whether they have responded to treatment when they complete the HRQOL instruments, has been considered a potential confounder in most longitudinal studies of HRQOL in chronic hepatitis C [33]. However, in this study we could not control patients' and health care providers' blindness to the PCR results at the time of data collection. Therefore, some of the patients did know their PCR results during data collection, which may have affected the patients' anxiety level as well as their HRQoL.

The participants were recruited from one centre largely due to the resources available to the research team. It was felt however, that a representative sample was obtained, as all the other centres were very similar in patient demographics, as well as clinic resources, policies and procedures. All these centres follow the same set of national guidelines for the treatment of patients with chronic HCV and are supervised by the NCCVH.

The limited sample size may have been one of the reasons that we found no significant association between some of the studied variables. Replicating this study with a larger sample of patients is needed to establish the reliability of these results.

Taking into consideration the real life nature of the treatment, losses in the availability of laboratory results during treatment and follow up did occur, which made it difficult to keep data consistency. Therefore, a future study should consider the haemoglobin levels during the follow up of the HRQoL.

Conclusions

This study found a significant change in HRQoL across the three different time periods among patients receiving DAAs. Only perceived support at baseline and anxiety during treatment were significantly higher among the triple therapy group than dual group when comparing the three different time points. At baseline, depression was the main variable that contributed to predicting change in HRQoL prior to therapy. During therapy, stress-T1, body mass index (BMI)-T1 and HRQoL-T0 significantly and respectively predicted HRQoL-T1. At the end of therapy, HRQoL-T1 and anxiety-T2 significantly predicted the variation in HRQoL-T2.

This study's findings highlight the critical importance of assessing HRQoL, mental health and perceived social support in patients receiving HCV antiviral therapy. These study's findings add value to what is important to healthcare providers by including outcomes from the patients' perspective. Therefore, the patient's perspective in terms of HRQoL, mental health and perceived social support should be fully considered by nurses and healthcare providers when planning care.

Abbreviations

BDI: Beck depression inventory; BMI: Body mass index; CASE-Index: Center for adherence support evaluation index; DAAs: Direct acting antivirals; DASS-21: The depression anxiety stress scale; HCV: Hepatitis C virus; HRQoL: Health-related quality of life; INDEXSCORE: Index score for the center for adherence support evaluation index; LDSI-2.0: The liver disease symptom index-2.0; MSPSS: The multidimensional scale of perceived social support; NHTMRI: National Hepatology and Tropical Medicine Research Institute; PCR: Polymerase Chain Reaction; Peg-IFN: Pegylated interferon; PROs: Patient reported outcomes; T0: Time 0 for data collection before/baseline data; T1: Time 1 after 4/5 weeks after therapy; T2: Time 2 at the end of therapy; WPAI-SHP: Work Productivity and Activity Impairment Questionnaire: Specific Health Problem

Acknowledgements

We are grateful to all the patients who participated in this study. We would also like to express our deep thanks to all the physicians and staff for their kind cooperation and support during the recruitment process. We also thank Stirling University APC Fund for publishing costs.

Funding

There was no external funding available to conduct this study. The only funding available to this research team was that provided by the Article Processing Charge (APC) Fund, University of Stirling, Stirling, UK for publishing charges.

Authors' contributions

All the authors designed the study. NY was responsible for data collection, statistical analysis, interpretation of data and drafting of the manuscript. AF shared in data entering. AS and MK revised the manuscript. All authors critically revised and approved the final manuscript.

Competing interests

The authors declare that they have no competing interests.

Consent for publication

Not applicable.

Author details

[1]Faculty of Nursing, Cairo University, Cairo 11562, Egypt. [2]Faculty of Medicine, Helwan University, Cairo, Egypt. [3]Faculty of Health Sciences and Sport, University of Stirling, Stirling FK9 4LA, Scotland, UK.

References

1. Mohd Hanafiah K, Groeger J, Flaxman AD, Wiersma ST. Global epidemiology of hepatitis C virus infection: New estimates of age-specific antibody to HCV seroprevalence. Hepatology. 2013;57(4):1333–42.
2. Lavanchy D. Evolving epidemiology of hepatitis C virus. Clin Microbiol Infect. 2011;17(2):107–15.
3. Guerra J, Garenne M, Mohamed MK, Fontanet A. HCV burden of infection in Egypt: results from a nationwide survey. J Viral Hepat. 2012;19(8):560–7.
4. Vietri J, Prajapati G, El Khoury AC. The burden of hepatitis C in Europe from the patients' perspective: a survey in 5 countries. BMC Gastroenterol. 2013; 13(1):1.
5. Younossi ZM, Stepanova M. Hepatitis C virus infection, age, and Hispanic ethnicity increase mortality from liver cancer in the United States. Clin Gastroenterol Hepatol. 2010;8(8):718–23.
6. Spiegel BM, Younossi ZM, Hays RD, Revicki D, Robbins S, Kanwal F. Impact of hepatitis C on health related quality of life: a systematic review and quantitative assessment. Hepatology. 2005;41(4):790–800.
7. Brook RA, Kleinman NL, Su J, Corey-Lisle PK, Iloeje UH. Absenteeism and productivity among employees being treated for hepatitis C. Am J Manag Care. 2011;17(10):657–64.
8. Marcellin F, Préau M, Ravaux I, Dellamonica P, Spire B, Carrieri MP. Self-reported fatigue and depressive symptoms as main indicators of the quality of life (QOL) of patients living with HIV and Hepatitis C: implications for clinical management and future research. HIV Clin Trials. 2007;8(5):320–7.
9. Hamlyn AN. Hepatitis C: tackling the silent epidemic. Br J Hosp Med (London, England: 2005). 2005;66(10):579–82.
10. Younossi ZM, Stepanova M, Afdhal N, Kowdley KV, Zeuzem S, Henry L, Hunt SL, Marcellin P. Improvement of health-related quality of life and work productivity in chronic hepatitis C patients with early and advanced fibrosis treated with ledipasvir and sofosbuvir. J Hepatol. 2015;63(2):337–45. US Food and Drug Administration.
11. Patient-reported outcome measures: Use in medical product development to support labeling claims. Guidance for industry. http://www.fda.gov/downloads/Drugs/Guidances/UCM193282.pdf. Accessed 01 June 2016.
12. Anderson KL, Burckhardt CS. Conceptualization and measurement of quality of life as an outcome variable for health care intervention and research. J Adv Nurs. 1999;29:298–306.
13. Younossi ZM, Singer ME, Mir HM, Henry L, Hunt S. Impact of interferon free regimens on clinical and cost outcomes for chronic hepatitis C genotype 1 patients. J Hepatol. 2014;60(3):530–7.
14. Smith-Palmer J, Cerri K, Valentine W. Achieving sustained virologic response in hepatitis C: a systematic review of the clinical, economic and quality of life benefits. BMC Infect Dis. 2015;15(1):1.
15. McHutchison JG, Ware JE, Bayliss MS, Pianko S, Albrecht JK, Cort S, Yang I, Neary MP. The effects of interferon alpha-2b in combination with ribavirin on health related quality of life and work productivity. J Hepatol. 2001;34(1):140–7.
16. Ghany MG, Nelson DR, Strader DB, Thomas DL, Seeff LB. An update on treatment of genotype 1 chronic hepatitis C virus infection: 2011 practice guideline by the American Association for the Study of Liver Diseases. Hepatology. 2011;54(4):1433–44.

17. Bernstein D, Kleinman L, Barker CM, Revicki DA, Green J. Relationship of health-related quality of life to treatment adherence and sustained response in chronic hepatitis C patients. Hepatology. 2002;35(3):704–8.

18. Ridruejo E. Safety of direct-acting antivirals in the treatment of chronic hepatitis C. Expert Opin Drug Saf. 2014;13(3):307–19.

19. Trembling PM, Tanwar S, Dusheiko GM. Boceprevir: an oral protease inhibitor for the treatment of chronic HCV infection. Expert Rev Anti-Infect Ther. 2012;10(3):269–79.

20. Lam BP, Jeffers T, Younoszai Z, Fazel Y, Younossi ZM. The changing landscape of hepatitis C virus therapy: focus on interferon-free treatment. Ther Adv Gastroenterol. 2015;8(5):298–312.

21. Gaetano JN. Benefit–risk assessment of new and emerging treatments for hepatitis C: focus on simeprevir and sofosbuvir. Drug Healthcare Patient Saf. 2014;6:37.

22. Velosa J, Serejo F, Ramalho F, Marinho R, Rodrigues B, Baldaia C, Raimundo M, Ferreira P. A practical guide for antiviral therapy of chronic Hepatitis C. GE Portuguese J Gastroenterol. 2014;21(6):221–30.

23. Lawitz E, Mangia A, Wyles D, Rodriguez-Torres M, Hassanein T, Gordon SC, Schultz M, Davis MN, Kayali Z, Reddy KR, Jacobson IM. Sofosbuvir for previously untreated chronic hepatitis C infection. N Engl J Med. 2013;368(20):1878–87.

24. Younossi ZM, Kanwal F, Saab S, Brown KA, El-Serag HB, Kim WR, Ahmed A, Kugelmas M, Gordon SC. The impact of hepatitis C burden: an evidence-based approach. Aliment Pharmacol Ther. 2014;39(5):518–31.

25. Younossi ZM, Stepanova M, Henry L, Gane E, Jacobson IM, Lawitz E, Nelson D, Gerber L, Nader F, Hunt S. Effects of sofosbuvir-based treatment, with and without interferon, on outcome and productivity of patients with chronic hepatitis C. Clin Gastroenterol Hepatol. 2014;12(8):1349–59.

26. Gaber M, HCV Treatment in Egypt: Why cost remains a challenge? Economic and Social Justice Unit, November 2014. http://www.eipr.org/sites/default/files/pressreleases/pdf/hcv_treatment_in_egypt.pdf. Accessed 20 May 2016.

27. Aroian K, Templin TN, Ramaswamy V. Adaptation and psychometric evaluation of the Multidimensional Scale of Perceived Social Support for Arab immigrant women. Health Care Women Int. 2010;31(2):153–69.

28. Taouk M, Lovibond PF, Laube R. Psychometric properties of an Arabic version of the Depression Anxiety Stress Scales (DASS21). Report for New South Wales Transcultural Mental Health Centre, Cumberland Hospital, Sydney. 2001.

29. Youssef NF. Health-related quality of life, symptoms experience and perceived social support among patients with liver cirrhosis: a cross-sectional study in Egypt. PhD thesis. Scotland: University of Stirling; 2013. http://hdl.handle.net/1893/15990. Accessed 24 June 2016.

30. Van Der Plas SM, Hansen BE, De Boer JB, Stijnen T, Passchier J, Rob A, Schalm SW. The Liver Disease Symptom Index 2.0; validation of a disease-specific questionnaire. Qual Life Res. 2004;13(8):1469–81.

31. Mannheimer SB, Mukherjee R, Hirschhorn LR, Dougherty J, Celano SA, Ciccarone D, Graham KK, Mantell JE, Mundy LM, Eldred L, Botsko M. The CASE adherence index: A novel method for measuring adherence to antiretroviral therapy. AIDS Care. 2006;18(7):853–61.

32. Field A. Discovering statistics using IBM SPSS statistics. Sage; 2013.

33. Bonkovsky HL, Snow KK, Malet PF, Back-Madruga C, Fontana RJ, Sterling RK, Kulig CC, Di Bisceglie AM, Morgan TR, Dienstag JL, Ghany MG. Health-related quality of life in patients with chronic hepatitis C and advanced fibrosis. J Hepatol. 2007;46(3):420–31.

34. Younossi Z, Kallman J, Kincaid J. The effects of HCV infection and management on health-related quality of life. Hepatology. 2007;45(3):806–16.

35. Manos MM, Ho CK, Murphy RC, Shvachko VA. Physical, social, and psychological consequences of treatment for hepatitis C. Patient-Patient-Centered Outcomes Res. 2013;6(1):23–34.

36. Younossi ZM, Stepanova M, Zeuzem S, Dusheiko G, Esteban R, Hezode C, Reesink HW, Weiland O, Nader F, Hunt SL. Patient-reported outcomes assessment in chronic hepatitis C treated with sofosbuvir and ribavirin: the VALENCE study. J Hepatol. 2014;61(2):228–34.

37. Younossi Z, Henry L. The impact of the new antiviral regimens on patient reported outcomes and health economics of patients with chronic hepatitis C. Dig Liver Dis. 2014;46:S186–96.

38. Younossi ZM, Stepanova M, Henry L, Gane E, Jacobson IM, Lawitz E, Nelson D, Nader F, Hunt S. Minimal impact of sofosbuvir and ribavirin on health related quality of life in Chronic Hepatitis C (CH-C). J Hepatol. 2014;60(4):741–7.

39. Modabbernia A, Poustchi H, Malekzadeh R. Neuropsychiatric and Psychosocial Issues of Patients With Hepatitis C Infection: A Selective Literature Review. Hepat Mon. 2013;13(1):e8340. doi:10.5812/hepatmon.8340.

40. Huckans M, Fuller B, Wheaton V, Jaehnert S, Ellis C, Kolessar M, Kriz D, Anderson JR, Berggren K, Olavarria H, Sasaki AW, Chang M, Flora KD, Loftis JM. A longitudinal study evaluating the effects of interferon-alpha therapy on cognitive and psychiatric function in adults with chronic hepatitis C. J Psychosom Res. 2015;78:184–92.

41. Erim Y, Tagay S, Beckmann M, Bein S, Cicinnati V, Beckebaum S, Senf W, Schlaak JF. Depression and protective factors of mental health in people with hepatitis C: a questionnaire survey. Int J Nurs Stud. 2010;47(3):342–9.

42. Bezemer G, Van Gool AR, Verheij-Hart E, Hansen BE, Lurie Y, Esteban JI, Lagging M, Negro F, Zeuzem S, Ferrari C, Pawlotsky JM. Long-term effects of treatment and response in patients with chronic hepatitis C on quality of life. An international, multicenter, randomized, controlled study. BMC Gastroenterol. 2012;12(1):1.

43. Kamal SM, Ahmed A, Mahmoud S, Nabegh L, Gohary IE, Obadan I, Hafez T, Ghoraba D, Aziz AA, Metaoei M. Enhanced efficacy of pegylated interferon alpha-2a over pegylated interferon and ribavirin in chronic hepatitis C genotype 4A randomized trial and quality of life analysis. Liver Int. 2011;31(3):401–11.

44. Younossi ZM, Stepanova M, Nader F, Jacobson IM, Gane E, Nelson D, et al. Patient-reported outcomes in chronic hepatitis C patients with cirrhosis treated with sofosbuvir-containing regimens. Hepatology. 2014;59:2161–9.

45. Dwight MM, Kowdley KV, Russo JE, Ciechanowski PS, Larson AM, Katon WJ. Depression, fatigue, and functional disability in patients with chronic hepatitis C. J Psychosom Res. 2000;49(5):311–7.

46. Patterson AL, Morasco BJ, Fuller BE, Indest DW, Loftis JM, Hauser P. Screening for depression in patients with hepatitis C using the Beck Depression Inventory-II: do somatic symptoms compromise validity? Gen Hosp Psychiatry. 2011;33(4):354–6.

12

Noninvasive assessment of liver steatosis in children: the clinical value of controlled attenuation parameter

Giovanna Ferraioli[1*†] (ID), Valeria Calcaterra[2†], Raffaella Lissandrin[1], Marinella Guazzotti[3], Laura Maiocchi[1], Carmine Tinelli[4], Annalisa De Silvestri[4], Corrado Regalbuto[2], Gloria Pelizzo[3], Daniela Larizza[2] and Carlo Filice[1]

Abstract

Background: To assess the clinical validity of controlled attenuation parameter (CAP) in the diagnosis of hepatic steatosis in a series of overweight or obese children by using the imperfect gold standard methodology.

Methods: Consecutive children referred to our institution for auxological evaluation or obesity or minor elective surgery were prospectively enrolled. Anthropometric and biochemical parameters were recorded. Ultrasound (US) assessment of steatosis was carried out using ultrasound systems. CAP was obtained with the FibroScan 502 Touch device (Echosens, Paris, France). Pearson's or Spearman's rank correlation coefficient were used to test the association between two study variables. Optimal cutoff of CAP for detecting steatosis was 249 dB/m. The diagnostic performance of dichotomized CAP, US, body mass indexes (BMI), fatty liver index (FLI) and hepatic steatosis index (HSI) was analyzed using the imperfect gold standard methodology.

Results: Three hundred five pediatric patients were enrolled. The data of both US and CAP were available for 289 children. Steatosis was detected in 50/289 (17.3%) children by US and in 77/289 (26.6%) by CAP. A moderate to good correlation was detected between CAP and BMI ($r = 0.53$), FLI ($r = 0.55$) and HSI ($r = 0.56$). In obese children a moderate to good correlation between CAP and insulin levels ($r = 0.54$) and HOMA-IR ($r = 0.54$) was also found. Dichotomized CAP showed a performance of 0.70 (sensitivity, 0.72 [0.64–0.79]; specificity, 0.98 [0.97–0.98], which was better than that of US (performance, 0.37; sensitivity, 0.46 [0.42–0.50]; specificity, 0.91 [0.89–0.92]), BMI (performance, 0.22; sensitivity, 0.75 [0.73–0.77]; specificity, 0.57 [0.55–0.60]) and FLI or HSI.

Conclusions: For the evaluation of liver steatosis in children CAP performs better than US, which is the most widely used imaging technique for screening patients with a suspicion of liver steatosis. A cutoff value of CAP of 249 dB/m rules in liver steatosis with a very high specificity.

Keywords: Liver steatosis, Pediatric series, NAFLD, Obesity, Controlled attenuation parameter, Ultrasound, Transient elastography

Background

Non-alcoholic fatty liver disease (NAFLD) is becoming a major health problem in children with an increasing incidence due to sedentary lifestyles and hyper-caloric diets that are the main factors of the obesity epidemics. Ten years ago, it was estimated that in Europe roughly one obese child out of three was affected by hepatic steatosis [1]. A recent review on the burden of liver disease in Europe has reported an even higher prevalence (36–44%) [2]. A study conducted in the United States has reported that children with NAFLD have an increased risk of liver-related mortality and a survival significantly shorter than that observed in the general population of the same age and sex [3]. Thus, the diagnosis and treatment of NAFLD at an early stage is of outmost importance for limiting the progression of the pathology. Liver biopsy is the reference standard for the assessment of liver steatosis, however the

* Correspondence: giovanna.ferraioli@unipv.it

†Equal contributors

[1]Ultrasound Unit, Department of Infectious Diseases, Fondazione IRCCS Policlinico San Matteo, University of Pavia, Viale Camillo Golgi 19, Pavia 27100, Italy

Full list of author information is available at the end of the article

procedure is invasive, has several limitations including intra and inter-observer variability in specimen's readings, and it's unpractical for screening purpose or to follow-up patients.

Ultrasound (US) is the imaging modality most widely used for the noninvasive assessment of liver steatosis. A good diagnostic accuracy of US for the detection of moderate to severe steatosis in children has been reported, with an area under the receiver operating characteristic (AUROC) curve of 0.87 [4]. However, US has a low sensitivity for the detection of mild steatosis [5].

Controlled attenuation parameter (CAP) is a method for the non-invasive assessment of liver steatosis. It measures the attenuation of the ultrasound beam that traverses the liver tissue, which increases in fatty liver, and is obtained by analyzing the ultrasound signal acquired by the transient elastography device (Fibroscan 502 Touch, Echosens, Paris, France) [6]. It has been shown that CAP has a good accuracy for quantifying liver steatosis also in pediatric patients [7].

The main aim of this study was to assess the clinical validity of CAP in the early diagnosis of hepatic steatosis in a series of overweight or obese children by using the imperfect gold standard methodology. Secondary aim was to analyze any association of CAP with liver stiffness values and with other indices of NAFLD.

Methods

Design of the study and patients

This was a single center cross-sectional study. From September 2012 to May 2016, consecutive children referred to our institution for auxological evaluation or obesity by their general practitioner or primary care pediatric consultant, scheduled for abdominal US examination and accepting to undergo also to CAP and liver stiffness measurements (LSM)s, were prospectively enrolled. Children referred to the outpatient clinic of the paediatric surgery department of our institution for minor elective surgery were also enrolled as controls.

The exclusion criteria were known secondary obesity conditions, the use of any medications, and concomitant chronic or acute illnesses.

According to the body mass indexes (BMI), the subjects were divided into three groups: obese subjects (group1): BMI that exceeded the 95th percentile for the age and sex; overweight subjects (group2): BMI 75th–95th percentile; normal weight subjects (group3): BMI < 75th percentile.

The study protocol was approved by the ethics committee of the Fondazione IRCCS Policlinico San Matteo (reference number 20120020673) and it was in accordance with the Helsinki Declaration of 1975, as revised in 2008. All the participants or their responsible guardians gave their written consent after being informed about the nature of the study.

Physical examination and biochemical parameters

The physical examination of the participants included evaluation of height, weight, body mass index (BMI), waist circumference, pubertal stage according to Marshall and Tanner, and measurement of the blood pressure.

Metabolic blood assays included fasting blood glucose, insulin, total cholesterol, high-density lipoprotein (HDL) cholesterol, triglycerides (TG), and transaminases. Insulin resistance was determined by the homeostasis model assessment for insulin resistance (HOMA-IR) using the formula: insulin resistance = (insulin × glucose)/22.5.

Abnormalities in lipid fasting levels were considered for TG values exceeding the 95th percentile and HDL cholesterol values below the fifth percentile for age and sex. Impaired insulin sensitivity was defined with HOMA-IR that exceeded the 97.5th percentile for age and sex.

Metabolic syndrome (MS) was diagnosed according to Weiss using the criteria modified from those of the National Cholesterol Education Program's Adult Treatment Panel III (NCEP-ATPIII) and the World Health Organization [8]. Patients were classified as having MS if they met three or more of the following criteria for age and sex: BMI > 95th percentile, TG levels > 95th percentile, HDL cholesterol level < 5th percentile, systolic and/or diastolic blood pressure > 95th percentile and fasting blood glucose >100 mg/dl and/or impaired insulin sensitivity with HOMA-IR > 97.5th percentile. In the definition by Weiss, BMI was chosen as a criterion for the MS because it correlates with visceral lipid depot, blood pressure and dyslipidemia. Although waist circumference is a good predictor of visceral adiposity in children, it might not detect differences in body proportions related to puberty and therefore no normative values exist for children and adolescents. Impaired insulin sensitivity was included because impaired fasting glucose is rare in childhood. Finally, blood pressure and fasting lipid levels were compared with population norms adjusted for age and sex.

Fatty liver index (FLI) and hepatic steatosis index (HSI) were obtained using the established formulas [9, 10]. FLI is an algorithm based on BMI, waist circumference, triglycerides and gamma-glutamyl-transferase and has been developed to detect steatosis [9], whereas HSI includes alanine aminotransferase (ALT)/aspartate aminotransferase (AST) ratio, BMI, diabetes mellitus and sex, and has been developed to detect NAFLD [10].

Ultrasound examination, controlled attenuation parameter and liver stiffness measurements

The US assessment of liver steatosis was performed using the iU22 system (Philips Medical Systems, Bothell, USA) or the HI VISION Ascendus system (Hitachi Ltd, Japan) equipped with convex multifrequency probes. The evaluation of liver steatosis was based on a series of

US findings including liver echogenicity, hepatorenal echo contrast, visualization of intrahepatic vessels, and visualization of liver parenchyma and the diaphragm. Steatosis was scored as follows: absent (score 0) steatosis was defined as normal liver echotexture; mild (score 1) steatosis as slight and diffuse increase in fine parenchymal echoes with normal visualization of diaphragm and portal vein borders; moderate (score 2) steatosis as moderate and diffuse increase in fine echoes with slightly impaired visualization of portal vein borders and diaphragm; severe (score 3) steatosis as fine echoes with poor or no visualization of portal vein borders, diaphragm, and posterior portion of the right lobe [4, 11]. The operators performing the examinations had at least 5 years of experience in US studies.

CAP was obtained by using the FibroScan 502 Touch device with the 3.5 MHz M probe or 2.5 MHz XL probes. CAP is a method for noninvasively quantifying the fat in the liver. The device estimates liver stiffness in kiloPascal (kPa) and liver steatosis in decibel/meter (dB/m). The principles of CAP have been described elsewhere [6]. CAP estimates the attenuation of the ultrasound waves at the central frequency of the probe of the Fibroscan device, and is guided by vibration-controlled transient elastography, ensuring that the operator automatically obtains the attenuation value of the liver. CAP was computed only when the associated LSM was valid and using the same signals as the one used to measure liver stiffness. As reported in the literature, only LSMs with 10 validated measurements and an interquartile range/median (IQR/M) <30% for values higher than 7.1 kPa were considered reliable [12]. There are no recommendations for successful CAP measurement. Examinations with no successful measurements after 10 attempts were deemed failures. Following a fast of at least 6 h, measurements were performed with the M probe when the skin to liver capsule distance, estimated with US, was ≤ 25 mm, otherwise the XL probe was used. In subjects with a thoracic perimeter less than 75 cm CAP measurements were not performed because the CAP is not available yet on the 5 MHz S probe, which is specifically designed for the assessment of these subjects. In each patient, the LSMs and CAP measurements were performed by the same physician who had performed the US exam.

Statistical analysis

Power considerations: The comparison between children with obesity and children non obese, was used to investigate the discriminant validity of CAP. In the hypothesis of a significant percentage of steatosis of 50 in the first group and 20 in the second [4], a sample size of 80 in each group will have more than 90% power to detect that difference using a the two-sided Z test with pooled variance with a 0.01 significance level. In view of the possibility of missing data, at least 100 patients and 100 controls should be enrolled.

Descriptive statistics were produced for demographic characteristics for this study sample of patients. The Shapiro-Wilk test was used to test the normal distribution of quantitative variables. When quantitative variables were normally distributed, the results were expressed as the mean value and standard deviation (SD), otherwise median and interquartile range (IQR; 25th–75th percentile) were reported. Qualitative variables were summarized as counts and percentages. Pearson's correlation coefficient was used to test the association between two quantitative continuous variables; while Spearman's rank correlation coefficient was used to test the association between two ranked variables, or one ranked variable and one quantitative continuous variable. The correlations were categorized as follows: 0.00 to 0.25 none or slight; 0.25 to 0.50 fair to moderate; 0.50 to 0.75 moderate to good; 0.75 to 1.00 almost perfect [13].

The results of blood tests were missed for about 20% of the subjects; thus in order to calculate FLI and HSI we performed a multiple imputation of missing data. Ten datasets were created fitting regression models with TG, GGT, AST, ALT, glycaemia, waist circumference as dependent and BMI, gender and age independent variables.

The diagnostic performance of CAP, BMI with AST and/or ALT abnormal, HSI and FLI on diagnosing liver steatosis compared to the US score (gold standard) was assessed using receiver operating characteristic (ROC) curves and the area under the ROC (AUROC) curve analysis.

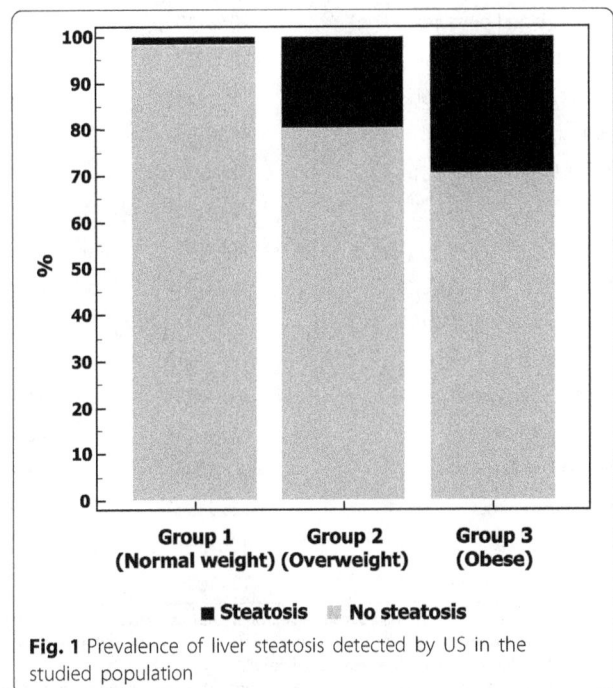

Fig. 1 Prevalence of liver steatosis detected by US in the studied population

As a subject's true disease status is seldom known with certainty, errors made by the gold standard mean that the sensitivity and specificity calculated for the new test are biased, and do not correctly estimate the new method's sensitivity and specificity. Therefore we fitted two-level Bayesian latent class models with discrete latent variables to estimate sensitivity, specificity, positive predictive value (PPV), and negative predictive value (NPV) of diagnostic tests (imperfect gold standard methodology), as previously reported [14]. Briefly, the observed results of the diagnostic tests are considered as a measure, prone to error, of an unobservable (latent) dichotomous variable, i.e. the true disease status of each subject.

To fit the model, the CAP was categorized as <249 dB/m and > =249 dB/m, i.e. the optimal cutoff obtained from our data (dichotomized CAP—dCAP), HSI and FLI as <0.3 and > =0.3, i.e. the value to rule out NAFLD or steatosis, respectively [9, 10]. To improve the performance of the models the BMI of patients (categorized according to age as normal vs overweight/obese and with AST and/or ALT abnormal) was added as

fourth test, since it has been previously used as an indicator of steatosis [15, 16].

$P < 0.05$ was considered statistically significant. All tests were two-sided. The data analysis was performed with the STATA statistical package (release 14.0, 2015, Stata Corporation, College (Station, Texas, USA)

Results

Overall 305 pediatric patients were enrolled of whom 199 (103 males, 96 females; mean age, 11.5 years ([SD: 2.7]; range, 4.1–17.4) were referred for auxological evaluation or obesity and 106 (64 males, 42 females; mean age, 9.9 [SD: 3.3 years] for minor elective surgery. 100/199 (50.3%) children referred for auxological evaluation or obesity were overweight (54 males, 46 females; mean age, 11.7 [SD: 2.6] years) and 99/199 (49.7%) children were obese (50 males, 49 females; mean age, 11.0 [SD: 2.9] years). The prevalence of liver steatosis estimated using US was 24.1%. 14/106 (13.2%) children referred for minor elective surgery were overweight (7 males, 7 females; mean age, 9.2 [SD: 2.5] years) and 2/106 (1.9%) children were obese

Table 1 Demographic, clinical and biochemical data of the studied population

Variabile	Overall N = 305	Group1 (Normal) N = 106	Group2 (Overweight) N = 100	Group3 (Obese) N = 99	P value #
Gender, female, N (%)	135 (44.8)	40 (38.5)	46 (46.9)	49 (49.4)	0.25
Age	10.9 (3.0)	10.1 (3.3)	11.8 (2.6)	11.0 (2.95)	<0.001[2]
Weight, kilograms	51.2 (19.9)	35.2 (12.2)	54.8 (13.8)	63.9 (20.4)	<0.001[*]
Height, meters	1.46 (0.16)	1.41 (0.17)	1.51 (0.14)	1.48 (0.16)	0.001[1,3]
BMI, kg/m^2	23.1 (5.7)	17.2 (2.8)	23.6 (2.3)	28.4 (4.4)	<0.001[*]
Waist circumference, cm	76.7 (17.2)	55.3 (11.5)	79.82 (9.1)	88.48 (11.8)	<0.001[*]
Systolic blood pressure, mmHg	107.8 (10.4)	110.9 (8.54)	106.3 (10.03)	106.9 (11.5)	0.02[1]
Diastolic blood pressure, mmHg	68.7 (8.3)	70.35 (7.63)	68.15 (7.83)	68.2 (9)	0.22
Total cholesterol, mg/dl	160.3 (29.5)	156.4 (29.4)	160.6 (28.3)	162.6 (30.5)	0.44
HDL cholesterol, mg/dl	48.9 (10.8)	52.7 (12.3)	49.4 (10.6)	46.2 (9.4)	0.001[1]
AST, IU/L	22.6 (8.69)	22.7 (6.45)	21.8 (9.01)	23.2 (9.9)	0.56
ALT, IU/L	20.8 (17.2)	15.1 (5.4)	21.4 (19.6)	25.0 (19.8)	0.001[3]
GGT, IU/L	16.5 (8.5)	13.3 (5.5)	16.7 (6.2)	18.9 (11.0)	<0.001[1,3]
Fasting blood glucose, mg/dl	76.6 (10.4)	76.0 (11.9)	76.7 (10.1)	77.1 (9.4)	0.78
Fasting insulin, microlU/ml	12.7 (9.1)	9.07 (6.1)	12.69 (8.5)	13.2 (10.0)	0.34
HOMA-IR, %	2.47 (1.9)	1.83 (1.22)	2.41 (1.71)	2.6 (2.17)	0.41
Triglycerides, mg/dl	72.2 (35.1)	63.6 (29.2)	75.3 (40.2)	74.8 (32.9)	0.09
Fatty liver index	0.18 (0.21)	0.03 (0.08)	0.14 (0.12)	0.3 (0.2)	<0.001[*]
Hepatic steatosis index	0.46 (0.34)	0.13 (0.18)	0.45 (0.26)	0.7 (0.2)	<0.001[*]
CAP, decibel/meter	228.5 (50.34)	200.5 (39.36)	231.6 (51.46)	254.6 (44.4)	<0.001[*]
LSM, kiloPascal	4.70 (.93)	4.59 (.96)	4.73 (.92)	4.80 (.9)	0.30
Metabolic syndrome, N (%)	12 (6.09)	0 (0)	7 (9.2)	5 (6.2)	0.143

BMI body mass index; *HDL* high-density lipoprotein; *AST* aspartate aminotransferase; *ALT* alanine aminotransferase; *GGT* gamma glutamyltransferase; *HOMA-IR* homeostasis model assessment for insulin resistance; *CAP* controlled attenuation parameter; *LSM* liver stiffness measurement. Values are reported as mean and standard deviation unless otherwise specified

P values refer to differences among three groups; [1] normal vs. overweight, [2]normal vs obese, [3]overweight vs obese: $p < 0.05$; [*] for all comparisons: $p < 0.01$

(2 females; mean age, 11.5 [SD: 6.5]). The prevalence of liver steatosis estimated using US was 2.8%.

The children of our cohort were assigned to group1, group2, or group3 according to their BMI. The prevalence of hepatic steatosis detected by US in the three groups is shown in Fig. 1. The demographic, clinical and biochemical data of our series are reported in Table 1.

Overall, MS occurred in five (6.2%) obese children, in seven (9.2%) overweight children and none child with normal weight ($p = 0.12$); no statistically significant difference was found between boys (9/99; 9.9%) and girls (3/98, 3.06%; $p = 0.08$).

One component of the MS was present in 46 (56.8%) obese children, 51 (67.1%) overweight children and 9 (22.5%) children with normal weight. Two components of the MS were found in 30 (37.0%) obese children, 18 (23.7%) overweight children and one (2.5%) child with normal weight.

Clinical and biochemical characteristics of the children with or without liver steatosis detected by US are reported in Table 2. Significant differences were found

Table 2 Clinical and biochemical characteristics of the children with and without liver steatosis detected with ultrasound

Variable	Liver steatosis [a]		P value
	Yes (N = 50)	No (N = 239)	
Age, years	11.6 (2.5)	10.8 (3.04)	0.06
Weight, kg	62.2 (16.0)	48.8 (19.7)	<0.001
Height, cm	1.54 (1.4–1.6)	1.47 (1.3–1.6)	.023
BMI, kg/m²	26.8 (4.1)	22.2 (5.5)	<0.001
Waist circumference, cm	86.58 (11.43)	74.1 (17.4)	<0.001
Systolic blood pressure, mmHg	107.65 (11.66)	108.0 (10.1)	0.85
Diastolic blood pressure, mmHg	69.38 (7.12)	68.8 (8.5)	0.67
Total cholesterol, mg/dl	159.1 (29.13)	160.6 (29.8)	0.75
HDL cholesterol, mg/dl	46.9 (10.34)	49.28 (11.0)	0.19
AST, IU/L	24.6 (10.2)	22.18 (8.3)	0.10
ALT, IU/L	32.6 (26.3)	18.16 (13.2)	<0.001
GGT, IU/L	15.2 (6.8)	22.4 (12.3)	<0.001
Fasting blood glucose, mg/dl	76.2 (9.1)	76.8 (10.6)	0.72
Fasting insulin, microIU/ml	15.7 (10.5)	11.8 (8.4)	0.012
HOMA-IR, %	3 (2.2)	2.3 (1.8)	0.04
Triglycerides, mg/dl	86.0 (49.4)	69.1 (30.6)	0.004
Fatty liver index	0.30 (0.20)	0.15 (0.19)	<0.001
Hepatic steatosis index	0.76 (0.24)	0.39 (0.32)	<0.001
CAP, decibel/meter	280.9 (54.1)	217.4 (41.8)	<0.001
LSM, kiloPascal	5.02 (1.03)	4.65 (0.89)	0.01

BMI body mass index; HDL high-density lipoprotein; AST aspartate aminotransferase; ALT alanine aminotransferase; GGT gamma glutamyltransferase; HOMA-IR homeostasis model assessment for insulin resistance; CAP: controlled attenuation parameter; LSM liver stiffness measurement
[a] Data [mean (SD)] of the 289 children for whom both US and CAP were available

for the anthropometric measures, ALT ($p < 0.001$), fasting insulin ($p = 0.01$), HOMA-IR ($p = 0.04$), triglycerides ($p = 0.004$), FLI ($p < 0.001$), HSI ($p < 0.001$), CAP ($p < 0.01$), and LSM ($p = 0.009$).

Controlled attenuation parameter

LSMs were obtained in 299/305 (98.0%) children. The six failures were due to narrow intercostal spaces. All LSMs were reliable. The M probe was used in 285/299 (95.3%) children, the XL probe in 10/299 (3.4%) children and the S probe in 4/299 (1.4%) children. In 4/299 (1.4%) the XL probe was used before the availability of CAP. Since CAP is not available yet on the S probe, only the data of 291 children examined with the M probe and XL probe were analyzed for the noninvasive assessment of liver steatosis with CAP. In two children US was not performed for technical reasons. Thus, the data of both CAP and US were available for 289 children. The mean LSM was 4.71 (SD: 0.93; range 2–7.8) kPa.

The distribution of CAP values in the three groups of children and in children without and with liver steatosis detected by US are reported in Figs. 2 and 3. CAP values were significantly lower in children with normal weight compared to overweight and obese children ($p < 0.001$). No differences were observed in LSM between the three groups (4.59 kPa [SD: 0.96], 4.73 kPa [SD: 0.92] and 4.79 kPa [SD: 0.90]; $p = 0.30$).

Steatosis was detected by US in 50/289 (17.3%) children and by CAP in 77/289 (26.6%).

A moderate to good correlation was detected between CAP and BMI ($r = 0.53$), FLI ($r = 0.55$) and HSI ($r = 0.56$). In the obese group a moderate to good correlation between CAP and insulin levels ($r = 0.54$) and HOMA-IR ($r = 0.54$) was also found. No significant correlation was found between CAP and the other study variables.

Diagnostic accuracy of noninvasive parameters of liver steatosis using US as the reference standard

The AUROCs of CAP, FLI, HSI, BMI + AST and/or ALT in the assessment of liver steatosis are reported in Fig. 4. The AUROC of CAP was 0.84 (95% CI:0.78–0.89, $p < 0.001$), which was higher than that of HSI (0.82; 95% CI:0.75–0.87), FLI (0.76; 95% CI:0.69–0.82), and BMI + AST and/or ALT (0.68; 95% CI:0.64–0.77).

Comparisons of AUROCs showed that CAP was significantly superior to BMI + AST and/or ALT ($p < 0.001$) whereas the differences between CAP and HSI, CAP and FLI were not statistically significant ($p = 0.58$ and $p = 0.10$, respectively).

Because several data for FLI and HSI calculation were missed, we compared FLI and HSI sensitivity/specificity calculated on complete cases and after

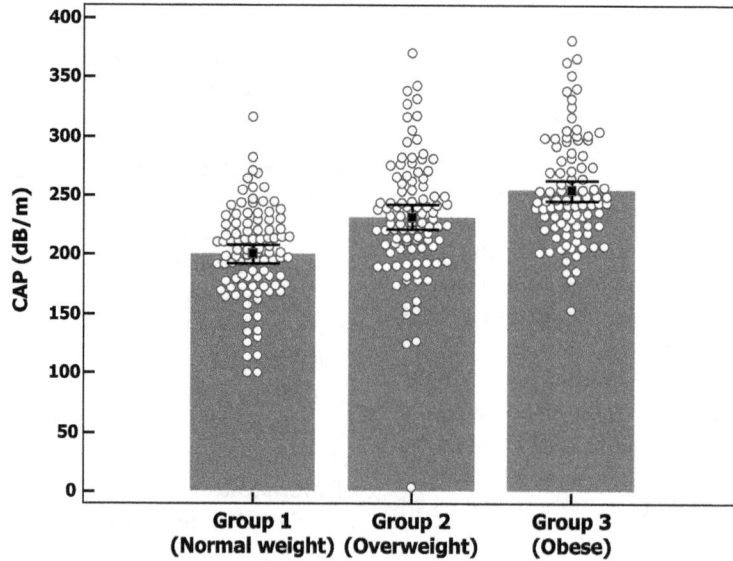

Fig. 2 Distribution of controlled attenuation parameter (CAP) values in the three groups of children

multiple imputation of missing data. On complete cases, FLI sensitivity and specificity were 0.44 (95% CI: 0.30–0.59) and 0.83 (95% CI: 0.78–0.87), whereas HSI sensitivity and specificity were 0.93 (95% CI: 0.84–0.99) and 0.48 (95% CI: 0.42–0.54). After multiple imputation of missing data FLI and HSI sensitivity/specificity were similar to those calculated on complete cases (FLI sensitivity 0.41 [95% CI: 0.27–0.55], specificity 0.84 (95% CI: 0.79–0.89); HSI sensitivity 0.88 (95% CI: 0.79–0.98), specificity 0.51 (95% CI: 0.44–0.57).

Performance of the noninvasive parameters of liver steatosis using the methodology without the gold standard and the Bayesian latent class model analysis

Because the models for the assessment of the performance without a gold standard require absolute independency of the diagnostic tests, we used two scenarios, one including dCAP, US, FLI, and BMI + AST and/or ALT, and the other one including the same parameters but with HSI instead of FLI. The results are reported in Table 3. In both scenarios dCAP showed the best performance with a sensitivity of 0.72 and a specificity of 0.98–1.00.

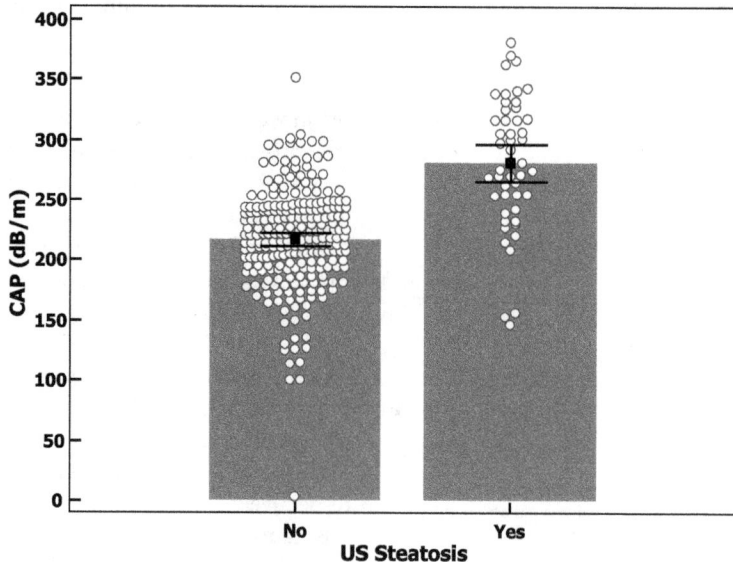

Fig. 3 Distribution of controlled attenuation parameter (CAP) values in children without and with liver steatosis detected by ultrasound

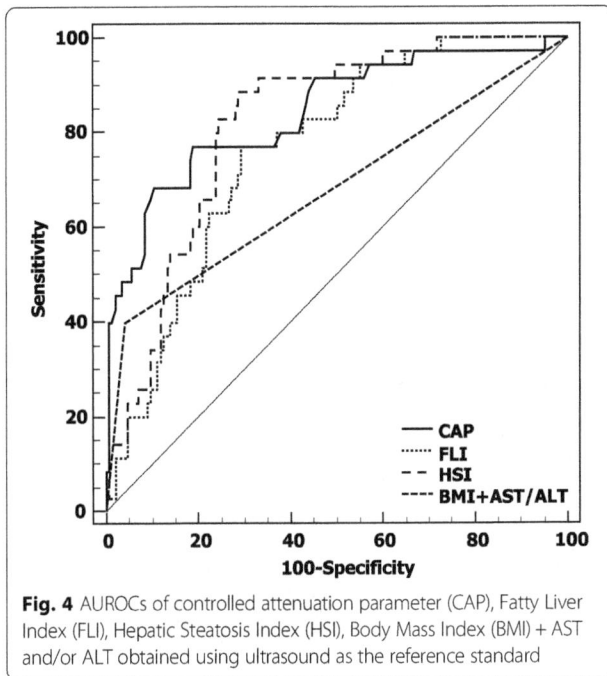

Fig. 4 AUROCs of controlled attenuation parameter (CAP), Fatty Liver Index (FLI), Hepatic Steatosis Index (HSI), Body Mass Index (BMI) + AST and/or ALT obtained using ultrasound as the reference standard

widely used technique for screening patients with a suspicion of liver steatosis. Over the years, the technological advancement of the US systems has led to an increase of the sensitivity of technique, which has been reported to be 0.90 in detecting steatosis involving at least 20% of the hepatocytes [17]. However, for lower levels of fat infiltration a negative US result does not rule out the presence of liver steatosis. Especially in children, it is of outmost importance to diagnose NAFLD at an early stage because a modification of the diet and of the lifestyle can avoid the progression to end-stage liver disease, whose incidence seems higher than in adults [18, 19]. Magnetic resonance spectroscopy is the most accurate method for the detection of fat in the liver, however the technique is costly and available only in few referral centers, and often requires sedation in children. CAP is a new noninvasive method that has shown promise in the assessment of steatosis also in pediatric patients. Recently, in a study performed in a small series of children in whom liver biopsy was carried out for clinical indications, a cut point of 225 dB/m for predicting steatosis has been identified, with 0.87 sensitivity, 0.83 specificity, and AUROC 0.93 [7]. The results of our study show that a CAP cutoff value of 249 dB/m rules in liver steatosis with a very high specificity. Moreover, steatosis was detected with CAP in 27 (9.3%) children with normal US findings. This finding suggests that CAP could be a useful tool for the diagnosis of liver steatosis at an early stage.

Discussion

The results of our study show that the diagnostic performance of CAP for the evaluation of liver steatosis was higher than that of US. Due to its noninvasiveness, availability, relatively low cost and repeatability because there is no exposition to ionizing radiation, US is the most

Table 3 Diagnostic accuracy of the noninvasive parameters of liver steatosis in the studied population using the imperfect gold standard methodology

Parameter	Sensitivity (95% CI)	Specificity (95% CI)	PPV (95% CI)	NPV (95% CI)	Performance [a]
Analysis with the imperfect gold standard methodology: scenario 1					
dCAP	0.72 (0.64–0.79)	0.98 (0.97–0.98)	0.93 (0.90–0.96)	0.89 (0.86–0.92)	0.70
Ultrasound	0.46 (0.42–0.50)	0.91 (0.89–0.92)	0.68 (0.62–0.73)	0.80 (0.78–0.81)	0.37
Fatty Liver index	0.73 (0.72–0.74)	0.27 (0.25–0.28)	0.30 (0.29–0.31)	0.7 (0.69–0.7)	0
BMI + AST and/or ALT	0.75 (0.73–0.77)	0.57 (0.55–0.60)	0.43 (0.41–0.45)	0.84 (0.82–0.86)	0.22
Analysis with the imperfect gold standard methodology: scenario 2					
dCAP	0.72 (0.69–0.78)	1.00 (1.00–1.00)	0.99 (0.99–1)	0.89 (0.88–0.91)	0.72
Ultrasound	0.43 (0.38–0.50)	0.99 (0.99–1.00)	0.96 (0.94–0.98)	0.8 (0.78–0.82)	0.42
Hepatic Steatosis Index	0.85 (0.84–0.85)	0.33 (0.32–0.35)	0.35 (0.34–0.36)	0.83 (0.82–0.84)	0.18
BMI + AST and/or ALT	0.73 (0.69–0.77)	0.73 (0.69–0.77)	0.54 (0.49–0.58)	0.86 (0.84–0.88)	0.54

PPV positive predictive value; *NPV* negative predictive value; *CI* 95% Credible Interval; *dCAP* dichotomized controlled attenuation parameter; *BMI* body mass index; *AST* aspartate aminotransferase; *ALT* alanine aminotransferase
[a] Performance = Sensitivity + Specificity - 100

In our series, children with liver steatosis showed LSMs significantly higher than those observed in children without steatosis by some 0.5 kPa. Although this difference was not relevant from a clinical point of view because these values were still in the normal range, we would like to underline that significant liver fibrosis was observed in one child with liver steatosis and in none child without. This finding confirms that liver steatosis is not always a benign condition, thus care should be taken to assess the disease at an early stage. On this regard, CAP seems a very useful tool.

FLI and HSI are biochemical indices of hepatic steatosis that have been derived and a currently used in the adult population, whereas data on children are scarce. In our series, similar to what observed in adults, a moderate to good correlation of CAP with these indices was detected, indicating that FLI and HSI could be used as noninvasive biomarkers of liver steatosis in the pediatric population as well. However, it has been reported that these indices have insufficient diagnostic accuracy for diagnosing or excluding NAFLD in severely obese children [20].

This study has limitations. First, we used the methodology without a gold standard since liver biopsy is not indicated for screening purpose even in a high risk population. The latent class analysis method for estimating test accuracy in the absence of a gold standard is well documented and has been applied in several studies [21]. Second, the biochemical data were not available for all children, thus we used the multiple imputation of missing data. However, the sensitivity and specificity were similar to those calculated with the complete data. Third, the children in our study were enrolled from pediatric patients referred to the hospital for auxological evaluation or obesity or elective minor surgery, therefore the results may not be applicable to the general population. Forth, since we used US as the reference standard to calculate the cutoff value of CAP for the detection of steatosis, we could have underestimated liver steatosis in our cohort. It is likely that with a lower cutoff, as the one obtained in the series of Desai et al [7] where liver biopsy was the reference standard, the performance of CAP would have been even higher than observed in our population.

Conclusions

For the evaluation of liver steatosis in children CAP performs better than US, which is the most widely used imaging technique for screening patients with a suspicion of liver steatosis. A cutoff value of CAP of 249 dB/m rules in liver steatosis with a very high specificity.

Abbreviations

ALT: Alanine aminotransferase; AST: Aspartate aminotransferase; AUROC: Area under the receiver operating characteristic; BMI: Body mass index; CAP: Controlled attenuation parameter; CI: Confidence interval; dB/ m: Decibel/meter; dCAP: Dichotomized CAP; FLI: Fatty liver index; HDL: High-density lipoprotein; HOMA-IR: Homeostasis model assessment for insulin resistance; HSI: Hepatic steatosis index; IQR: Interquartile range; IQR/ M: Interquartile range/median; kPa: kiloPascal; LSM: Liver stiffness measurements; MS: Metabolic syndrome; NAFLD: Non-alcoholic fatty liver disease; NCEP-ATP: National Cholesterol Education Program's Adult Treatment Panel; NPV: Negative predictive value; PPV: Positive predictive value; ROC: Receiver operating characteristic; SD: Standard deviation; TG: Triglycerides; US: Ultrasound

Acknowledgements

The authors would like to thank Ms. Nadia Locatelli, Secretary of the Ultrasound Unit, for her valuable help in complying with the study protocol.

Funding

This work has been supported by a grant given by the Italian Ministry of Health [RF-2011-02347402]. Carlo Filice is the recipient of the grant. The funding body had no role in the design of the study and collection, analysis, and interpretation of data and in writing the manuscript.

Authors' contributions

GF and CF developed the study protocol; VC, RL, MG, LM, CR performed the study and collected the data; CT and ADS analyzed and interpreted the patients' data; GF wrote the manuscript; VC, RL, MG, LM, CT, ADS, CR, GP, DL, CF critically revised the draft of the manuscript for important intellectual content; all authors read and approved the final manuscript and agreed to be accountable for all aspects of the work in ensuring that questions related to the accuracy or integrity of any part of the work are appropriately investigated and resolved.

Competing interests

GF has served as a speaker for Philips Healthcare, Hitachi Ltd., Toshiba Medical Systems. CF has served as a speaker for Philips Healthcare, Hitachi Ltd., Esaote S.p.A., and has received research funding from Esaote S.p.A., Bracco Imaging, Hitachi Ltd., Toshiba Medical Systems. VC, RL, MG, LM, CT, ADS, CR, GP, DL have no conflict of interest to declare.

Consent for publication

Not applicable.

Author details

[1]Ultrasound Unit, Department of Infectious Diseases, Fondazione IRCCS Policlinico San Matteo, University of Pavia, Viale Camillo Golgi 19, Pavia 27100, Italy. [2]Pediatric Unit, Department of the Mother and Child Health, Fondazione IRCCS Policlinico San Matteo, University of Pavia, Pavia, Italy. [3]Pediatric Surgery Unit, Department of the Mother and Child Health, Fondazione IRCCS Policlinico San Matteo, University of Pavia, Pavia, Italy. [4]Clinical Epidemiology and Biometric Unit, Fondazione IRCCS Policlinico San Matteo, Pavia, Italy.

References

1. Lobstein T, Jackson-Leach R. Estimated burden of paediatric obesity and co-morbidities in Europe. Part 2. Numbers of children with indicators of obesity-related disease. Int J Pediatr Obes. 2006;1(1):33–41. doi:10.1080/17477160600586689.
2. Blachier M, Leleu H, Peck-Radosavljevic M, Valla DC, Roudot-Thoraval F. The burden of liver disease in Europe: a review of available epidemiological data. J Hepatol. 2013;58(3):593–608. doi:10.1016/j.jhep.2012.12.005.
3. Feldstein AE, Charatcharoenwitthaya P, Treeprasertsuk S, Benson JT, Enders FB, Angulo P. The natural history of non-alcoholic fatty liver disease in children: a follow-up study for up to 20 years. Gut. 2009;58(11):1538–44. doi:10.1136/gut.2008.171280.
4. Shannon A, Alkhouri N, Carter-Kent C, Monti L, Devito R, Lopez R, et al. Ultrasonographic quantitative estimation of hepatic steatosis in children with NAFLD. J Pediatr Gastroenterol Nutr. 2011;53(2):190–5. doi:10.1097/MPG.0b013e31821b4b61.
5. Lee SS, Park SH, Kim HJ, Kim SY, Kim MY, Kim DY, et al. Non-invasive

assessment of hepatic steatosis: prospective comparison of the accuracy of imaging examinations. J Hepatol. 2010;52(4):579–85. doi:10.1016/j.jhep.2010. 01.008.

6. Sasso M, Beaugrand M, de Ledinghen V, Douvin C, Marcellin P, Poupon R, et al. Controlled attenuation parameter (CAP): a novel VCTE guided ultrasonic attenuation measurement for the evaluation of hepatic steatosis: preliminary study and validation in a cohort of patients with chronic liver disease from various causes. Ultrasound Med Biol. 2010;36(11):1825–35. doi: 10.1016/j.ultrasmedbio.2010.07.005.

7. Desai NK, Harney S, Raza R, Al-Ibraheemi A, Shillingford N, Mitchell PD, et al. Comparison of controlled attenuation parameter and liver biopsy to assess hepatic steatosis in pediatric patients. J Pediatr. 2016;173:160–4. doi:10.1016/ j.jpeds.2016.03.021. e161.

8. Weiss R, Dziura J, Burgert TS, Tamborlane WV, Taksali SE, Yeckel CW, et al. Obesity and the metabolic syndrome in children and adolescents. N Engl J Med. 2004;350(23):2362–74. doi:10.1056/NEJMoa031049.

9. Bedogni G, Bellentani S, Miglioli L, Masutti F, Passalacqua M, Castiglione A, et al. The Fatty Liver Index: a simple and accurate predictor of hepatic steatosis in the general population. BMC Gastroenterol. 2006;6:33. doi:10. 1186/1471-230X-6-33.

10. Lee JH, Kim D, Kim HJ, Lee CH, Yang JI, Kim W, et al. Hepatic steatosis index: a simple screening tool reflecting nonalcoholic fatty liver disease. Dig Liver Dis. 2010;42(7):503–8. doi:10.1016/j.dld.2009.08.002.

11. Kim SH, Lee JM, Kim JH, Kim KG, Han JK, Lee KH, et al. Appropriateness of a donor liver with respect to macrosteatosis: application of artificial neural networks to US images-initial experience. Radiology. 2005;234(3):793–803. doi:10.1148/radiol.2343040142.

12. Boursier J, Zarski JP, de Ledinghen V, Rousselet MC, Sturm N, Lebail B, et al. Determination of reliability criteria for liver stiffness evaluation by transient elastography. Hepatology. 2013;57(3):1182–91. doi:10.1002/hep.25993.

13. Colton T, editor. Statistics in medicine. Boston: Little, Brown and Company; 1974.

14. Ferraioli G, Tinelli C, De Silvestri A, Lissandrin R, Above E, Dellafiore C, et al. The clinical value of controlled attenuation parameter for the noninvasive assessment of liver steatosis. Liver Int. 2016;36(12):1860–6. doi:10.1111/liv.13207.

15. Peng CJ, Yuan D, Li B, Wei YG, Yan LN, Wen TF, et al. Body mass index evaluating donor hepatic steatosis in living donor liver transplantation. Transplant Proc. 2009;41(9):3556–9. doi:10.1016/j.transproceed.2009.06.235.

16. Rinella ME, Alonso E, Rao S, Whitington P, Fryer J, Abecassis M, et al. Body mass index as a predictor of hepatic steatosis in living liver donors. Liver Transpl. 2001;7(5):409–14. doi:10.1053/jlts.2001.23787.

17. Dasarathy S, Dasarathy J, Khiyami A, Joseph R, Lopez R, McCullough AJ. Validity of real time ultrasound in the diagnosis of hepatic steatosis: a prospective study. J Hepatol. 2009;51(6):1061–7. doi:10.1016/j.jhep.2009.09.001.

18. Berardis S, Sokal E. Pediatric non-alcoholic fatty liver disease: an increasing public health issue. Eur J Pediatr. 2014;173(2):131–9. doi:10. 1007/s00431-013-2157-6.

19. Rashid M, Roberts EA. Nonalcoholic steatohepatitis in children. J Pediatr Gastroenterol Nutr. 2000;30(1):48–53. doi:10.1097/00005176-200001000-00017.

20. Koot BG, van der Baan-Slootweg OH, Bohte AE, Nederveen AJ, van Werven JR, Tamminga-Smeulders CL, et al. Accuracy of prediction scores and novel biomarkers for predicting nonalcoholic fatty liver disease in obese children. Obesity (Silver Spring). 2013;21(3):583–90. doi:10.1002/oby.20173.

21. Rutjes AW, Reitsma JB, Coomarasamy A, Khan KS, Bossuyt PM. Evaluation of diagnostic tests when there is no gold standard. A review of methods. Health Technol Assess. 2007;11(50):iii. doi:10.3310/hta11500. ix-51.

13

A rare cause of acute liver failure

Sónia Bernardo*, Sofia Carvalhana, Teresa Antunes, Paula Ferreira, Helena Cortez-Pinto and José Velosa

Abstract

Background: Acute liver failure (ALF) induced by diffuse metastatic disease has rarely been reported.

Case presentation: We present a 51-years-old woman with relevant clinical history for breast cancer. The patient was admitted in the emergency department with jaundice, dark urine and pale stools. She was on the 10th day of hormonotherapy for recurrence of breast cancer, diagnosed 7 years previously. Usual causes of acute liver failure were excluded, all drugs were stopped and the imaging studies performed were positive only for steatosis. Nonetheless, ALF progressed and the patient died 4 days later. Autopsy demonstrated a massive intrasinusoidal infiltration of the liver by breast cancer cells.

Conclusion: We highlight a rare cause of ALF. Although uncommon, physicians should be alert for this situation as the diagnosis can be challenging and the imaging studies can remain normal.

Keywords: Acute liver failure, Diffuse malignant infiltration

Background

ALF is defined by acute liver dysfunction manifesting as coagulopathy (INR ≥ 1.5) and presence of hepatic encephalopathy of any degree with less than 26 weeks duration, in a patient without preexisting liver disease [1].

The incidence of ALF is 2000 cases/year in USA [1]. The etiology varies broadly throughout the world and the most common causes of ALF are drug toxicity (50%), viral hepatitis (9%) and autoimmune hepatitis (7%) [2, 3]. However, in 20-40% of the cases the etiology remains unknown after an extensive workup [2].

The liver is a common target for metastasis, with 40% of autopsies in adults with malignant tumors, identifying liver metastases [4]. Nonetheless, a significant number of cases are asymptomatic with mild abnormal liver tests.

Malignancy is an uncommon cause of ALF and in very rare cases (0.44-1.4%) [3, 5] can occur due to a diffuse pattern of metastatic infiltration to the liver [3]. Different cancers have been associated with ALF [4]. Hematologic malignancies are the most common (41%), especially non-Hodgkin lymphoma [3, 4] but it also occurs with solid tumors, including breast (30%) [3], lung, pancreatic and gastric cancers for example.

The diagnosis of wide infiltration of the liver can be challenging because imaging studies are not able to detect this type of infiltration pattern and just 25% of the cases are diagnosed *premortem* [6]. Most cases have a poor prognostic, with death occurring in the majority and within several days of clinical presentation [2].

We report a case of ALF induced by metastatic infiltration of a breast cancer diagnosed 7 years before. We appraise the clinical and laboratorial findings, discuss treatment and prognosis, and review the available literature.

Case presentation

We report a case of a 51 years-old woman with medical relevant story of ductal breast carcinoma, submitted to mastectomy followed by adjuvant radio and chemotherapy. She had remained disease-free for 7 years following treatment. After this period, due to tumor recurrence, the patient was started on hormonotherapy with Fulvestrant (estrogen receptor antagonist). Three days later, she developed asthenia, anorexia, nausea and vomiting. On day 10 of therapy she was admitted in the emergency department with jaundice, dark urine and pale stools. There was no history of alcohol, drugs or natural products consumption. The patient also denied recent travels. On admission, she was hemodynamically stable

* Correspondence: soniamcb@hotmail.com
Departament of Gastroenterology and Hepatology, Hospital de Santa Maria, CHLN.Av. Prof. Egas Moniz, 1649-028 Lisbon, Portugal

and with no fever, abdominal pain or pruritus. Physical examination was positive only for icteric sclera. No other relevant findings including hepatosplenomegaly, ascites or hepatic encephalopathy were found. Also, there were no lymphadenopathies or rash. Blood tests revealed leukopenia of 3.1×10^9 ($4.0\text{-}11.0 \times 10^9$) with normal eosinophil value and thrombocytopenia of 82.000 (150.000-450.000). Immunoglobulin IgE level was normal. Liver tests demonstrated a cytocholestase pattern, with elevated aminotransferases: AST 3170 IU/L (<34 IU/L), ALT 908 IU/L (<49 IU/L), GGT 1132 IU/L (<38 IU/L), alkaline phosphatase (AP) 109 IU/L (<104 IU/L), TB 5.1 mg/dl (<1.0 mg/dl) and DB 4.46 mg/dl (<0.2 mg/dl), as well as prolonged prothrombin time: 20s. (<11,6 s.) and APTT 53 s. (< 31 s.) Abdominal ultrasound showed a homogeneous liver, with regular borders. Only steatosis was evident and no nodular or mass lesions were observed.

An extensive workup diagnosis including chest CT, viral serologies (HAV, HBV, HCV, CMV), and autoimmune and metabolic studies failed to show an etiology for the disease. A presumptive diagnosis of liver toxicity to Fulvestrant was assumed. Although the drug was immediately withdrawn, clinical worsening occurred with the development of hepatic encephalopathy and rapid progression of acute liver failure (factor V 35%, AST 5530 IU/L, ALT 1810 IU/L, TB 8.6 mg/dl, APTT 55 s. and PT 23.4 s.) associated with bleeding diathesis. Because the patient had an active tumor recurrence which is a contraindication for liver transplant and chemotherapy wasn't possible because of severe abnormal liver function, a transjugular liver biopsy wasn't considered as

it wouldn't change the management of the patient. There was no response to medical support treatment and the patient died. Post-mortem examination revealed a wide hepatic infiltration by neoplastic tissue with morphologic characteristics compatible with adenocarcinoma (Fig. 1a). The carcinoma cells were arranged singly in small clusters (Fig. 1b) with a high proliferation index (Fig. 1c). Immunohistochemical stains were positive for estrogens receptor but negative for progesterone and Herb2 receptors (Fig. 2), consistent with the diagnosis of primary breast carcinoma. Unfortunately, E-cadherin and CD44 stains weren't tested.

Discussion and conclusions

Although Fulvestrant is a steroidal antiestrogen and it can be associated with liver enzyme elevations, there is no cases of ALF described in literature. In case described liver biopsy excluded this hypothesis. Although liver metastasizing is a common phenomenon, ALF from the spread of the tumor is rare and can be a diagnostic challenge. Clinical, laboratory and radiologic findings are often nonspecific and inconclusive, as it were the case with our patient [1]. According to the largest review of ALF, only 32 cases induced by diffuse metastatic breast cancer have been reported between 1950 and 2014 [6]. The average age described is 47.9 ± 9.9 years such as in the case reported [6]. Most of reported cases have occurred in patients with a previous history of known and treated breast cancer. Ductal carcinoma, like in the present case, is the most frequent one [6]. Our patient had non-specific prodromal symptoms, such malaise and nausea 2 weeks prior to the onset of liver failure, as it

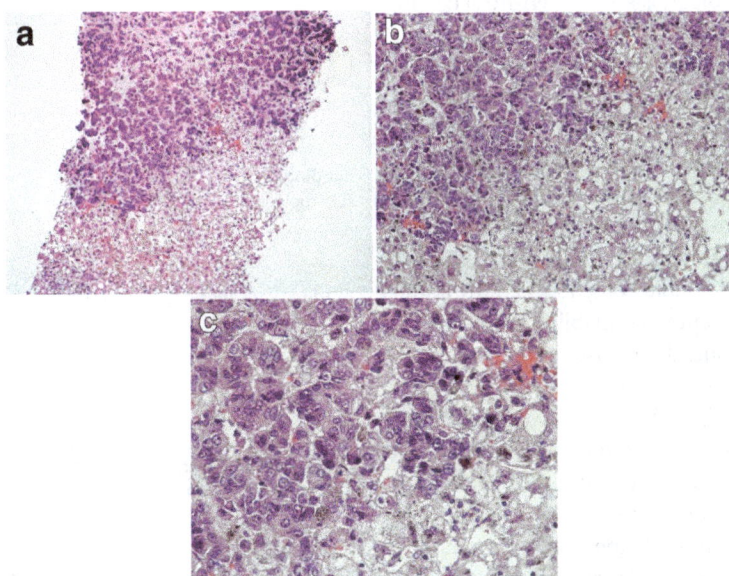

Fig. 1 Liver histological findings. **a** Diffuse infiltration by a poorly differentiated adenocarcinoma. **b** The carcinoma cells were arranged singly, in small clusters. **c** Evidence of nucleoli and multiple mitosis suggesting a high proliferation index

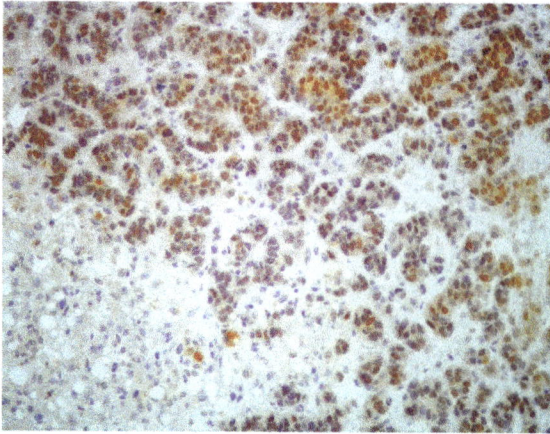

Fig. 2 Positive immunohistochemical stains for estrogen receptor and negative for progesterone and Herb-2 receptors

has been described [4]. Typically, liver metastases are asymptomatic with a focal/target pattern of parenchymal infiltration on ultrasonography and contrast-CT [2]. However, in ALF, as in case reported, imaging may be not specific, without any focal abnormality of the liver parenchyma. In contrast, in such cases tumor cells invade diffusely liver sinusoids, without involving the parenchyma. Thus, liver surface is smooth, with a preserved shape and with no nodularity, despite an important degree of tumor infiltration. Hence, due to diffuse nature of spread typical findings are not seen on radiologic imaging [2] and the majority of the cases of ALF induced by metastatic infiltration are diagnosed after death [2, 7]. In a recent review of literature only 25% of cases were diagnosed premortem [6]. However, a significant trend for increased *premortem* diagnosis has been noticed [6]. Several mechanisms have been proposed to explain the molecular mechanism of massive liver infiltration and hepatocellular injury that occur in such cases. First, loss of cellular adhesion molecules expression as E-cadherin and CD44 can be involved in this process. The first one, being a cell-to-cell and cell-to-extracellular-matrix adhesion protein, when absent allows cell detachment from the primary tumor and single-cell infiltration. On the other hand, CD44 is responsible for endothelium adhesion and its absence may reflect an inability of the metastatic cells to invade beyond the sinusoidal endothelium preventing the formation of a mass in the parenchyma (intrasinusoidal pattern) [5, 8, 9]. Also, invasion of hepatic vessels by tumor cells may result in ischemia with neoplastic cells exerting a pressure effect on hepatocytes competing for nutrients and oxygen, finally leading to liver cell necrosis [2]. Hepatic metastases, including from breast cancer, can also mimic cirrhosis [7, 9]. This "pseudocirrhosis" or carcinomatous cirrhosis is the result of a desmoplastic response of the liver. Due to the

infiltrating tumor and the associated inflammation, stellate cells are activated and produce collagen, causing an extensive fibrosis that results in the atrophy of hepatocytes [5–9].

Most cases of ALF from neoplastic invasion have an extremely poor prognosis, with death occurring from 3 days to 6 months after presentation [2]. The mortality rate of breast carcinoma with diffuse hepatic infiltration is 3 days to 2 months after presentation in 90% of the cases. [2]. *Premortem* diagnosis is important because it affects therapy. Hepatic transplantation is contraindicated for this etiology and chemotherapy is limited by severally abnormal liver function and multiorganic failure [5]. Nonetheless, there are a few clinical cases of patients with metastatic disease unrecognized prior to transplantation that underwent liver transplantation and adjuvant chemotherapy with success [3]. There are also two cases of short-term reversal of ALF from metastatic breast cancer after chemotherapy with longer survival (9 months) [5, 10].

In conclusion, we report a case of a rare cause of ALF induced by metastatic breast cancer. Although rare, physicians must have a high index of suspicion to consider this etiology when approaching a case of ALF, as diffuse intrasinusoidal hepatic metastases of breast cancer can infiltrate the liver with imaging studies remaining normal. There may be a role for liver transplantation in strict selected patients.

Abbreviations

ALF: Acute liver failure; CMV: Cytomegalovirus; HAV: Hepatitis A virus; HBV: Hepatitis B virus; HCV: Hepatitis C virus

Acknowledgements

Not applicable.

Funding

Not applicable.

Authors' contributions

SRF, SF TA, PH, HCP - Preparation and critical review of the manuscript; JV - Critical review of the manuscript. All authors read and approved the final manuscript.

Consent for publication

Written informed consent was obtained from the patient next of kin for the publication of this case report.

Competing interests

The authors declare that they have no competing interests.

References
1. Lee WM. Acute liver failure in the United States. Liver Dis. 2003;23(3):217–26.
2. Goswani R, Babich M, Farah KF. Occult breast malignancy masquerading as acute hepatic failure. Gastroenterol Hepatol. 2011;7:62–4.
3. Rich NE, Sanders C, Hughes RS, et al. Malignant infiltration of the liver presenting as acute liver failure. Clin Gastroenterol Hepatol. 2015;13(5):1025–8.
4. Sanghay N, Hanmornroongruang S. Acute liver failure associated with diffuse liver infiltration by metastatic breast carcinoma: a case report. Oncol Lett. 2013;5:1250–2.
5. Rowbotham D, Wendow J, Williams R. Acute liver failure secondary to hepatic infiltration: a single centre experience of 18 cases. Gut. 1998;42:576–80.
6. Mogrovejo E, Manickam P, Amin M, et al. Characterization of the syndrome of acute liver caused by metastases from breast carcinoma. Dig Dis Sci. 2014;59:724–36.
7. Sass DA, Clark K, Grzybicki D, et al. Diffuse desmoplastic metastatic breast cancer simulating cirrhosis with severe portal hypertension: a case of "pseudocirrhosis". Dig Dis Sci. 2007;52:749–52.
8. Myszor MF, Recor CO. Primary and secondary malignant disease of the liver and fulminant hepatic failure. J Clin Gastroenterol. 1990;12(4):441–6.
9. Nazario HE, Lepe R, Trotter JF. Metastatic breast cancer presenting as acute liver failure. Gastroenterol Hepatol. 2011;7:65–6.
10. Bonetti A, Giuliani J. Acute liver failure caused by metastatic breast cancer: can we expect some results from chemotherapy? Dig Dis Sci. 2015;60:2541–3.

14

Prediction of posthepatectomy liver failure using transient elastography in patients with hepatitis B related hepatocellular carcinoma

Jie-wen Lei[1†], Xiao-yu Ji[2†], Jun-feng Hong[1,3†], Wan-bin Li[4], Yan Chen[1], Yan Pan[5] and Jia Guo[1*] (iD)

Abstract

Background: It is essential to accurately predict Postoperative liver failure (PHLF) which is a life-threatening complication. Liver hardness measurement (LSM) is widely used in non-invasive assessment of liver fibrosis. The aims of this study were to explore the application of preoperative liver stiffness measurements (LSM) by transient elastography in predicting postoperative liver failure (PHLF) in patients with hepatitis B related hepatocellular carcinoma.

Methods: The study included 247 consecutive patients with hepatitis B related hepatocellular carcinoma who underwent hepatectomy between May 2015 and September 2015. Detailed preoperative examinations including LSM were performed before hepatectomy. The endpoint was the development of PHLF.

Results: All of the patients had chronic hepatitis B defined as the presence of hepatitis B surface antigen (HBsAg) for more than 6 months and 76 (30.8%) had cirrhosis. PHLF occurred in 37 (14.98%) patients. Preoperative LSM (odds ratio, OR, 1.21; 95% confidence interval, 95% CI: 1.13–1.29; $P < 0.001$) and international normalized ratio (INR) (OR, 1.07; 95% CI: 1.01–1.12; $P < 0.05$) were revealed to be independent risk factors for PHLF, and a new model was defined as LSM-INR index (LSM-INR index = 0.191*LSM + 6.317*INR-11.154). The optimal cutoff values of LSM and LSM-INR index for predicting PHLF were 14 kPa (AUC 0.86, 95% CI: 0.811–0.901, $P < 0.001$) and −1.92 (AUC 0.87, 95% CI: 0.822–0.909, $P < 0.001$), respectively.

Conclusions: LSM can be helpful for surgeons to make therapeutic decisions in patients with hepatitis B related hepatocellular carcinoma.

Keywords: Hepatocellular carcinoma, Hepatectomy, Posthepatectomy liver failure, Liver stiffness measurement, Hepatitis B

Background

Hepatocellular carcinoma (HCC) is one of the common malignant tumors worldwide. Surgical resection is the most effective treatment for patients with localized HCC [1, 2]. However, postoperative liver failure (PHLF) is a life-threatening complication and intrinsic risk of mortality [3]. It is not only correlated with the volumes of liver resection, but also the insufficient function of hepatic reserve (FHR) [4].

More than 80% of HCCs arise in patients with hepatic fibrosis or cirrhosis [5], which has a very important impact on liver function [4]. Hence, we attempted to determine whether FHR can be indirectly predicted by assessing the degree of liver fibrosis.

LSM is a technology involving obtaining the liver instantaneous elastic modulus to estimate the degree of liver fibrosis by transient elastography (TE), an easy and noninvasive method with high accuracy [6–8].

Recently, several studies reported that liver stiffness is associated with posthepatectomy outcomes [10–12].

* Correspondence: jia_guo@163.com
Jie-wen Lei, Xiao-yu Ji and Jun-feng Hong contributed equally to this work.
†Equal contributors
[1]Department of Ultrasound, Eastern Hepatobiliary Surgery Hospital (EHBH), Second Military Medical University, Shanghai, China
Full list of author information is available at the end of the article

However, baseline characteristics of patients differed greatly among these studies, and few of the studies focused on PHLF. Unlike those in the western countries, about 80% HCC patients in China had hepatitis B virus infection [13].

Aim of the study
In this study, we aimed to assess the usefulness of liver stiffness measured by transient elastography Fibro Touch® (Wuxi HISKY Medical Technologies Co., Ltd. Beijing, China) for predicting PHLF in patients with hepatitis B-related hepatocellular carcinoma.

Methods
Patients
This study was approved by the Institutional Ethics Committee of the Eastern Hepatobiliary Surgery Hospital (EHBH).

HCC patients who underwent liver resection at EHBH were prospectively recruited between May 2015 and September 2015. The exclusion criteria were as follows: (i) patients with hepatolithiasis or patients who will receive hepatectomy because of intrahepatic cholangiocarcinoma (ICC) or hepatic maligancies other than HCC; (ii) patients with cirrhosis due to schistosomiasis, alcoholic liver disease or non-alcoholic fatty liver disease (NAFLD); (iii) patients undergoing preoperative transhepatic arterial chem otherapy and embolization (TACE).

Transient elastography
All patients fasted for at least 6 h before receiving LSM examination by transient elastography FibroTouch®. The examination was performed by two trained and certified operators who were blinded to the patients' clinical data, according to the operation manual and the Liver Stiffness Study Group "Elastica" of the Italian Association for the Study of the Liver [14]. LSM was expressed in kiloPascals (kPa) and was considered reliable only if 10 successful measurements were obtained, with an IQR/median of LSM of < 30% and a success rate of > 60% [15].

Liver surgery
During surgery, right costal margin incision was chosen and the fluid infusion was minimal to keep central venous pressure lower than 5 mmHg to reduce bleeding from hepatic veins [16, 17]. Intraoperative ultrasound (US) was performed systematically to detect the presence of any additional nodules not detected preoperatively. Major hepatectomy was defined as removal of 3 or more Couinaud segments [18, 19]. Diuretics and Ampicillin were used for routine postoperative care.

PHLF was defined as the presence of at least one of the following variables: 1) occurrence of refractory ascites causing a delay in the removal of surgical drainages and/or postoperative drainage exceeding 500 ml/day, a continuous elevation of total serum bilirubin concentration (≥60umol/l) beyond postoperative day 7; 2) alteration of coagulation factors requiring fresh frozen plasma infusion with an International Normalized Ratio (INR) of more than 1.50 [20]. The endpoint of this study is the presence of PHLF.

Statistical analysis
Continuous variables were expressed as the mean and standard deviation. Differences between the subgroups were compared by t-test or Mann-Whitney U test.

Table 1 Baseline characteristics of patients (N = 247)

Variables	n (%), mean ± SD, or median (range)
Age (years)	53.3 ± 10.3
Gender (Male /Female)	213/34(86%/14%)
BMI (kg /m2)	29.9 ± 16.5
Complications[a]	43(17%)
Cirrhosis (yes /no)	76/171(30.8%/69.2%)
White blood cell (10⁹/l)	5.2 ± 2.0
Hemoglobin (g/l)	143.9 ± 14.1
Platelet Count (10⁹/l)	145(41–466)
Child–Pugh class A	247
Total bilirubin (umol/l)	16.0 ± 11.8
Albumin (g/l)	41.7 ± 3.3
Prealbumin (mg/l)	238.6 ± 62.6
Alanine transaminase (u/l)	39.2 ± 34.2
Aspartate aminotransferase (u/l)	36.99 ± 31.3
Gamma-glutamyl transpeptidase (u/l)	47(11–866)
Alkaline phosphatase (u/l)	81(34–250)
PT(s)	11.5(9.4–15.4)
INR	1.0(0.8–1.3)-
APTT(s)	27.2(16.7–52.9)
LSM(Kpa)	12.7(3.8–38.5)
Intraoperative blood infusion (yes / no)	19/228(8%/92%)
Portal vein occlusion (yes / no)	194/53(79%/21%)
Esophageal varices (yes / no)	18/229(7.3%/92.7%)
Tumor capsule (yes / no)	174/73(70%/30%)
Number of tumors (Single / multiple)	217/30(88%/12%)
Anti-viral medication(Positive / negative)	71/176(28.7%/71.2%)
HBV DNA levels (>1.0E + 04iu/ml/<1.0E + 04iu/ml)	73/174(30%/70%)
Major hepatectomy	40 (16%)
Median main tumor size(cm)	5.02 ± 3.18
Tumor location (right lobe /left lobe/ both)	158/79/10(64%/32%/4%)

[a]Complications include one or more of the following: hypertension, heart disease (myocardial ischemia, cardiomyopathy, arrhythmia), chronic obstructive pulmonary disease, diabetes, etc.

Categorical variables were compared using χ^2 test with Yates' correction or Fisher's exact test. Factors with significant impact on PHLF upon univariate analysis were explored with multivariate forward logistic regression as hypothetical independent predictors of PHLF. A significance level of 0.05 was used in all analyses. The prognostic value of PHLF prediction model and the LSM only were assessed using receiver operating characteristic (ROC) curve analysis (MedCalc Software bvba, Ostend, Belgium). The area under the ROC curve (AUC), the sensitivity, the specificity, the positive and negative predictive values, and the positive and negative likelihood ratio for cutoff values were obtained.

Data analysis was performed using SPSS, version 19.0 for Windows (SPSS, Inc., Chicago, IL) and R software 2.10.1 (R Foundation for Statistical Computing, Vienna, Austria; www.r-project.org). All reported p values were two-sided, and $p < 0.05$ was considered to be statistically significant.

Results

Characteristics of the study population

The demographic and clinicopathologic characteristics of these patients were shown in Table 1.

All the patients (213 men and 34 women), with a mean age of 53.27 ± 10.33 years, had postive HBsAg lasting for >6 months. All of them were Child-Pugh class A, and a small proportion had complications (17%). As shown by the pathological results, 76 (31%) patients had cirrhosis and 18 (7%) had esophageal varices consistent with gastroscopy results. 37 (14.98%) patients developed PHLF postoperatively, and they had a significantly higher preoperative mean LSM (21.4 ± 6.3 kPa) than those without PHLF (12.7 ± 5.7 kPa, $P < 0.001$).

Table 2 Univariate analysis and multivariate linear regression analysis of the variables associated with PHLF

Variables	Univariate analysis			Multivariate analysis		
	PLF(+)($n = 37$)	PLF(−)($n = 210$)	p	Exp(B)	OR95%CI	p
Age (years)	54.9 ± 10.9	53.0 ± 10.2	0.286			
Gender (Male /Female)	33/4 (89%/11%)	180/30 (86%/14%)	0.572			
BMI (kg /m2)	23.7 ± 3.1	23.3 ± 3.0	0.423			
White blood cell (10^9/l)	4.9 ± 1.5	5.3 ± 2.1	0.275			
Hemoglobin (g/l)	144.2 ± 12.3	143.8 ± 14.4	0.881			
Platelet Count (10^9/l)	139.0 ± 79.9	155.3 ± 56.9	0.037			
Total bilirubin (umol/l)	19.1 ± 8.8	15.4 ± 12.2	0.079			
Albumin (g/l)	41.0 ± 3.6	41.9 ± 3.2	0.123			
Prealbumin (mg/l)	218.2 ± 67.9	242.2 ± 61.0	0.032			
Alanine transaminase (u/l)	43.2 ± 31.3	38.5 ± 34.7	0.449			
Aspartate aminotransferase (u/l)	41.2 ± 23	36.1 ± 32.4	0.366			
Gamma-glutamyl transpeptidase (u/l)	104.8 ± 148.6	68.6 ± 69.2	0.027			
Alkaline phosphatase (u/l)	100.0 ± 47.4	83.2 ± 23.3	0.173			
PT(s)	12.1 ± 1.2	11.6 ± 0.8	0.005			
INR	1.0 ± 0.1	1.0 ± 0.1	0.005	1.065	1.014–1.119	0.013
APTT(s)	28.9 ± 5.9	27.1 ± 5.2	0.067			
LSM(kpa)	21.4 ± 6.3	12.7 ± 5.7	<0.001	1.211	1.134–1.293	<0.001
Intraoperative blood infusion (yes /no)	7/30 (18.9%/81.1%)	12/198 (5.7%/94.3%)	0.005			
Portal vein occlusion (yes/no)	24/13 (64.9%/35.1%)	160/50 (76.2%/23.8%)	0.145			
Number of tumors (Single/multiple)	32/5 (86.5%/13.5%)	185/25 (88.1%/11.9%)	0.782			
Tumor capsule (yes/no)	24/13 (64.9%/35.1%)	150/60 (71.4%/28.6%)	0.420			
HBV DNA levels (>1.0E + 04iu/ml/<1.0E + 04iu/ml)	13/24 (35.1%/64.9%)	60/150 (28.6%/71.4%)	0.422			
Cirrhosis (yes/no)	22/15 (59.5%/40.5%)	54/156 (27.7%/74.3%)	<0. 001			
Esophageal varices (yes/no)	7/30 (18.9%/81.1%)	11/199 (5.2%/94.8%)	0.003			
Major hepatectomy	8 (22%)	32 (15%)	0.331			
Median main tumor size (cm)	5.6 ± 4.0	4.9 ± 3	0.687			
Tumor location (right lobe/left lobe/both)	29/6/2 (78.4%/16.2%/5.4%)	129/73/8 (61.4%/34.8%/3.8%)	0.082			

Independent predictors for PHLF in HCC patients

Univariate and multivariate analysis were used for analyzing the potential influencing factors associated with PHLF, and the results were reported in Table 2.

Univariate analysis revealed that the factors including platelet count ($p = 0.037$), prealbumin ($p = 0.032$), gamma-glutamyl transpeptidase ($p = 0.027$), prothrombin time ($p = 0.005$) and INR ($p = 0.005$), LSM ($p < 0.001$), the use of intraoperative blood transfusions ($p = 0.005$), the presence of cirrhosis ($p < 0.001$) and esophageal varices ($p = 0.003$) were significant predictors for PHLF.

Multivariate analysis showed that only LSM (odds ratio, OR, 1.2; 95% confidence interval, 95% CI, 1.134–1.293, $P < 0.001$) and INR (OR, 1.1; 95% CI, 1.014–1.119, $p < 0.05$) remained in a binary logistic regression model, and revealed they were independent risk factors for PHLF. Meanwhile, a new algorithm was defined for predicting PHLF: the LSM-INR index = 0.191*LSM + 6.317*INR-11.154.

Diagnostic performance of LSM for predicting PHLF

The diagnostic performance and corresponding ROC curves of LSM are shown in Fig. 1. The optimal cutoff value of LSM is 14 kPa for predicting PHLF [AUC 0.860 95% CI: 0.811–0.901, $p < 0.001$; sensitivity (Se) 94.6%, specificity (Sp) 67.6%, positive predictive values (PPV) 34%, negative predictive values (NPV) 98.6%, positive likelihood ratio (LR$^+$) 2.9, negative likelihood ratio (LR$^-$) 0.1].

When considering cirrhotic patients only, ROC curve analysis identified the best cutoff value of LSM is 17.0 kPa for predicting PHLF (AUC 0.825, 95% CI: 0.721–0.903, $p < 0.001$; Se 81.8%, Sp 70.4%, PPV 52.9%, NPV 90.5%, LR$^+$ 2.86, LR$^-$ 0.3) (Fig. 2).

Meanwhile, the optimal cutoff value of LSM is 12.8 kPa for predicting the presence of cirrhosis (AUC 0.789, 95% CI: 0.727–0.834, $p < 0.001$; Se 79.0%, Sp 65.5%, PPV 50.4%, NPV 87.5%, LR$^+$ 2.3, LR$^-$ 0.3) (Fig. 3).

Diagnostic performance of INR for predicting PHLF

The optimal cutoff value of INR is 1.0 for predicting PHLF (AUC 0.646, 95% CI: 0.583–0.706, $p < 0.001$; Se 54.1%, Sp 71.9%, PPV 25.3%, NPV 89.9%, LR$^+$ 1.9, LR$^-$ 0.6) (Fig. 4).

Diagnostic performance of the LSM-INR index for predicting PHLF

The diagnostic performance and corresponding ROC curves of the LSM-INR index are shown in Fig. 5. The optimal cutoff value of the LSM-INR index is –1.9 for predicting the presence of PHLF (AUC 0.865, 95% CI: 0.822–0.909, $p < 0.001$; Se 86.5%, Sp 74.8%, PPV 37.6%, NPV 96.9%, LR$^+$ 3.4 LR$^-$ 0.2).

Discussion

Surgical resection is the first-line therapeutic option for early HCC [21]. However, insufficient FHR may result in postoperative complications and even PHLF (4), which is a major cause of postoperative morbidity and mortality after elective hepatic resection [22, 23].

Liver resection for HCC patients with chronic liver diseases still carries higher risk of PHLF than normal liver resection [22, 24].To the best of our knowledge, this

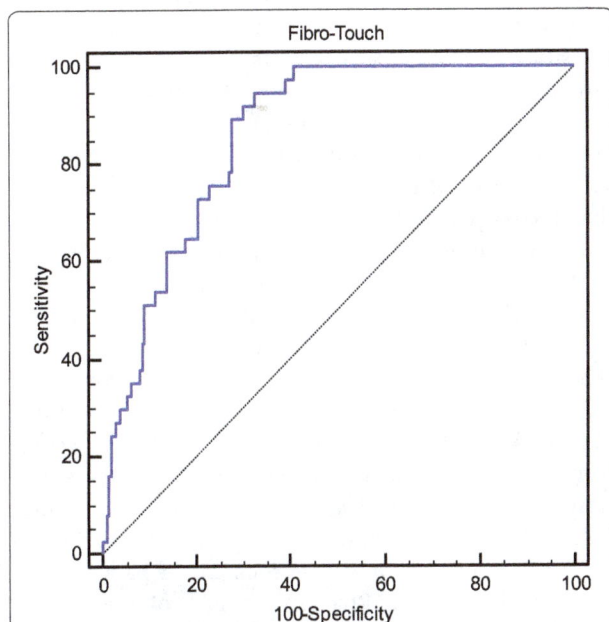

Fig. 1 ROC analysis of liver stiffness measurement for predicting PHLF

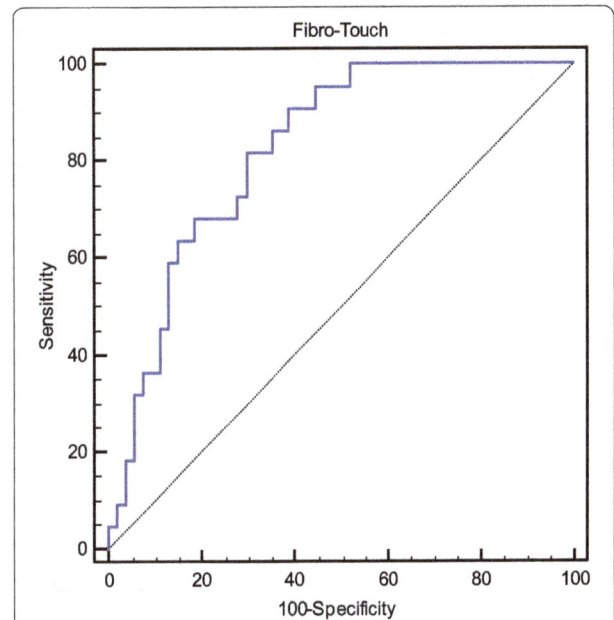

Fig. 2 ROC analysis of liver stiffness measurement with only cirrhotic patients for predicting PHLF

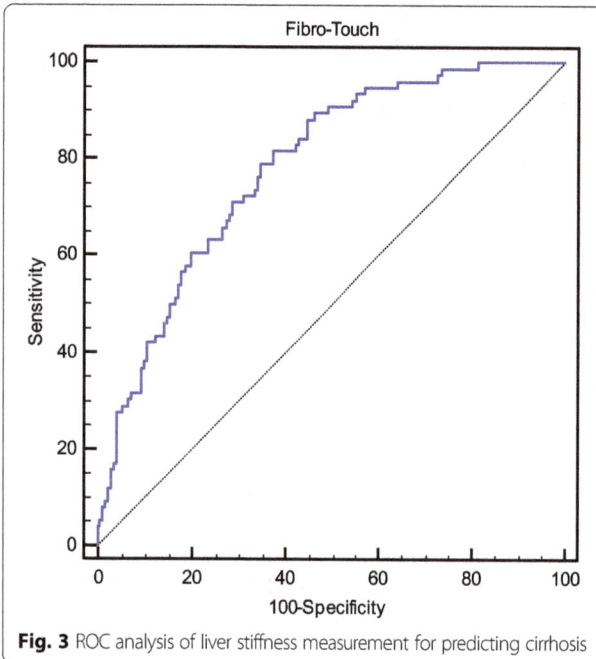

Fig. 3 ROC analysis of liver stiffness measurement for predicting cirrhosis

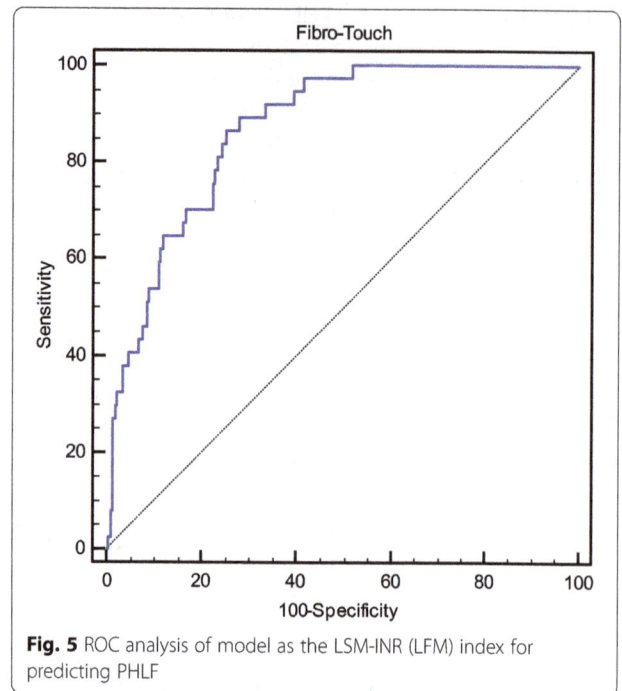

Fig. 5 ROC analysis of model as the LSM-INR (LFM) index for predicting PHLF

is the first published study on the effectiveness of LSM measurement in predicting PHLF in patients with hepatitis B related hepatocellular carcinoma since previous studies only suggested a potential role of LSM in predicting post-resection hepatic insufficiency. Furthermore, in those previous studies [10, 25], the background hepatic conditions causing HCC showed a great variability and included HCV, alcoholic and nonalcoholic steatohepatitis in addition to HBV. The baseline characteristics of patients differed by studies and it may result in a selection bias.

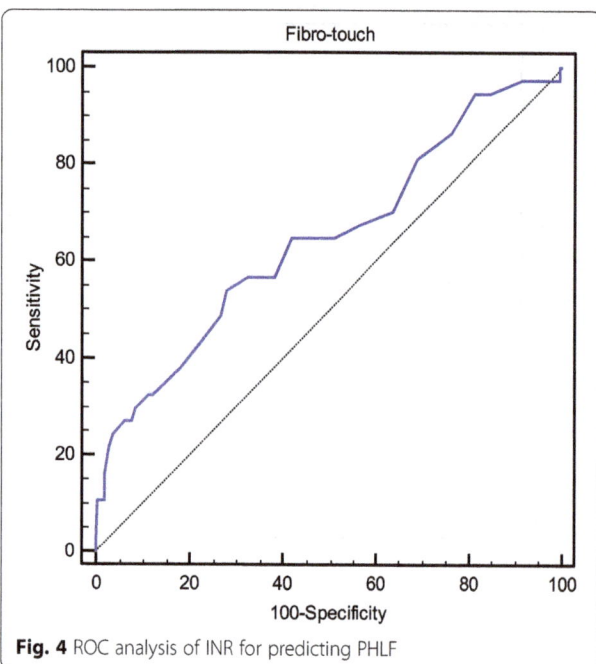

Fig. 4 ROC analysis of INR for predicting PHLF

In this study, we used a new generation transient elastography, FibroTouch® for liver stiffness measurement (LSM) [9, 26], which has enhanced 2D–image-guided positioning function. It's particularly advantageous for precise preoperative examination, because the examiners are able to set the the region of interest(ROI) in the non-tumor area. It may also explain why the optimal cut-off LSM value (14.0 Kpa) in this study is lower than that in previous studies [10, 12]. Although the conclusions of their studies were similar to that of this study, some differences have to be pointed out. First, although the study population was very similar to ours, the background of the population was not homogenous. Secondly, their definition of PHLF was only based on postoperative serum bilirubin levels, which configures a very high risk of irreversible PHLF (5 mg/dL for more than 5 days post operation) [27]. Perhaps for this reason, their LSM cutoff was higher and may miss milder grades of PHLF [25].

Using the calculated cutoff value of 14.0 Kpa, LSM had high specificity and negative predictive value for predicting PHLF. The value in liver failure group was significantly higher than that in non-liver failure group (21.4 Kpa vs. 12.7Kpa). It implied that FHR may become worse with the increase of LSM value. While the effectiveness of LSM for diagnosing cirrhosis is not high (AUC = 0.78, 95% confidence interval: 0.727–0.834), it may be confounded by the enrollment of patients with Child-Pugh Class A. Precisely because of this reason, one interesting result of this study is that the degree of resection is not a significant predictor of PHLF.

In our study, HBV DNA showed no statistical differences, which is not in line with a previous report [28], and a possible explanation is the inclusion of patients with HBV DNA higher than 10^4 IU/ml. For such patients, we will first use antiviral drugs to control the amount of HBV, and then choose surgery. Univariate analysis showed that platelet count, LSM and others were significant prognostic factors for PHLF. This is consistent with the previous finding of risk factors for postoperative complications [29].

We must acknowledge this study has several potential limitations. Compared to similar articles, LSM was significantly better than ICG-15 and MELD score in the prediction of postoperative complications [10, 12], we do not routinely use ICG-15 or MELD to assess liver function. The number of the outcome of PHLF was relatively small, and further acquisition of cases and the external validation should be accomplished in the future. Second, our analysis did not include other variables that may affect the outcomes of surgery, such as the resected liver volume which is closely correlated with the functional liver reserve and postoperative results [11]. A well-designed, well-controlled, randomized study of a large population is required.

Conclusions

In summary, our study showed that the preoperative LSM is a valid tool for surgeons in making therapeutic decisions in patients with hepatitis B related hepatocellular carcinoma. We also established a new index, LSM-INR index, which quantitatively evaluated the risk of the INR and LSM that should be useful for surgeons in making therapeutic decisions in patients with hepatitis B related hepatocellular carcinoma before hepatectomy.

Abbreviations
AUC: The area under the ROC curve; EHBH: Eastern Hepatobiliary Surgery Hospital; FHR: Function of hepatic reserve; HBsAg: Hepatitis B surface antigen; HCC: Hepatocellular carcinoma; ICC: Intrahepatic cholangiocarcinoma; LR⁻: Negative likelihood ratio; LR⁺: Positive likelihood ratio; LSM: Liver stiffness measurements; NPV: Negative predictive values; PHLF: Postoperative liver failure; PPV: Positive predictive values; ROC: Receiver operating characteristic; Se: Sensitivity; Sp: Specificity; TACE: Transhepatic arterial chem otherapy and embolization; TE: Transient elastography

Acknowledgements
Not applicable.

Funding
This study was funded by the Shanghai Shenkang Hospital development Center Clinical Science and Technology Innovation Project (NO. SHDC22015004) and by the leading project of the Science and Technology Department of Fujian province (2015Y01010204).

Availability of data and materials
The data that support the findings of this study are available from [Department of Ultrasound, Eastern Hepatobiliary Surgery Hospital (EHBH), Third Affiliated Hospital of Second Military Medical University, Shanghai, China] but restrictions apply to the availability of these data, which were used under license for the current study, we will use this data for another direction and so are not publicly available. Data are however available from the authors upon reasonable request and with permission of [Department of Ultrasound, Eastern Hepatobiliary Surgery Hospital (EHBH), Third Affiliated Hospital of Second Military Medical University, Shanghai, China].

Authors' contributions
Tables and Figures were produced by JL and XJ who also drafted the manuscript with equal contribution to the article; WL reviewed the literature, collected and interpreted the clinical data; JL assembled and interpreted the clinical data; XJ conducted the data analysis; JL, JH, YC, YP and JG made the revision; All authors finalized the manuscript and have read and approved the final manuscript.

Consent for publication
Not applicable.

Competing interests
The authors declare that they have no competing interests.

Author details
[1]Department of Ultrasound, Eastern Hepatobiliary Surgery Hospital (EHBH), Second Military Medical University, Shanghai, China. [2]People's Liberation Army Military Academy, Second Military Medical University, Shanghai, China. [3]Department of Ultrasound, FuZhou General Hospital (Dongfang Hospital), Xiamen University, Fuzhou, Fujian, China. [4]Department of Ultrasound, Shanghai First People's Hospital, Shanghai, China. [5]Department of Ultrasound, Yuhuangding Hospital, Yantai, Shandong, China.

References
1. Shimada M, Matsumata T, Akazawa K, Kamakura T, Itasaka H, Sugimachi K, et al. Estimation of risk of major complications after hepatic resection. Am J Surg. 1994;167(4):399–403. doi:10.1016/0002-9610(94)90124-4. [PubMed: 8179084]
2. Fan ST, Lai EC, Lo CM, Ng IO, Wong J. Hospital mortality of major hepatectomy for hepatocellular carcinoma associated with cirrhosis. Arch Surg. 1995;130(2):198–203. doi:10.1001/archsurg.1995.01430020088017. [PubMed: 7848092]
3. Schroeder RA, Marroquin CE, Bute BP, Khuri S, Henderson WG, Kuo PC. Predictive indices of morbidity and mortality after liver resection. Ann Surg. 2006;243(3):373–9. doi:10.1097/01.sla.0000201483.95911.08. [PubMed: 16495703]
4. Fan ST. Liver functional reserve estimation: state of the art and relevance for local treatments: the Eastern perspective. J Hepatobiliary Pancreat Sci. 2010; 17(4):380–4. doi:10.1007/s00534-009-0229-9. [PubMed: 19865790]
5. Matsumura H, Moriyama M, Goto I, Tanaka N, Okubo H, Arakawa Y. Natural course of progression of liver fibrosis in Japanese patients with chronic liver disease type C–a study of 527 patients at one establishment. J Viral Hepat. 2000;7(4):268–75. doi:10.1046/j.1365-2893.2000.00235.x. [PubMed: 10886535]
6. Castéra L, Vergniol J, Foucher J, Darriet M, Couzigou P, De Lédinghen V. Prospective comparison of transient elastography, Fibrotest, APRI, and liver biopsy for the assessment of fibrosis in chronic hepatitis C. Gastroenterology. 2005;128(2):343–50. doi:10.1053/j.gastro.2004.11.018. [PubMed: 15685546]
7. Fraquelli M, Rigamonti C, Casazza G, Conte D, Donato MF, Ronchi G, et al. Reproducibility of transient elastography in the evaluation of liver fibrosis in patients with chronic liver disease. Gut. 2007;56(7):968–73. doi:10.1136/gut.2006.111302. [PubMed: 17255218]
8. Friedrich-Rust M, Ong MF, Martens S, Sarrazin C, Bojunga J, Zeuzem S, et al. Performance of transient elastography for the staging of liver fibrosis: a meta-analysis. Gastroenterology. 2008;134(4):960–74. doi:10.1053/j.gastro.2008.01.034. [PubMed: 18395077]
9. Deng H, Wang CL, Lai J, Yu SL, Xie DY, Gao ZL. Noninvasive diagnosis of hepatic steatosis using fat attenuation parameter measured by FibroTouch and a new algorithm in CHB patients. Hepat Mon. 2016;16(9):e40263. doi:10.5812/hepatmon.40263. [PubMed: 27822268]
10. Wong JS, Wong GL, Chan AW, Wong VW, Cheung YS, Chong CN, et al. Liver stiffness measurement by transient elastography as a predictor on posthepatectomy outcomes. Ann Surg. 2013;257(5):922–8. doi:10.1097/SLA.0b013e318269d2ec. [PubMed: 23001077]
11. Du ZG, Li B, Wei YG, Yin J, Feng X, Chen X. A new scoring system for

assessment of liver function after successful hepatectomy in patients with hepatocellular carcinoma. Hepatobiliary Pancreat Dis Int. 2011;10(3):265–9. doi:10.1016/S1499-3872(11)60044-1. [PubMed: 21669569]

12. Kim SU, Ahn SH, Park JY, Kim DY, Chon CY, Choi JS, et al. Prediction of postoperative hepatic insufficiency by liver stiffness measurement (FibroScan((R))) before curative resection of hepatocellular carcinoma: a pilot study. Hepatol Int. 2008;2(4):471–7. doi:10.1007/s12072-008-9091-0. [PubMed: 19669322]

13. Patanwala IY, Bauer HM, Miyamoto J, Park IU, Huchko MJ, Smith-McCune KK. A systematic review of randomized trials assessing human papillomavirus testing in cervical cancer screening. Am J Obstet Gynecol. 2013;208(5):343–53. https://doi.org/10.1016/j.ajog.2012.11.013. [PubMed: 23159693]

14. Bonino F, Arena U, Brunetto MR, Coco B, Fraquelli M, Oliveri F, et al. Liver stiffness, a non-invasive marker of liver disease: a core study group report. Antivir Ther. 2010;15(Suppl 3):69–78. doi:10.3851/IMP1626. [PubMed: 21041906]

15. Sandrin L, Fourquet B, Hasquenoph JM, Yon S, Fournier C, Mal F, et al. Transient elastography: a new noninvasive method for assessment of hepatic fibrosis. Ultrasound Med Biol. 2003;29(12):1705–13. [PubMed: 14698338]

16. Cucchetti A, Siniscalchi A, Ercolani G, Vivarelli M, Cescon M, Grazi GL, et al. Modification of acid-base balance in cirrhotic patients undergoing liver resection for hepatocellular carcinoma. Ann Surg. 2007;245(6):902–8. doi:10.1097/01.sla.0000256356.23026.9f. [PubMed: 17522516]

17. Melendez JA, Arslan V, Fischer ME, Wuest D, Jarnagin WR, Fong Y, et al. Perioperative outcomes of major hepatic resections under low central venous pressure anesthesia: blood loss, blood transfusion, and the risk of postoperative renal dysfunction. J Am Coll Surg. 1998;187(6):620–5. doi:10.1016/S1072-7515(98)00240-3. [PubMed: 9849736]

18. Pang YY. The Brisbane 2000 terminology of liver anatomy and resections. HPB 2000; 2:333-39. HPB (Oxford). 2002;4(2):99. author reply 99-100. [PubMed: 18332933]

19. Jarnagin WR, Gonen M, Fong Y, DeMatteo RP, Ben-Porat L, Little S, et al. Improvement in perioperative outcome after hepatic resection: analysis of 1,803 consecutive cases over the past decade. Ann Surg. 2002;236(4):397–406; discussion 406–7. [PubMed: 12368667]. doi:10.1097/00000658-200210000-00001.

20. Sugimoto H, Okochi O, Hirota M, Kanazumi N, Nomoto S, Inoue S, et al. Early detection of liver failure after hepatectomy by indocyanine green elimination rate measured by pulse dye-densitometry. J Hepato-Biliary-Pancreat Surg. 2006; 13(6):543–8. doi:10.1007/s00534-006-1114-4. [PubMed: 17139429]

21. Bruix J. M. Sherman. Management of hepatocellular carcinoma. Hepatology. 2005;42(5):1208–36. doi:10.1002/hep.20933. [PubMed: 16250051]

22. Belghiti J, Hiramatsu K, Benoist S, Massault P, Sauvanet A, Farges O. Seven hundred forty-seven hepatectomies in the 1990s: an update to evaluate the actual risk of liver resection. J Am Coll Surg. 2000;191(1):38–46. [PubMed: 10898182]

23. Wang Q, Lau WY, Zhang B, Zhang Z, Huang Z, Luo H, et al. Preoperative total cholesterol predicts postoperative outcomes after partial hepatectomy in patients with chronic hepatitis B- or C-related hepatocellular carcinoma. Surgery. 2014; 155(2):263–70. doi:10.1016/j.surg.2013.08.017. [PubMed: 24569301]

24. Fan ST. ProbLSM-INR indexs of hepatectomy in cirrhosis. Hepato-Gastroenterology. 1998;45(Suppl 3):1288–90. [PubMed: 9730390]

25. Cescon M, Colecchia A, Cucchetti A, Peri E, Montrone L, Ercolani G, et al. Value of transient elastography measured with FibroScan in predicting the outcome of hepatic resection for hepatocellular carcinoma. Ann Surg. 2012; 256(5):706–712; discussion 712-3. [PubMed: 23095613]. doi:10.1097/SLA.0b013e3182724ce8.

26. Yuan L, Shao J, Hao M, Li C, Wang G, Wang T, et al. Correlation between liver hardness testing results obtained by FibroTouch and FibroScan and liver pathological stage. Zhonghua Gan Zang Bing Za Zhi. 2014;22(6):425–9. [PubMed: 25203705]

27. Balzan S, Belghiti J, Farges O, Ogata S, Sauvanet A, Delefosse D, et al. The "50-50 criteria" on postoperative day 5: an accurate predictor of liver failure and death after hepatectomy. Ann Surg. 2005;242(6):824–828, discussion 828-9. [PubMed: 16327492]. doi:10.1097/01.sla.0000189131.90876.9e.

28. Huang G, Lau WY, Shen F, Pan ZY, Fu SY, Yang Y, et al. Preoperative hepatitis B virus DNA level is a risk factor for postoperative liver failure in patients who underwent partial hepatectomy for hepatitis B-related hepatocellular carcinoma. World J Surg. 2014;38(9):2370–6. doi:10.1007/s00268-014-2546-7. [PubMed: 24696061]

29. Capussotti L, Muratore A, Amisano M, Polastri R, Bouzari H, Massucco P. Liver resection for hepatocellular carcinoma on cirrhosis: analysis of mortality, morbidity and survival–a European single center experience. Eur J Surg Oncol. 2005;31(9):986–93. doi:10.1016/j.ejso.2005.04.002. [PubMed: 15936169]

15

Hepatocellular carcinoma is the most common liver-related complication in patients with histopathologically-confirmed NAFLD in Japan

Norio Akuta[1][*], Yusuke Kawamura[1], Yasuji Arase[1], Satoshi Saitoh[1], Shunichiro Fujiyama[1,1], Hitomi Sezaki[1], Tetsuya Hosaka[1], Masahiro Kobayashi[1], Mariko Kobayashi[2], Yoshiyuki Suzuki[1], Fumitaka Suzuki[1], Kenji Ikeda[1] and Hiromitsu Kumada[1]

Abstract

Background: The incidence of liver-related events, cardiovascular events and type 2 diabetes mellitus in patients with histopathologically confirmed NAFLD remains unclear.

Methods: We retrospectively investigated the incidence of liver events, cardiovascular events, malignancy, and type 2 diabetes mellitus in 402 Japanese patients with histopathologically confirmed NAFLD for a median follow-up of 4.2 years. We also investigated predictors of the development of hepatocellular carcinoma and type 2 diabetes mellitus in these patients.

Results: The rate of liver-related events per 1000 person years was 4.17 (hepatocellular carcinoma, 3.67; hepatic encephalopathy, 1.60; esophago-gastric varices, 2.43; ascites, 0.80; and jaundice, 0.40). The rate of cardiovascular events and type 2 diabetes mellitus was 5.73 and 9.95, respectively. Overall mortality was 3.33 (liver-related events, 1.25; cardiovascular events, 0.42; and malignancies other than hepatocellular carcinoma, 0.83), in patients free of previous or current malignancies. Multivariate analyses identified old age (≥70 years) and advanced fibrosis stage 4 as significant determinants of hepatocellular carcinoma development, and hepatocyte steatosis (> 33%), female sex, and serum ferritin (≤80 μg/l) as significant determinants of type 2 diabetes mellitus development in these patients.

Conclusions: Our results highlighted the importance of cardiovascular and liver-related events in Japanese patients with histopathologically-confirmed NAFLD. Hepatocellular carcinoma was the most common liver-related event, and the incidence of hepatocellular carcinoma was more than half of that of cardiovascular events.

Keywords: Nonalcoholic fatty liver disease, Nonalcoholic steatohepatitis, Hepatocellular carcinoma, Liver-related events, Cardiovascular events, Type 2 diabetes mellitus, Malignancy, Mortality, Fibrosis stage, Hepatocyte steatosis

Background

The most common liver disease worldwide is non-alcoholic fatty liver disease (NAFLD) [1–6]. Liver pathology ranges from the typically benign non-alcoholic fatty liver to non-alcoholic steatohepatitis (NASH), which may progress to liver cirrhosis, hepatocellular carcinoma (HCC), and liver failure [7].

The incidence of liver events, cardiovascular events, malignancy, and type 2 diabetes mellitus (T2DM) in patients with histopathologically confirmed NAFLD remains unclear. T2DM and fibrosis stage are significant and independent risk factors for HCC in patients with NAFLD [5]. Results of recent prospective studies have shown that antidiabetic drugs may improve histological features, including fibrosis stage [8–10]. Thus, it may be important to identify predictors of the development of

* Correspondence: akuta-gi@umin.ac.jp; norioakuta@toranomon.gr.jp
[1]Department of Hepatology, Toranomon Hospital and Okinaka Memorial Institute for Medical Research, 2-2-2 Toranomon, Minato-ku, Tokyo 105-0001, Japan
Full list of author information is available at the end of the article

HCC and T2DM to improve the prognosis of patients with NAFLD.

It has been suggested that fibrosis stage may be more reliable than the NAFLD activity score (NAS) for the prediction of liver-specific mortality [11]. Fibrosis stage, but not other histopathological features of steatohepatitis, was reported to be an independent and significant predictor of overall mortality, liver transplantation, and liver-related events [12].

The purpose of the present study was to determine the incidence of liver-related events, cardiovascular events, and T2DM, and the predictors of development of HCC and T2DM in patients with NAFLD by retrospectively analyzing the outcome of 402 Japanese patients with histopathologically confirmed NAFLD.

Methods

Patients

This is a retrospective cohort study of patients with histopathologically-confirmed NAFLD. Between 1976 and 2017, liver biopsy was performed at our hospital for patients with liver dysfunction and/or fatty liver diagnosed by abdominal ultrasonography. Of those, the diagnosis of NAFLD was confirmed in 402 patients by histopathology. The median duration of follow-up, from diagnosis to death or last visit, was 4.2 years (range, 0.0–41.4 years), and the total sum of person-years was 2625 years. The characteristics of the patients at the time of histopathological diagnosis of NAFLD are summarized in Table 1. Patients with histopathological changes of steatosis in at least 5% of hepatocytes and alcohol intake < 20 g/day were included in the analysis. We excluded patients with 1) underlying liver disease (e.g., viral hepatitis, autoimmune hepatitis, drug-induced liver disease, or primary biliary cirrhosis); 2) systemic autoimmune diseases (e.g., systemic lupus erythematosus and rheumatoid arthritis); and 3) metabolic diseases (e.g., hemochromatosis, α-1-antitrypsin deficiency, or Wilson disease).

The study was conducted in compliance with the International Conference on Harmonisation guidelines for Good Clinical Practice (E6) and the 2013 Declaration of Helsinki. The protocol was approved by the institutional review board at Toranomon Hospital (number 953). Written informed consent was provided by all patients prior to liver biopsy.

Diagnosis and follow-up

Liver-related events included HCC, hepatic encephalopathy, esophago-gastric varices with bleeding, ascites, and jaundice. Cardiovascular events included coronary artery disease, heart valve disease, arrhythmia, heart failure, hypertension, orthostatic hypotension, shock, endocarditis, diseases of the aorta and its branches, disorders of

Table 1 Patient characteristics at the time of histological diagnosis of NAFLD

Demographic data	
Numbers of patients	402
Gender, Male / Female, n	245 / 157
Age, y[a]	51 (20–87)
Body mass index, kg/m^{2a}	26.1 (18.1–42.4)
Presence of previous and current malignancy	
None / Hepatocellular carcinoma / Other malignancy, n	351 / 26 / 30
Type 2 diabetes mellitus, Absence / Presence, n	276 / 126
Hypertension, Absence / Presence, n	230 / 172
Hyperlipidemia, Absence / Presence, n	274 / 128
Histological findings	
Steatosis, 5–33% / > 33–66% / > 66%, n	152 / 149 / 98
Lobular inflammation	
No foci / < 2 foci / 2–4 foci / > 4 foci per 200× field, n	28 / 242 / 116 / 13
Ballooning, None / Few cells / Many cells, n	39 / 252 / 108
Stage, 0 / 1 / 2 / 3 / 4, n	48 / 165 / 63 / 98 / 28
NAFLD activity score, ≤2 / 3, 4 / ≥5, n	34 / 181 / 184
Diagnosis according to FLIP algorithm, NASH / non-NASH, n	349 / 50
Laboratory data[a]	
Serum aspartate aminotransferase, IU/l	44 (3–378)
Serum alanine aminotransferase, IU/l	69 (15–783)
Gamma-glutamyl transpeptidase, IU/l	72 (11–990)
Platelet count, ×10^3/mm^3	213 (40–471)
Fasting plasma glucose, mg/dl	101 (65–287)
HbA1c, %	5.9 (4.4–12.6)
Uric acid, mg/dl	5.9 (1.9–11.1)
Total cholesterol, mg/dl	204 (101–370)
Triglycerides, mg/dl	140 (31–1088)
High-density lipoprotein cholesterol, mg/dl	45 (14–85)
Low-density lipoprotein cholesterol, mg/dl	120 (27–243)
Serum ferritin, μg/l	227 (< 10–2067)
High sensitive C-reactive protein, mg/dl	0.095 (0.006–2.240)
Alpha-fetoprotein, μg/l	4 (1–10,930)
PIVKA-II, AU/l	18 (1–157,050)

Data are number of patients, except those denoted by [a], which represent the median (range) values

the peripheral vascular system, and stroke. Furthermore, the incidence of T2DM and other malignancies, apart from HCCs, were also evaluated. The incidence of T2DM was assessed at least twice a year after baseline examination. T2DM was diagnosed as the presence of elevated fasting plasma glucose (≥126 mg/dl), elevated

HbA1c (≥6.5%) or self-reported history of clinical diagnosis.

Hematological and biochemical data were collected at least twice yearly after the diagnosis of NAFLD. Ultrasonography, computed tomography, or magnetic resonance imaging studies were performed at least once annually.

The clinical details of the events of 3 patients were missing. The rate of cancer development was evaluated only in patients confirmed to have no previous or existing HCC at the time of diagnosis of NAFLD, and no previous or current other malignancies apart from HCCs. The rates of development of hepatic encephalopathy, esophago-gastric varices, ascites, and jaundice were evaluated in patients confirmed to have no previous or current hepatic encephalopathy, esophago-gastric varices, ascites, jaundice or HCC at the time of NAFLD

diagnosis, respectively. Mortality was evaluated in patients, who had no previous or present malignancies at the time of NAFLD diagnosis. Details of patient enrolment are shown in Fig. 1.

Liver histopathology

Liver specimens were obtained with a 14-gauge modified Vim Silverman needle (Tohoku University style, Kakinuma Factory, Tokyo, Japan), a 16-gauge core tissue biopsy needle (Bard Peripheral Vascular Inc., Tempe, AZ) or surgical resection. Specimen was fixed in 10% formalin, and the prepared sections were stained with hematoxylin-eosin, Masson trichrome, silver impregnation, or periodic acid-Schiff after diastase digestion. Four pathologists (K.K., F.K., T.F., and T.F.), who were blinded to the clinical findings, evaluated each specimen, and the final assessment was reported by consensus. An

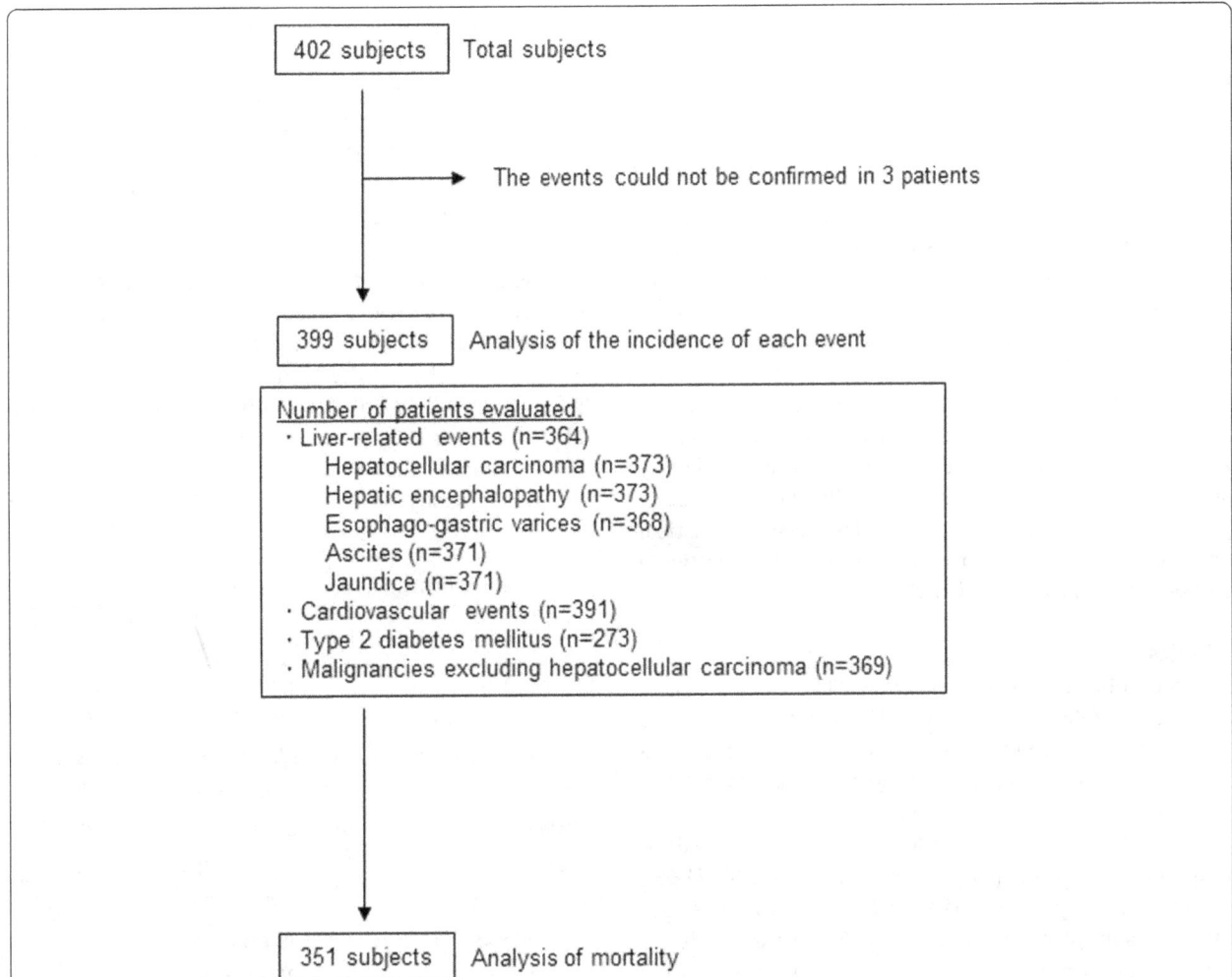

Fig. 1 Between 1976 and 2017, liver biopsy was performed at our hospital, for patients with liver dysfunction and/or fatty liver, as confirmed by abdominal ultrasonography. NAFLD was confirmed histopathologically in 402 Japanese consecutive patients. Follow-up was missing in 3 patients, and 399 patients were evaluated in sub-cohorts in which patients who had experienced an event were excluded from that specific analysis. Mortality was evaluated in 351 patients, without previous or current malignancies at the time of NAFLD diagnosis

adequate liver biopsy sample was defined as a specimen longer than 1.5 cm and/or containing more than 11 portal tracts.

Steatosis grade 0, 1, 2, and 3 corresponded to steatosis of < 5%, ≥5 to < 33%, ≥33 to < 66%, and ≥ 66% of hepatocytes, respectively. Lobular inflammation with no foci, < 2 foci, 2–4 foci, and ≥ 4 foci per 200× field was scored as 0, 1, 2, and 3, respectively. Hepatocyte ballooning of none, few, and many cells was scored as 0, 1, and 2, respectively. The sum of the steatosis, lobular inflammation, and hepatocyte ballooning scores (range, 0–8 points) was the NAS [13]. Fibrosis stage was defined as 0, 1, 2, 3, and 4 [13, 14]. NASH was defined according to the Fatty Liver Inhibition of Progression (FLIP) algorithm [15].

Clinical parameters

We analyzed clinicopathological parameters that could affect NAFLD prognosis. At our hospital, the normal range of aspartate aminotransferase (AST) was 13–33 IU/l, and the normal range of alanine aminotransferase (ALT) was 8–42 IU/l for males and 6–27 IU/l for females. Obesity was defined as body mass index of > 25.0 kg/m^2.

Statistical analysis

The incidence of each event was analyzed during the period from the time of histopathological diagnosis of NAFLD until the last visit or occurrence of event. Stepwise Cox regression analysis was used to determine independent predictive factors associated with the development of HCC and T2DM. The hazard ratio (HR) and 95% confidence interval (95% CI) were also calculated. Variables that were statistically significant on univariate analysis were tested by multivariate analysis to identify significant independent factors. Significance was set at p value < 0.05 by the two-tailed test. Statistical comparisons were performed with the SPSS software (SPSS Inc., Chicago, IL, USA).

Results

Incidence of liver-related events in NAFLD

During the follow-up, 9/373 (2.4%) patients developed HCC (rate per 1000 person years, 3.67), and 21/369 (5.7%) patients developed malignancies other than HCC (rate per 1000 person years, 8.93).

4/373 (1.1%) patients developed hepatic encephalopathy (rate per 1000 person years, 1.60). 6/368 (1.6%) patients developed esophago-gastric varices (rate per 1000 person years, 2.43). 2/371 (0.5%) patients developed ascites (rate per 1000 person years, 0.80). 1/371 (0.3%) patient developed jaundice (rate per 1000 person years, 0.40).

Hence, 10 of 364 patients (2.8%) confirmed to have no previous or current liver-related events at NAFLD

diagnosis developed liver-related events (rate per 1000 person years, 4.17) (Table 2).

Predictors of development of HCC in patients with NAFLD

The characteristics of the 373 patients confirmed to have no previous or current HCC at the time of NAFLD diagnosis were evaluated for prediction of HCC development. Twenty-seven potential predictive factors of the clinicopathological parameters were analyzed (Table 3). Univariate analysis identified the following five parameters that correlated significantly with HCC development: age, fibrosis stage, platelet count, total cholesterol, and α-fetoprotein. These factors were entered into multivariate analysis, which identified two factors that significantly and independently influenced HCC development: advanced age (≥70 years; HR 9.54, 95% CI = 1.63–55.9, P = 0.012) and advanced fibrosis stage (stage 4; HR 7.14, 95% CI = 1.29–39.5, P = 0.024) (Table 3).

Rate of development of cardiovascular events in NAFLD

The characteristics of the 391 patients confirmed to have no previous or current cardiovascular events at NAFLD diagnosis were evaluated for the rate of development of cardiovascular events. During the follow-up, 14 patients (3.6%) developed cardiovascular events, and the development rate per 1000 person years was 5.73 (Table 2).

Rate and predictors of development of T2DM in NAFLD

The incidence of type 2 diabetes mellitus was evaluated in patients confirmed to have no previous or current T2DM (n = 273) at the time of NAFLD diagnosis. During the follow-up, 19 (7.0%) patients developed T2DM (rate per 1000 person years, 9.95) (Table 2).

The characteristics of the 273 patients confirmed to have no previous or current T2DM at the time of

Table 2 Incidence of liver events, cardiovascular events and type 2 diabetes mellitus in patients with NAFLD

Events	n/N (%)[a]	1000 person years
Liver-related events[b]	10/364 (2.8%)	4.17
Hepatocellular carcinoma	9/373 (2.4%)	3.67
Hepatic encephalopathy	4/373 (1.1%)	1.60
Esophago-gastric varices	6/368 (1.6%)	2.43
Ascites	2/371 (0.5%)	0.80
Jaundice	1/371 (0.3%)	0.40
Cardiovascular events	14/391 (3.6%)	5.73
Type 2 diabetes mellitus	19/273 (7.0%)	9.95
Malignancies except for hepatocellular carcinoma	21/369 (5.7%)	8.93

[a]n; number of events. N; number of patients, not having, or having had, the respective event simultaneously or previously to the time of NAFLD diagnosis
[b]Liver-related events were evaluated in patients, without previous or current hepatocellular carcinoma at the time of NAFLD diagnosis

Table 3 Predictors of development of hepatocellular carcinoma in patients with NAFLD

Factor	Category	Univariate Hazard ratio	(95% CI)	P value*	Multivariate Hazard ratio	(95% CI)	P value*
Demographic data							
Gender	Male	1					
	Female	0.24	(0.03–1.97)	0.186			
Age	< 70 y	1			1		
	≥70 y	18.6	(3.74–92.6)	< 0.001	9.54	(1.63–55.9)	0.012
Body mass index	< 25.0 kg/m^2	1					
	≥25.0 kg/m^2	0.46	(0.11–1.88)	0.276			
Type 2 diabetes mellitus	Absence	1					
	Presence	3.64	(0.95–14.0)	0.060			
Hypertension	Absence	1					
	Presence	1.06	(0.28–3.95)	0.932			
Hyperlipidemia	Absence	1					
	Presence	0.36	(0.05–2.91)	0.339			
Histological findings							
Steatosis	5–33%	1					
	> 33%	0.40	(0.10–1.63)	0.201			
Lobular inflammation	< 2 foci per 200× field	1					
	≥2 foci per 200× field	0.31	(0.04–2.50)	0.272			
Ballooning	None / Few cells	1					
	Many cells	0.47	(0.05–3.84)	0.482			
Stage	0–3	1			1		
	4	33.9	(7.14–161)	< 0.001	7.14	(1.29–39.5)	0.024
NAFLD activity score	< 5	1					
	≥5	0.19	(0.02–1.50)	0.114			
Diagnosis according to FLIP algorithm	non-NASH	1					
	NASH	1.34	(0.17–10.8)	0.784			
Laboratory data							
Serum aspartate aminotransferase	< 2 × ULN IU/l	1					
	≥2 × ULN IU/l	2.74	(0.73–10.2)	0.134			
Serum alanine aminotransferase	< 2 × ULN IU/l	1					
	≥2 × ULN IU/l	0.85	(0.22–3.22)	0.810			
Gamma-glutamyl transpeptidase	< 110 IU/l	1					
	≥110 IU/l	1.29	(0.34–4.86)	0.706			
Platelet count	< 200 × 10^3/mm^3	1			1		
	≥200 × 10^3/mm^3	0.06	(0.01–0.50)	0.009	0.14	(0.01–1.33)	0.086
Fasting plasma glucose	< 110 mg/dl	1					
	≥110 mg/dl	3.61	(0.85–15.3)	0.081			
HbA1c	< 5.8%	1					
	≥5.8%	56.2	(0.01–634,349)	0.397			
Uric acid	< 7.1 mg/dl	1					
	≥7.1 mg/dl	0.03	(0.00–21.0)	0.298			
Total cholesterol	< 200 mg/dl	1					
	≥200 mg/dl	0.18	(0.04–0.87)	0.033			

Table 3 Predictors of development of hepatocellular carcinoma in patients with NAFLD *(Continued)*

Factor	Category	Univariate Hazard ratio	(95% CI)	P value*	Multivariate Hazard ratio	(95% CI)	P value*
Triglycerides	< 150 mg/dl	1					
	≥150 mg/dl	0.46	(0.09–2.28)	0.342			
High-density lipoprotein cholesterol	< 41 mg/dl	1					
	≥41 mg/dl	0.58	(0.15–2.25)	0.428			
Low-density lipoprotein cholesterol	< 136 mg/dl	1					
	≥136 mg/dl	0.24	(0.03–2.06)	0.191			
Serum ferritin	< 81 μg/l	1					
	≥81 μg/l	0.71	(0.14–3.61)	0.674			
High sensitive C-reactive protein	< 0.2 mg/dl	1					
	≥0.2 mg/dl	1.02	(0.11–10.0)	0.984			
Alpha-fetoprotein	< 5 μg/l	1			1		
	≥5 μg/l	7.15	(1.44–35.6)	0.016	4.44	(0.84–23.4)	0.079
PIVKA-II	< 21 AU/l	1					
	≥21 AU/l	0.47	(0.06–4.05)	0.495			

*Significance was determined using a Cox proportional hazard model. *CI* confidence interval, *ULN* upper limit of normal

histopathological diagnosis of NAFLD were evaluated for prediction of T2DM development. Twenty-six potential predictive factors of the clinicopathological parameters were analyzed (Table 4). Univariate analysis identified the following five parameters that correlated significantly with T2DM development: gender, hepatocyte steatosis, γ-glutamyl transpeptidase, low-density lipoprotein cholesterol, and serum ferritin. These factors were entered into multivariate analysis, which identified three factors that significantly and independently influenced T2DM development: gender (female; HR 5.83, 95% CI = 1.47–23.1, $P = 0.012$), hepatocyte steatosis (> 33%; HR 9.52, 95% CI = 1.57–57.6, $P = 0.014$), and serum ferritin (≥81 μg/l; HR 0.18, 95% CI = 0.06–0.56, $P = 0.003$) (Table 4).

Mortality in NAFLD, without previous or current malignancies

In patients without previous or present malignancies at the time of NAFLD diagnosis, the overall mortality per 1000 person years was 3.33. The rate was 1.25 for those who died of liver-related events, 0.42 for those who died of cardiovascular events, and 0.83 for those who died of malignancies events other than HCC (Table 5). In the 3 patients who died from liver-related events, 2 of 3 patients and 1 of 3 patients had HCC and liver failure, respectively.

Discussion

The incidence of liver-related and cardiovascular events in patients with histopathologically confirmed NAFLD remains unclear. Furthermore, it is important to identify

the predictors of development of HCC and T2DM to improve the prognosis of patients with NAFLD. There is limited information on the long-term development rate of these events in patients with histopathologically confirmed NAFLD [16, 17].

We found that patients with NAFLD were at increased risk of HCC (HR 6.55, $P = 0.001$) and cardiovascular diseases (HR 1.55, $P = 0.01$) [18]. In the present study, cardiovascular events had the highest incidence (5.73 per 1000 person years), with liver-related events the second highest incidence (4.17 per 1000 person years). Interestingly, among liver-related events, HCC was the event with the highest incidence (3.67 per 1000 person years). The incidence of HCC was more than half of that of cardiovascular events (3.67 vs. 5.73 per 1000 person years). In the present study, the mortality of liver-related events per 1000 person years (1.25) was not lower than that of cardiovascular events (0.42) and malignancies other than HCC (0.83). Hence, liver-related events accounted for about one-third of mortality in NAFLD patients who presented with no previous or present malignancies at the time of NAFLD diagnosis.

The present study has certain limitations. First, only a small number of deaths (8 patients) were recorded during the study period. Further studies of larger number of patients with NAFLD and longer follow-up period should be performed to investigate the impact of each event on mortality.

In another study, the incidence of HCC among all malignancies reported in 1600 patients with NAFLD diagnosed based on the presence of fatty liver by ultrasonography, was 6.0%, and the rate per 1000 person

Table 4 Predictors of development of type 2 diabetes mellitus in patients with NAFLD

Factor	Category	Univariate Hazard ratio	(95% CI)	P value*	Multivariate Hazard ratio	(95% CI)	P value*
Demographic data							
Gender	Male	1			1		
	Female	5.59	(2.07–15.1)	0.001	5.83	(1.47–23.1)	0.012
Age	< 70 y	1					
	≥70 y	0.05	(0.00–5618)	0.606			
Body mass index	< 25.0 kg/m^2	1					
	≥25.0 kg/m^2	1.41	(0.56–3.57)	0.472			
Hypertension	Absence	1					
	Presence	1.53	(0.62–3.77)	0.357			
Hyperlipidemia	Absence	1					
	Presence	1.20	(0.43–3.56)	0.732			
Histological findings							
Steatosis	5–33%	1			1		
	> 33%	3.30	(1.09–10.0)	0.035	9.52	(1.57–57.6)	0.014
Lobular inflammation	< 2 foci per 200× field	1					
	≥2 foci per 200× field	1.70	(0.63–4.57)	0.296			
Ballooning	None / Few cells	1					
	Many cells	0.57	(0.13–2.49)	0.452			
Stage	0–3	1					
	4	1.47	(0.20–11.0)	0.711			
NAFLD activity score	< 5	1					
	≥5	1.30	(0.51–3.26)	0.583			
Diagnosis according to FLIP algorithm	non-NASH	1					
	NASH	1.42	(0.41–4.90)	0.579			
Laboratory data							
Serum aspartate aminotransferase	< 2 × ULN IU/l	1					
	≥2 × ULN IU/l	1.19	(0.45–3.13)	0.730			
Serum alanine aminotransferase	< 2 × ULN IU/l	1					
	≥2 × ULN IU/l	1.47	(0.59–3.64)	0.408			
Gamma-glutamyl transpeptidase	< 110 IU/l	1					
	≥110 IU/l	0.28	(0.08–0.96)	0.043			
Platelet count	< 200 × 10^3/mm^3	1					
	≥200 × 10^3/mm^3	1.94	(0.64–5.87)	0.239			
Fasting plasma glucose	< 110 mg/dl	1					
	≥110 mg/dl	1.31	(0.37–4.62)	0.672			
HbA1c	< 5.8%	1					
	≥5.8%	2.33	(0.32–16.9)	0.404			
Uric acid	< 7.1 mg/dl	1					
	≥7.1 mg/dl	1.28	(0.49–3.38)	0.615			
Total cholesterol	< 200 mg/dl	1					
	≥200 mg/dl	2.43	(0.80–7.34)	0.116			
Triglycerides	< 150 mg/dl	1					
	≥150 mg/dl	0.78	(0.31–1.97)	0.594			

Table 4 Predictors of development of type 2 diabetes mellitus in patients with NAFLD *(Continued)*

Factor	Category	Univariate Hazard ratio	(95% CI)	P value*	Multivariate Hazard ratio	(95% CI)	P value*
High-density lipoprotein cholesterol	< 41 mg/dl	1					
	≥41 mg/dl	0.49	(0.20–1.20)	0.117			
Low-density lipoprotein cholesterol	< 136 mg/dl	1					
	≥136 mg/dl	3.20	(1.06–9.69)	0.040			
Serum ferritin	< 81 µg/l	1			1		
	≥81 µg/l	0.26	(0.10–0.70)	0.008	0.18	(0.06–0.56)	0.003
High sensitive C-reactive protein	< 0.2 mg/dl	1					
	≥0.2 mg/dl	1.84	(0.57–5.97)	0.312			
Alpha-fetoprotein	< 5 µg/l	1					
	≥5 µg/l	1.08	(0.38–3.04)	0.887			
PIVKA-II	< 21 AU/l	1					
	≥21 AU/l	0.23	(0.03–1.79)	0.160			

*Significance was determined using a Cox proportional hazard model. *CI* confidence interval, *ULN* upper limit of normal

years was 0.78, [19]. However, the results of our study indicated that the rate per 1000 person years was 3.67, and rate of HCC was higher compared to the above studies. The discrepant results could reflect patient selection bias, as all patients had histopathologically confirmed NAFLD, with elevated aminotransferases (indicators of high activity) and/or low levels of platelet counts (indicator of advanced fibrosis stage). Furthermore, patients treated with anti-platelet agents and anticoagulants for the prevention of cardiovascular events, did not undergo liver biopsy, and were thus not included. Also, patients who visit the hospital regularly tend to receive treatments for hypertension, hyperlipidemia, and diabetes mellitus, which are as risk factors of cardiovascular events. As previously reported [5], multivariate analysis identified advanced fibrosis stage and old age as significant and independent determinants of HCC development.

Seko and colleagues [20] reported that 13 of 89 (14.6%) patients with biopsy-confirmed NAFLD developed T2DM, and multivariate analysis identified the presence of insulin resistance as an independent risk factor for the development of T2DM. The present study showed that 19 of 273 (6.96%) patients developed T2DM, which is a lower rate compared to the above study. The discrepant results could be due to differences in the diagnostic methods for T2DM; patients in the previous study were diagnosed with a 75-g oral glucose tolerance test. The other reasons for the low frequency of T2DM development is probably that many patients had diabetes at the time of liver biopsy and the follow-up time was short, i.e. selection bias and short follow-up. Interestingly, multivariate analysis in the present study identified higher frequencies of hepatocyte steatosis, lower levels of serum ferritin, and female sex as significant and independent determinants of the incidence of T2DM. Previous reports showed that the incidence of T2DM is higher in postmenopausal female patients with hepatocyte steatosis [17, 21]. However, at this stage, we do not known why lower levels of serum ferritin influence the incidence of T2DM. This finding must be further explored and validated in a larger independent cohort.

Other limitations of the present study included the retrospective study design and the fact that the patients in our study were inpatients. We could not investigate whether factors during the course of observation, such as weight loss and exercise, might affect the development of HCC and T2DM. Furthermore, all participants were Japanese, and thus the results might not be applicable to patients of other races or ethnic groups. Also, the study did not address the epidemiological burden and complexity of the natural history of NAFLD [22, 23]. Identification of predictors of development of HCC and T2DM in patients with NAFLD is a clinical priority due to the currently available suboptimal surveillance criteria [5, 24].

Table 5 Mortality in patients with NAFLD, without previous and current malignancies

Cause of death	n/N (%)[a]	1000 person years
Overall	8/351 (2.3%)	3.33
Liver-related events	3/351 (0.9%)	1.25
Cardiovascular events	1/351 (0.3%)	0.42
Malignancies events except for hepatocellular carcinoma	2/351 (0.6%)	0.83
Other events	2/351 (0.6%)	0.83

[a]n; number of events. N; number of patients, not having, or having had, the respective event simultaneously or previously to the time of NAFLD diagnosis

In conclusion, the results of the present study suggest that cardiovascular and liver-related events are important in Japanese patients with histopathologically-confirmed NAFLD. Especially, HCC was the most common liver-related event, and the incidence of HCC was more than half of that of cardiovascular events. It may be important to identify fibrosis stage and hepatocyte steatosis as determinants of HCC and T2DM, respectively. Further large-scale prospective studies should be performed to identify the predictors of development of HCC and T2DM to improve the prognosis of patients with NAFLD.

Conclusions

Hepatocellular carcinoma was the most common liver-related event in Japanese patients with histopathologically-confirmed NAFLD.

Abbreviations

ALT: alanine aminotransferase; AST: aspartate aminotransferase; CI: confidence interval; FLIP: Fatty Liver Inhibition of Progression; HbA1c: Glycated hemoglobin type A1c; HCC: hepatocellular carcinoma; HR: hazard ratio; NAFLD: non-alcoholic fatty liver disease; NAS: NAFLD activity score; NASH: non-alcoholic steatohepatitis; T2DM: type 2 diabetes mellitus

Acknowledgments

The authors thank Drs. Keiichi Kinowaki and Takeshi Fujii (Department of Pathology, Toranomon Hospital) and also Drs. Fukuo Kondo and Toshio Fukusato (Department of Pathology, Teikyo University School of Medicine) for assistance in histopathological diagnosis.

Disclaimers

This paper has not been published or presented elsewhere in part or in entirety, and is not under consideration by another journal.

Funding

This study was supported in part by Grant-in-Aid from Japan Agency for Medical Research and Development (17fk0210304h0003).

Authors' contributions

N.A., Y.K., Y.A., S.S., S.F., H.S., T.H., M.K. (Masahiro Kobayashi), M.K. (Mariko Kobayashi), Y.S., F.S., K.I., and H.K. contributed to this work. N.A., Y.K., and Y.A. analyzed the data. N.A. wrote the manuscript. All authors read and approved the final manuscript.

Consent for publication

Not Applicable.

Competing interests

(1) Hiromitsu Kumada has received honoraria from MSD K.K., Bristol-Myers Squibb, Gilead Sciences, AbbVie Inc., and Dainippon Sumitomo Pharma. (2) Norio Akuta has received an honorarium from Bristol-Myers Squibb and AbbVie Inc. (3) Yoshiyuki Suzuki has received an honorarium from Bristol-Myers Squibb and AbbVie Inc. All other authors declare no conflict of interest.

Author details

[1]Department of Hepatology, Toranomon Hospital and Okinaka Memorial Institute for Medical Research, 2-2-2 Toranomon, Minato-ku, Tokyo 105-0001, Japan. [2]Liver Research Laboratory, Toranomon Hospital, Tokyo, Japan.

References

1. Angulo P. Nonalcoholic fatty liver disease. N Engl J Med. 2002;346:1221–31.
2. Williams R. Global changes in liver disease. Hepatology. 2006;44:521–6.
3. Torres DM, Harrison SA. Diagnosis and therapy of nonalcoholic steatohepatitis. Gastroenterology. 2008;134:1682–98.
4. Vuppalanchi R, Chalasani N. Nonalcoholic fatty liver disease and nonalcoholic steatohepatitis: selected practical issues in their evaluation and management. Hepatology. 2009;49:306–17.
5. Kawamura Y, Arase Y, Ikeda K, Seko Y, Imai N, Hosaka T, et al. Large-scale long-term follow-up study of Japanese patients with non-alcoholic fatty liver disease for the onset of hepatocellular carcinoma. Am J Gastroenterol. 2012;107:253–61.
6. Sumida Y, Nakajima A, Itoh Y. Limitations of liver biopsy and non-invasive diagnostic tests for the diagnosis of nonalcoholic fatty liver disease/nonalcoholic steatohepatitis. World J Gastroenterol. 2014;20:475–85.
7. Kleiner DE, Brunt EM. Nonalcoholic fatty liver disease: pathologic patterns and biopsy evaluation in clinical research. Semin Liver Dis. 2012;32:3–13.
8. Sanyal AJ, Chalasani N, Kowdley KV, McCullough A, Diehl AM, Bass NM, et al. Pioglitazone, vitamin E, or placebo for nonalcoholic steatohepatitis. N Engl J Med. 2010;362:1675–85.
9. Armstrong MJ, Gaunt P, Aithal GP, Barton D, Hull D, Parker R, et al. Liraglutide safety and efficacy in patients with non-alcoholic steatohepatitis (LEAN): a multicentre, double-blind, randomised, placebo-controlled phase 2 study. Lancet. 2016;387:679–90.
10. Akuta N, Watanabe C, Kawamura Y, Arase Y, Saitoh S, Fujiyama S, et al. Effects of a sodium - glucose cotransporter 2 inhibitor in nonalcoholic fatty liver disease complicated by diabetes mellitus: preliminary prospective study based on serial liver biopsies. Hepatol Commun. 2017;1:46–52.
11. Younossi ZM, Stepanova M, Rafiq N, Makhlouf H, Younoszai Z, Agrawal R, et al. Pathologic criteria for nonalcoholic steatohepatitis: Interprotocol agreement and ability to predict liver-related mortality. Hepatology. 2011;53:1874–82.
12. Angulo P, Kleiner DE, Dam-Larsen S, Adams LA, Bjornsson ES, Charatcharoenwitthaya P, et al. Liver fibrosis, but no other histologic features, is associated with long-term outcomes of patients with nonalcoholic fatty liver disease. Gastroenterology. 2015;149:389–97.
13. Kleiner DE, Brunt EM, Van Natta M, Behling C, Contos MJ, Cummings OW, et al. Design and validation of a histological scoring system for nonalcoholic fatty liver disease. Hepatology. 2005;41:1313–21.
14. Brunt EM, Janney CG, Di Bisceglie AM, Neuschwander-Tetri BA, Bacon BR. Nonalcoholic steatohepatitis: a proposal for grading and staging the histological lesions. Am J Gastroenterol. 1999;94:2467–74.
15. Bedossa P. Utility and appropriateness of the fatty liver inhibition of progression (FLIP) algorithm and steatosis, activity, and fibrosis (SAF) score in the evaluation of biopsies of nonalcoholic fatty liver disease. Hepatology. 2014;60:565–75.
16. Hagström H, Nasr P, Ekstedt M, Hammar U, Stål P, Hultcrantz R, et al. Fibrosis stage but not NASH predicts mortality and time to development of severe liver disease in biopsy-proven NAFLD. J Hepatol. 2017;67:1265–73.
17. Björkström K, Stål P, Hultcrantz R, Hagström H. Histologic scores for fat and fibrosis associate with development of type 2 diabetes in patients with nonalcoholic fatty liver disease. Clin Gastroenterol Hepatol. 2017;15:1461–8.
18. Ekstedt M, Hagström H, Nasr P, Fredrikson M, Stål P, Kechagias S, et al. Fibrosis stage is the strongest predictor for disease-specific mortality in NAFLD after up to 33 years of follow-up. Hepatology. 2015;61:1547–54.
19. Arase Y, Kobayashi M, Suzuki F, Suzuki Y, Kawamura Y, Akuta N, et al. Difference in malignancies of chronic liver disease due to non-alcoholic fatty liver disease or hepatitis C in Japanese elderly patients. Hepatol Res. 2012;42:264–72.

20. Seko Y, Sumida Y, Tanaka S, Mori K, Taketani H, Ishiba H, et al. Insulin resistance increases the risk of incident type 2 diabetes mellitus in patients with non-alcoholic fatty liver disease. Hepatol Res. 2017 Jun 19. [Epub ahead of print].

21. Gaspard U. Hyperinsulinaemia, a key factor of the metabolic syndrome in postmenopausal women. Maturitas. 2009;62:362–5.

22. Lonardo A, Bellentani S, Argo CK, Ballestri S, Byrne CD, Caldwell SH, et al. Epidemiological modifiers of non-alcoholic fatty liver disease: focus on high-risk groups. Dig Liver Dis. 2015;47:997–1006.

23. Lonardo A, Sookoian S, Chonchol M, Loria P, Targher G. Cardiovascular and systemic risk in nonalcoholic fatty liver disease - atherosclerosis as a major player in the natural course of NAFLD. Curr Pharm Des. 2013;19:5177–92.

24. Della Corte C, Colombo M. Surveillance for hepatocellular carcinoma. Semin Oncol. 2012;39:384–98.

16

Prevalence of and risk factors for fatty liver in the general population of Northern Italy: the Bagnacavallo Study

Francesco Giuseppe Foschi[1†], Giorgio Bedogni[2†], Marco Domenicali[3], Pierluigi Giacomoni[4], Anna Chiara Dall'Aglio[1], Francesca Dazzani[1], Arianna Lanzi[1], Fabio Conti[3,5*], Sara Savini[1], Gaia Saini[1], Mauro Bernardi[3], Pietro Andreone[5], Amalia Gastaldelli[6], Andrea Casadei Gardini[7], Claudio Tiribelli[2], Stefano Bellentani[8] and Giuseppe Francesco Stefanini[1]

Abstract

Background: The estimation of the burden of disease attributable to fatty liver requires studies performed in the general population.

Methods: The Bagnacavallo Study was performed between October 2005 and March 2009. All the citizens of Bagnacavallo (Ravenna, Italy) aged 30 to 60 years as of January 2005 were eligible. Altered liver enzymes were defined as alanine transaminase > 40 U/l and/or aspartate transaminase > 37 U/l.

Results: Four thousand and thirty-three (58%) out of 6920 eligible citizens agreed to participate and 3933 (98%) had complete data. 393 (10%) of the latter had altered liver enzymes and 3540 had not. After exclusion of subjects with HBV or HCV infection, liver ultrasonography was available for 93% of subjects with altered liber enzymes and 52% of those with normal liver enzymes. The prevalence of fatty liver, non-alcoholic fatty liver disease (NAFLD) and alcoholic fatty liver disease (AFLD) was 0.74 (95%CI 0.70 to 0.79) vs. 0.35 (0.33 to 0.37), 0.46 (0.41 to 0.51) vs. 0.22 (0.21 to 0.24) and 0.28 (0.24 to 0.33) vs. 0.13 (0.11 to 0.14) in citizens with than in those without altered liver enzymes. Ethanol intake was not associated and all the components of the metabolic syndrome (MS) were associated with fatty liver. All potential risk factors were associated with a lower odds of normal liver vs. NAFLD while they were unable to discriminate AFLD from NAFLD.

Conclusions: Fatty liver as a whole was highly prevalent in Bagnacavallo in 2005/9 and was more common among citizens with altered liver enzymes.

Keywords: epidemiology, cross-sectional study, prevalence, risk factors, fatty liver, chronic liver disease

Background

Fatty liver (FL), the most common liver disease worldwide, is usually classified into non-alcoholic fatty liver disease (NAFLD) and alcoholic fatty liver disease (AFLD) [1, 2]. After the exclusion of hepatitis B and C and steatogenic drugs, NAFLD is currently diagnosed when FL is associated with an ethanol intake ≤20 g/day in women and ≤ 30 g/day in men [1, 2]. The NAFLD vs. AFLD dichotomization is useful in clinical practice because ethanol is unlikely to be toxic at quantities ≤30 g/day but hides the important fact that ethanol and obesity do interact to determine the burden of liver disease in the general population [2–4]. FL is commonly considered the hepatic manifestation of the metabolic syndrome (MS) but the formal testing of the hypothesis that FL is the hepatic component of MS has led to conflicting results [2, 5–7].

In the early 2000s, the Dionysos Study reported the first data on the prevalence and incidence of FL in the

* Correspondence: fabio.conti2@studio.unibo.it
†Francesco Giuseppe Foschi and Giorgio Bedogni contributed equally to this work.
[3]Department of Medical and Surgical Sciences, University of Bologna, Via Massarenti 9, 40138 Bologna, Italy
[5]Research Center for the Study of Hepatitis, Department of Medical and Surgical Sciences, University of Bologna, Bologna, Italy
Full list of author information is available at the end of the article

general population [8, 9]. In the Dionysos Nutrition & Liver Study, the citizens of Campogalliano (Modena, Emilia-Romagna, Italy) with suspected liver disease were matched with randomly chosen citizens without suspected liver disease to obtain estimates of the prevalence of and the risk factors for NAFLD and AFLD in the general population [8]. Many epidemiological studies on FL have been published since the Dionysos Nutrition & Liver Study findings were made available [10]. The worldwide prevalence of NAFLD was estimated to be 0.25 (95%CI 0.22 to 0.28) by a recent meta-analysis of 45 studies [10]. Eleven of these 45 studies were performed in Europe and yielded an estimate of 0.24 (0.16 to 0.33) for the prevalence of NAFLD. Five of these 11 studies used imaging techniques to diagnose FL and were performed in the general population [3, 8, 11–13], with one of them being a nested case-control study [3].

The so-called "ecology of medical care" model provides a strong rationale to expect that the estimates of illness made in the general population will differ from those obtained in other settings and this has indeed been repeatedly shown in practice [14, 15]. The inescapable conclusion is that the real burden attributable to a given disease cannot be estimated without epidemiological data obtained from the general population [15]. There is also mounting evidence that within a given level of the ecology of medical care [14], the individuals actually studied are often not representative of the persons making up that level, e.g. the patients enrolled in trials of NAFLD drugs are not representative of those treated in everyday practice [16].

It was with the aim of providing data on the epidemiology of FL in the general population that we performed the Bagnacavallo Study of liver disease. In detail, the aim of the Bagnacavallo Study was threefold: 1) to evaluate the prevalence of and the risk factors for FL in a cross-section of the general population of a Northern Italy town; 2) to develop a cohort of subjects from the general population where the association between FL and incident health outcomes could be studied; 3) to develop a cohort of subjects from the general population where nested case-control studies of potential risk factors for FL could be performed (taking the advantage of a purposely built serum bank) [17].

The present report deals with the first aim of the Bagnacavallo Study, i.e. the estimation of the prevalence of and the risk factors for FL in a general population. We also report the prevalence of and the risk factors for FL dichotomized into NAFLD and AFLD.

Methods
Study design
The Bagnacavallo Study was performed between October 2005 and March 2009. All citizens of Bagnacavallo

(Ravenna, Emilia-Romagna, Italy) aged 30 to 60 years as of January 2005 were eligible and were invited by written letter to participate to the study. Public encounters were also held to promote participation to the study. Altered liver enzymes (ALE) were defined as alanine transaminase (ALT) > 40 U/l and/or aspartate transaminase (AST) > 37 U/l. These cut-points were the upper normal limits of ALT and AST applied by the laboratory that performed all the analyses of the Bagnacavallo study. The study protocol specified that all ALE+ and at least 50% of ALE- citizens had to undergo liver ultrasonography (LUS). ALE- citizens were chosen consecutively on the basis of their surname starting from a randomly chosen letter of the alphabet. The study was approved by the Ethical Committee of Area Vasta Romagna - IRST (reference number 112). All citizens gave written informed consent.

Clinical and anthropometric assessment
All participants underwent a detailed clinical history and physical examination following the model of the Dionysos Study [8, 18]. Current alcohol intake was assessed by trained interviewers by measuring the quantity (grams) of beer, wine and liquor drunk in the week prior to the enrollment [19]. Such quantity was divided by 7 to obtain a daily estimate and converted into alcohol units with rounding to the next integer. The conversion was done using an alcohol unit corresponding to 10 g of ethanol. Weight and height were measured following international guidelines [20]. Body mass index (BMI) was calculated and classified following the NIH guidelines [21]. Waist circumference (WC) was measured at the midpoint between the last rib and the iliac crest [22].

Laboratory assessment
Venous blood samples were obtained after 12-h fasting. The performed blood tests included: 1) glucose; 2) triglycerides; 3) total cholesterol; 4) high-density lipoprotein (HDL) cholesterol; 5) low-density lipoprotein (LDL) cholesterol; 6) ALT; 7) AST; 8) gamma-glutamyl-transferase (GGT); 9) bilirubin; 10) hepatitis B surface antigen (HBsAg); 11) antibodies against hepatitis C virus (anti-HCV).

Metabolic syndrome
The MS was diagnosed using the harmonized international definition [23]. In detail, large WC was defined as WC ≥ 102 cm in men and ≥ 88 cm in women; high triglycerides as triglycerides ≥150 mg/dl or use of triglyceride-lowering drugs; low HDL as HDL < 40 mg/dl in men and < 50 mg/dl in women or use of HDL-increasing drugs; high blood pressure as systolic blood pressure ≥ 130 mmHg or diastolic blood pressure ≥ 85 mmHg or use or blood pressure-lowering drugs; high glucose as glucose ≥100 mg/dl or use of glucose lowering drugs; and MS as ≥3 of the above.

Liver ultrasonography

LUS was performed by five experienced physicians (ACDA, GS, FD, AL and FC) using the same methodology of the Dionysos Nutrition & Liver Study [9, 24]. Normal liver was defined as the absence of liver steatosis or other liver abnormalities. Light FL was defined as the presence of slight "bright liver" or hepatorenal echo contrast without intrahepatic vessels blurring and no deep attenuation; moderate FL as the presence of mild "bright liver" or hepatorenal echo contrast without intrahepatic vessel blurring and with deep attenuation; and severe FL as diffusely severe "bright liver" or hepatorenal echo contrast, with intrahepatic vessels blurring (no visible borders) and deep attenuation without visibility of the diaphragm. NAFLD was defined as FL associated with ethanol intake ≤2 alcohol units (20 g) / day in women and ≤ 3 alcohol units (30 g) / day in men testing negative for HBsAg and anti-HCV and not treated with steatogenic drugs [2]. AFLD was defined as FL associated with ethanol intake ≥2 alcohol units / day in women and ≥ 3 alcohol units / day in men testing negative for HBsAg and anti-HCV and not treated with steatogenic drugs [2].

Statistical analysis

Most continuous variables were not Gaussian-distributed and all are reported as median and interquartile range. Discrete variables are reported as the number and proportion of subjects with the characteristic of interest. Between-group comparisons of discrete variables were performed using Pearson's Chi-square test and those of continuous variables using median regression with heteroskedasticity-robust standard errors [25].

Binary logistic regression was used to evaluate the association between FL and potential risk factors by means of six pre-specified models [26, 27]. The outcome of all the logistic regression models was FL (discrete; 0 = no; 1 = yes). Model 1 had ALE (0 = no; 1 = yes) as predictor; Model 2 added sex (0 = female, 1 = male) and age (continuous, years/10) to Model 1; Model 3 added BMI (continuous, kg/m²/5) and ethanol intake (continuous, alcohol units) to Model 2; Model 4 replaced BMI in Model 3 with WC (continuous, cm/10); Model 5 added MS (discrete, 0 = no; 1 = yes) and ethanol intake (continuous, alcohol units) as predictors to Model 2; Model 6 replaced MS in Model 5 with its single components, i.e. large WC (discrete, 0 = no; 1 = yes), high triglycerides (discrete, 0 = no; 1 = yes), low HDL (discrete, 0 = no; 1 = yes), high blood pressure (discrete, 0 = no; 1 = yes) and high glucose (discrete, 0 = no; 1 = yes). Before fitting the logistic regression models, we used univariable and multivariable scatterplot smoothers to get an idea of the functional form and shape of the continuous predictors and found no evidence of deviation from linearity for any predictor [28]. We also checked that the multivariable

logits of the continuous predictors were linear using multivariable fractional polynomials [29]. Because alcohol intake as quantified by the present study is strictly speaking an ordinal and not a continuous variable, we tested whether its multivariable relationship with FL was linear by modeling it as both continuous and discrete in the same model [30]. We found that the relationship was linear in all models (data not shown). We also tested whether age and gender interacted in the models involving them (Models 2 to 6) and found that they did not (data not shown). Even if ethanol was not associated with FL, we nonetheless evaluated its interaction with BMI and WC because of its potential clinical significance [3]. We found no evidence of interaction of ethanol with both BMI and WC (data not shown). We evaluated the presence of collinearity among predictors in all models using the Belsley-Kuh-Welsch condition number [31]. We compared models using Akaike information criterion (AIC) and the Bayesian information criterion (BIC) and additionally calculated Nagelkerke pseudo-R^2 and the area the under the receiver-operating characteristic curve (-ROC-AUC) [26]. We used Model 3 to calculate and plot the sex-specific marginal probabilities of FL corresponding to the 5th, 25th, 50th, 75th and 95th internal percentiles of age and BMI at the median intake of ethanol [27, 32].

Multinomial logistic regression was used to evaluate the association between FL type and potential predictors by means of six pre-specified models [26, 27]. The outcome of all the multinomial logistic regression models was FL type (discrete; 0 = NAFLD; 1 = normal liver; 2 = AFLD). The prediction models were the same described above under binary logistic regression with the exception that ethanol was not entered into any model. We set NAFLD as the reference category in order to obtain estimates of effect sizes for the normal liver vs. NAFLD and the AFLD vs. AFLD comparisons. We performed the same tests of model assumptions described above under binary logistic regression. We compared models using Akaike information criterion (AIC) and the Bayesian information criterion (BIC) and additionally calculated Nagelkerke pseudo-R^2. ROC-AUC were calculated for the two binary logistic models underlying the multinomial logistic model. Statistical analysis was performed using Stata 15.1 (Stata Corporation, College Station, TX, USA).

Results
Flow of the citizens through the study

The flow of the citizens through the study is depicted in Fig. 1. Four thousand and thirty-three (58%) of the 6920 citizens aged 30 to 60 years who resided in Bagnacavallo as of January 2005 agreed to participate to the study and 3933 (98%) of them had all the data required for analysis. The citizens were consecutively studied during the first three days of every week (except for holidays)

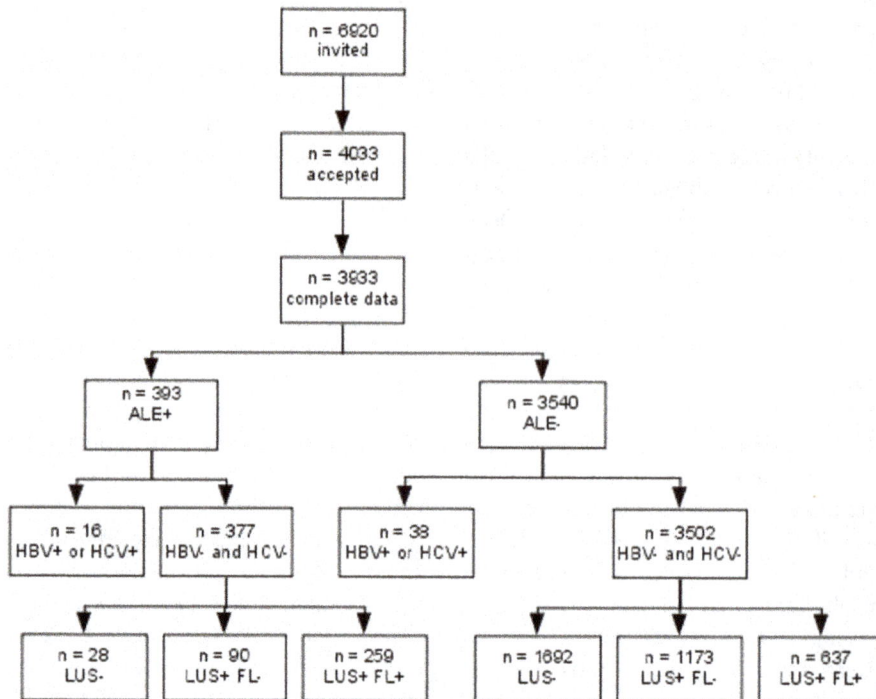

Fig. 1 Flow of the subjects through the study. Abbreviations: ALE = altered liver enzymes; HBV = Hepatitis B virus; HCV = hepatitis C virus; LUS = liver ultrasonography; FL = fatty liver

between October 2005 and March 2009. The study protocol required that all ALE+ and at least 50% of ALE- citizens were recalled to undergo LUS.

Comparison of the subjects with and without liver ultrasonography among the citizens with altered liver enzymes

Three hundred ninety-three (10%) of the 3933 citizens with complete data were ALE+. Sixteen (4.1%) of them had HBV or HCV infection and will not be considered here. Of the remaining 377 ALE+ citizens, 349 (93%) underwent LUS. Additional file 1: Table S1 compares the 349 ALE+ citizens with LUS to the 28 ALE+ citizens without LUS. As compared to ALE+ citizens without LUS, ALE+ citizens with LUS had higher values of triglycerides, ALT and GGT ($p < 0.05$). Besides not being of great interest in itself [33], the lack of statistical significance should be taken with an additional degree of caution here owing to the low number of ALE+ subjects without LUS ($n = 28$).

Comparison of the subjects with and without liver ultrasonography among the citizens with normal liver enzymes

Among the 3540 (90%) ALE- citizens, 38 had HBV or HCV infection (1.1%) and will not be considered here. Of the remaining 3502 ALE- citizens, 1810 (52%) underwent LUS. Additional file 2: Table S2 compares the 1810 ALE- citizens with LUS to the 1692 ALE- citizens

without LUS. As compared to ALE- citizens without LUS, ALE- citizens with LUS were more likely to be male and had higher values of age, weight, BMI, WC, glucose, triglycerides, cholesterol, LDL-cholesterol, systolic blood pressure, ALT, GGT and bilirubin ($p \leq 0.05$). Besides not being of great interest in itself [33], the presence of statistical significance should be taken with an additional degree of caution here owing to the high number of ALE- subjects with ($n = 1810$) and without LUS ($n = 1692$).

Comparison of the citizens with and without altered liver enzymes among those with liver ultrasonography

Table 1 compares the ALE+ and ALE- citizens with availability of LUS. ALE+ citizens were more frequently male and slightly younger than ALE- citizens. ALE+ citizens had greater values of BMI, WC, glucose, triglycerides, total cholesterol, LDL-cholesterol, systolic blood pressure and diastolic blood pressure and lower values of HDL-cholesterol.

Prevalence and risk factors for fatty liver

The prevalence of FL was 0.74 (95%CI 0.70 to 0.79) among ALE+ and 0.35 (0.33 to 0.37) among ALE- citizens ($p < 0.001$). The severity of FL (light vs. moderate vs. severe) was also higher among ALE+ than ALE- citizens. All the components of the MS and the MS itself were more prevalent among ALE+ than ALE- subjects.

Table 1 Comparison of citizens with and without altered liver enzymes

	ALE-	ALE+	p-value[*]
	n = 1810	n = 349	
Age (years)	49 (41–56)	47 (40–55)	0.03
Male sex	812 (44.9%)	267 (76.5%)	< 0.001
Weight (kg)	72.0 (61.0–82.0)	84.0 (74.0–95.0)	< 0.001
Height (m)	1.68 (1.60–1.74)	1.73 (1.67–1.79)	< 0.001
BMI (kg/m^2)	25.1 (22.6–28.1)	27.9 (25.4–30.9)	< 0.001
BMI class (NIH)			< 0.001
Underweight	19 (1.0%)	0 (0.0%)	
Normal	871 (48.1%)	66 (18.9%)	
Overweight	607 (33.5%)	170 (48.7%)	
Obesity class 1	230 (12.7%)	81 (23.2%)	
Obesity class 2	65 (3.6%)	28 (8.0%)	
Obesity class 3	18 (1.0%)	4 (1.1%)	
Fatty liver	637 (35.2%)	259 (74.2%)	< 0.001
Fatty liver degree			< 0.001
Light	428 (67.2%)	107 (41.3%)	
Moderate	151 (23.7%)	102 (39.4%)	
Severe	58 (9.1%)	50 (19.3%)	
Fatty liver type			< 0.001
None	1173 (64.8%)	90 (25.8%)	
NAFLD	407 (22.5%)	160 (45.8%)	
AFLD	230 (12.7%)	99 (28.4%)	
Waist circumference (cm)	100.0 (93.0–107.0)	105.0 (100.0–113.0)	< 0.001
Large waist circumference	1236 (68.3%)	259 (74.2%)	0.028
Glucose (mg/dl)	89 (83–96)	93 (87–102)	< 0.001
High fasting glucose	307 (17.0%)	109 (31.2%)	< 0.001
Triglycerides (mg/dl)	97 (68–139)	138 (98–206)	< 0.001
High triglycerides	405 (22.4%)	159 (45.6%)	< 0.001
Total cholesterol (mg/dl)	207 (184–234)	215 (192–240)	0.005
HDL cholesterol (mg/dl)	61 (51–73)	50 (44–61)	< 0.001
Low HDL	219 (12.1%)	64 (18.3%)	0.002
LDL cholesterol (mg/dl)	126 (104–150)	138 (117–159)	< 0.001
Systolic blood pressure (mm Hg)	125 (120–140)	130 (120–140)	< 0.001
Diastolic blood pressure (mm Hg)	80 (80–90)	85 (80–90)	< 0.001
High blood pressure	1053 (58.2%)	270 (77.4%)	< 0.001
Metabolic syndrome	444 (24.5%)	171 (49.0%)	< 0.001
Metabolic syndrome score			< 0.001
0	216 (11.9%)	19 (5.4%)	
1	595 (32.9%)	59 (16.9%)	
2	555 (30.7%)	100 (28.7%)	
3	294 (16.2%)	97 (27.8%)	
4	117 (6.5%)	59 (16.9%)	
5	33 (1.8%)	15 (4.3%)	

Table 1 Comparison of citizens with and without altered liver enzymes *(Continued)*

	ALE-	ALE+	p-value*
	n = 1810	n = 349	
ALT (U/l)	20 (15–26)	50 (44–63)	< 0.001
AST (U/l)	20 (18–24)	33 (29–41)	< 0.001
GGT (U/l)	17 (12–26)	42 (27–69)	< 0.001
Total bilirubin (mg/dl)	0.60 (0.40–0.81)	0.62 (0.49–0.90)	0.003
Alcohol intake (alcohol units/day)	2 (0–4)	3 (1–5)	< 0.001
Wine intake (alcohol units/day)	2 (0–2)	2 (1–3)	< 0.001
Beer intake (alcohol units/day)	0 (0–1)	0 (0–1)	0.52
Liquor intake (alcohol units/day)	0 (0–0)	0 (0–1)	< 0.001

Values are given as median (interquartile range) for continuous variables and number (proportion) for dichotomous variables
Abbreviations: ALE altered liver enzymes, *BMI* body mass index, *NAFLD* non-alcoholic fatty liver disease, *AFLD* alcoholic fatty liver disease, *NIH* National Institutes of Health, *HDL* high-density lipoprotein, *LDL* low-density lipoprotein, *ALT* alanine transaminase, *AST* aspartate transaminase, *GGT* gamma-glutamyl transferase
*Median regression for continuous variables and Pearson's Chi-square test for binary categorical variables

Lastly, alcohol intake was higher in ALE+ than in ALE- subjects.

Table 2 reports the logistic regression models used to investigate the association between FL and potential risk factors.

Model 1 shows that the odds of FL was 5.3 (95%CI 4.1 to 6.9) times higher in ALE+ than in ALE- citizens. The corresponding probabilities of FL estimated from the logistic regression model are 74% (95%CI 70 to 79%) for ALE+ and 35% (95%CI 33 to 37%) for ALE- citizens.

Model 2 evaluates whether sex and age are associated with FL independently from ALE. While both sex (OR = 2.1, 95%CI 1.7 to 2.5 for males) and age (OR = 1.8, 95%CI 1.6 to 2.0 per decade) show an independent effect on FL, the OR of ALE changed only slightly (4%) compared to Model 1.

Model 3, obtained by adding BMI and alcohol intake as predictors to Model 2, shows that BMI is associated with FL (OR = 3.9, 95%CI 3.3 to 4.5 per 5 kg/m²) with modest changes of the OR of sex (5%) and age (11%) and with a moderate change of the OR of ALE (23%).

Table 2 Logistic regression models used to investigate the association between fatty liver and potential risk factors

	M1	M2	M3	M4	M5	M6
ALE	5.3** [4.1 to 6.9]	5.1** [3.9 to 6.7]	3.9** [2.9 to 5.2]	4.0** [3.0 to 5.4]	4.2** [3.2 to 5.6]	3.7** [2.8 to 5.0]
Male	–	2.1** [1.7 to 2.5]	2.0** [1.6 to 2.5]	2.1** [1.7 to 2.6]	2.0** [1.6 to 2.4]	2.4** [1.9 to 3.0]
Age (years) / 10	–	1.8** [1.6 to 2.0]	1.6** [1.4 to 1.8]	1.5** [1.4 to 1.7]	1.5** [1.4 to 1.7]	1.4** [1.3 to 1.6]
BMI (kg/m²) / 5	–	–	3.9** [3.3 to 4.5]	–	–	–
Alcohol intake (units)	–	–	1.0 [0.9 to 1.0]	1.0 [1.0 to 1.1]	–	–
Waist circumference (cm) / 10	–	–	–	2.5** [2.3 to 2.8]	–	–
Metabolic syndrome	–	–	–	–	5.1** [4.1 to 6.3]	–
Large waist circumference	–	–	–	–	–	2.9** [2.3 to 3.8]
High triglycerides	–	–	–	–	–	3.1** [2.4 to 3.9]
Low HDL	–	–	–	–	–	1.6* [1.2 to 2.2]
High blood pressure	–	–	–	–	–	1.9** [1.5 to 2.3]
High glucose	–	–	–	–	–	2.0** [1.5 to 2.6]
n	2159	2159	2159	2159	2159	2159
AIC	2750	2595	2131	2244	2376	2266
BIC	2762	2618	2165	2278	2405	2317
ROC-AUC	0.61	0.72	0.83	0.81	0.79	0.81
Pseudo-R² (Nagelkerke)	0.11	0.20	0.42	0.37	0.31	0.36

Values are odds ratios and 95% confidence intervals (logistic regression)
Abbreviations: M# model number, *ALE* altered liver enzymes, *BMI* body mass index, *HDL* high-density lipoprotein, *AIC* Akaike information criterion, *BIC* Bayesian information criterion, *ROC-AUC* area under the ROC curve, *pseudo-R²* pseudo-squared R
*p < 0.01; **p < 0.001

Importantly, this model shows that ethanol intake is not associated with FL (OR = 1.0, 95%CI 1.0 to 1.1 per alcohol unit). All the employed metrics of model fit identified Model 3 as the best of all models (lowest AIC, lowest BIC, highest ROC-AUC and highest pseudo-R^2).

Model 4, obtained by replacing BMI in Model 3 with WC, shows that WC is associated with FL (OR = 2.5, 95%CI 2.3 to 2.8) independently of ALE, sex and alcohol intake. The effect sizes of ALE, sex and age are similar to those of Model 3 using BMI as predictor and ethanol intake is again not associated with FL. (We did not evaluate BMI and WC together in Model 4 because of the evidence of collinearity as determined by a Belsley-Kuh-Welsch condition number of 31).

Model 5 evaluates the association of MS with FL taking into account ALE, sex and age. Having MS is associated with an odds of FL equal to 5.1 (95%CI 4.1 to 6.3). (Neither BMI nor WC were entered into this model because WC is already included in the definition of MS and BMI and WC were collinear as explained above.)

Model 6 evaluates the independent contribution of each component of the MS (large WC, high triglycerides, low HDL, high blood pressure and high glucose) to FL. Not only was each component of the MS associated with FL, but all the measures of model fit were better for Model 6 than for Model 5 (lower AIC, lower BIC, higher ROC-AUC and higher pseudo-R^2), showing that there is some advantage in considering the single components of the MS instead of the MS as its association with FL is concerned.

Figure 2 plots the prevalence of FL in men and women with and without ALE as estimated by Model 3 with ethanol intake set at the median value [32]. In both sexes, the prevalence of FL increases with age and BMI.

Prevalence of and risk factors for NAFLD and AFLD

The prevalence of NAFLD and AFLD in ALE+ and ALE- subjects was 0.46 (0.41 to 0.51) vs. 0.22 (95%CI 0.21 to 0.24) and 0.28 (0.24 to 0.33) vs. 0.13 (CI 0.11 to 0.14).

Table 3 reports the multinomial logistic regression models used to investigate the association between FL type and potential risk factors.

Not unexpectedly, all potential risk factors were associated with a lower odds of normal liver vs. NAFLD. All

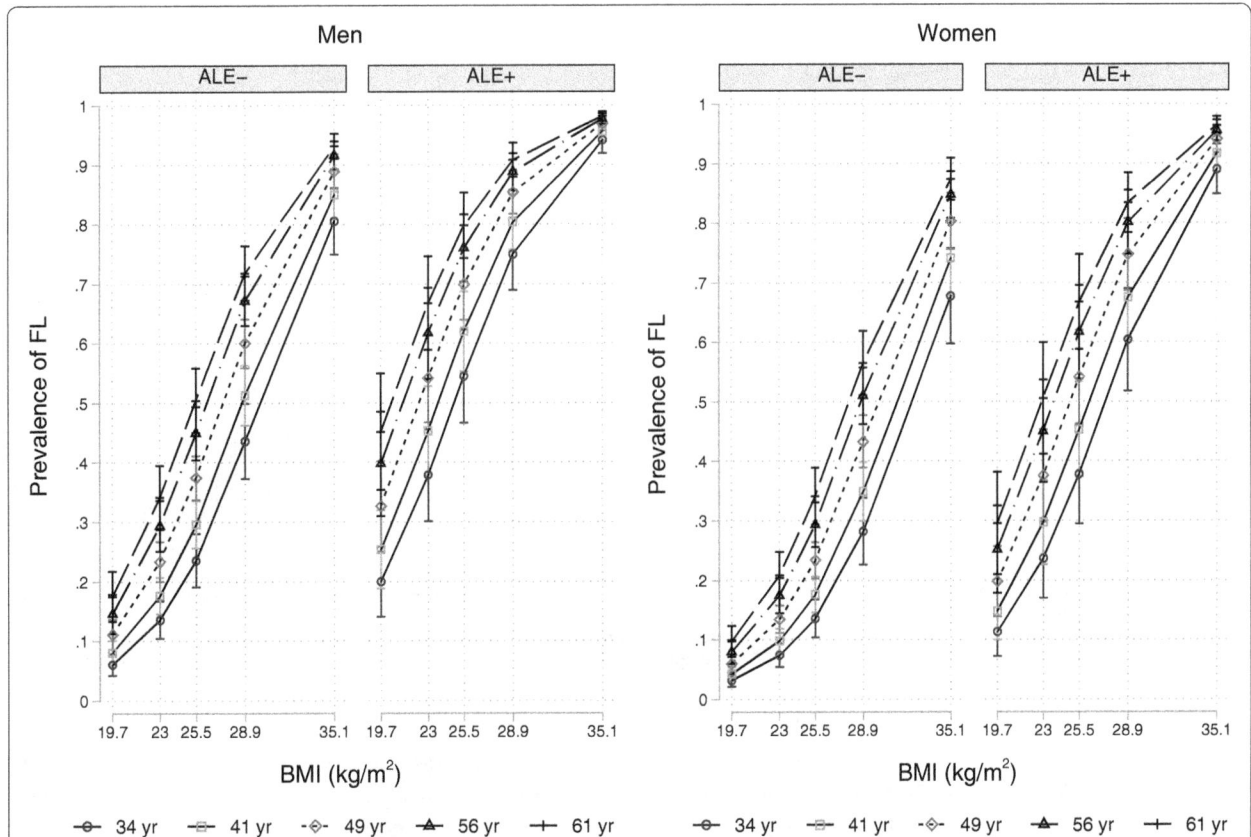

Fig. 2 Prevalence of fatty liver in men and women with and without altered liver enzymes as estimated by Model 3 of Table 2. Values are proportions and pointwise 95% confidence intervals. Abbreviations: ALE = altered liver enzymes; FL = fatty liver; BMI = body mass index. The values of age correspond to the 5th (34 yr), 25th (41 yr), 50th (49 yr), 75th (56 yr) and 95th (61 yr) internal percentiles. The values of BMI correspond to the 5th (19.7 kg/m²), 25th (23.0 kg/m²), 50th (25.5 kg/m²), 75th (28.9 kg/m²) and 95th (35.1 kg/m²) internal percentiles and alcohol intake is set to the median value

Table 3 Multinomial logistic regression models used to investigate the association between fatty liver type and potential risk factors

	M1	M2	M3	M4	M5	M6
Normal liver vs. NAFLD						
Altered liver enzymes	0.20*** [0.15,0.26]	0.19*** [0.14,0.25]	0.25*** [0.18,0.34]	0.24*** [0.17,0.33]	0.23*** [0.17,0.31]	0.26*** [0.19,0.35]
Male sex	–	0.61*** [0.49,0.75]	0.65*** [0.51,0.82]	0.58*** [0.46,0.73]	0.64*** [0.51,0.81]	0.49*** [0.37,0.64]
Age (years) / 10	–	0.53*** [0.46,0.60]	0.60*** [0.52,0.69]	0.61*** [0.53,0.70]	0.61*** [0.53,0.70]	0.65*** [0.56,0.75]
BMI (kg/m^2) / 5	–	–	0.26*** [0.22,0.30]	–	–	–
WC (cm) / 10	–	–	–	0.39*** [0.34,0.43]	–	–
Metabolic syndrome	–	–	–	–	0.20*** [0.16,0.26]	–
High waist circumference	–	–	–	–	–	0.29*** [0.21,0.39]
High triglycerides	–	–	–	–	–	0.38*** [0.29,0.50]
Low HDL	–	–	–	–	–	0.54*** [0.39,0.76]
High blood pressure	–	–	–	–	–	0.56*** [0.43,0.72]
High fasting glucose	–	–	–	–	–	0.52*** [0.39,0.69]
n	1830	1830	1830	1830	1830	1830
ROC-AUC	0.61	0.72	0.83	0.82	0.78	0.81
AFLD vs. NAFLD						
Altered liver enzymes	1.09 [0.81,1.48]	0.89 [0.65,1.21]	0.87 [0.64,1.20]	0.91 [0.66,1.24]	0.87 [0.63,1.19]	0.87 [0.63,1.20]
Male sex	–	1.95*** [1.44,2.63]	1.96*** [1.44,2.65]	1.89*** [1.39,2.56]	1.95*** [1.44,2.64]	1.52* [1.09,2.13]
Age (years) / 10	–	0.82* [0.70,0.97]	0.83* [0.70,0.97]	0.84* [0.71,0.99]	0.82* [0.69,0.97]	0.80* [0.67,0.96]
BMI (kg/m^2) / 5	–	–	1.01 [0.87,1.17]	–	–	–
WC (cm) / 10	–	–	–	0.92 [0.81,1.03]	–	–
Metabolic syndrome	–	–	–	–	1.05 [0.79,1.39]	–
High waist circumference	–	–	–	–	–	0.68* [0.47,0.97]
High triglycerides	–	–	–	–	–	1.58** [1.17,2.13]
Low HDL	–	–	–	–	–	0.64* [0.44,0.93]
High blood pressure	–	–	–	–	–	1.10 [0.78,1.56]
High fasting glucose	–	–	–	–	–	1.12 [0.82,1.53]
n	896	896	896	896	896	896
ROC-AUC	0.51	0.60	0.60	0.61	0.61	0.63
Whole model						
N	2159	2159	2159	2159	2159	2159
AIC	3932	3754	3290	3402	3537	3419
BIC	3955	3800	3347	3459	3594	3521
Pseudo-R^2 (Nagelkerke)	0.10	0.19	0.38	0.34	0.28	0.34

Values are odds ratios and 95% confidence intervals (multinomial logistic regression). ROC-AUC were calculated for the two binary logistic models underlying the multinomial logistic model

Abbreviations: M# model number, *NAFLD* non-alcoholic fatty liver disease, *BMI* body mass index, *WC* waist circumference, *HDL* high-density lipoprotein, *AFLD* alcoholic fatty liver disease, *AIC* Akaike information criterion, *BIC* Bayesian information criterion, *ROC-AUC* area under the ROC curve, *pseudo-R^2* pseudo-squared R
* $p < 0.05$; ** $p < 0.01$; *** $p < 0.001$

odds ratios were in fact < 1 for all predictors (Models 1–6). More interestingly, the same predictors were unable to discriminate AFLD from NAFLD as made clear by the unsatisfactory ROC-curves of the binary ALFD vs. NAFLD model.

In detail, ALE (Models 1–6), BMI (Model 3), WC (Model 4) and MS (Model 5) were not associated with the odds of having AFLD vs. NAFLD. Although male gender and lower age were associated with a greater odds of AFLD vs. NAFLD in all models (Models 1–6), their 95%CI are wide. It is of some interest that high WC and low HDL made AFLD less likely than NAFLD and that high triglycerides made AFLD more likely than NAFLD (Model 6) but the 95%CI of these estimates are again wide.

Discussion

Although much more epidemiological data are presently available on FL as compared to when the Dionysos Study was performed [3, 8], there are still few studies performed in representative samples of the general population [10]. FL has a different course in the general population than in primary, secondary and tertiary care centers, where most of the presently available studies on FL were performed [34]. This is in line with the so-called "ecology of medical care" model, according to which only a minority of citizens with a given illness will actually search for and get medical care [14]. Thus, the real burden attributable to FL cannot be estimated without epidemiological data obtained from the general population [15].

The strengths of the present study are that it was performed in a representative sample of the general population, that it enrolled a high number of subjects, and that it built a serum bank that we plan to use in future studies. The most important limitation of the study is the suboptimal response rate (58%). Although this response rate is the same of the Dionysos Nutrition & Liver Study [8] and is higher than that reported by most studies [35], it is possible that the citizens who refused to participate to the Bagnacavallo Study differed systematically from those who accepted to participate with an ensuing selection bias. Another limitation of the present study is the use of LUS to diagnose FL. Although LUS is virtually the only feasible option to diagnose FL in population studies, it is known to offer an accurate assessment of FL only starting from an intrahepatic triglyceride content of 10% [5, 36]. Thus, lesser degrees of FL may have gone undetected in the present study and our estimates of FL prevalence may be conservative.

In the present study, 74% of ALE+ citizens had FL compared to 35% of ALE- citizens. In the Dionysos Nutrition & Liver Study, performed in the same region of Northern Italy during 2002/3, 44% of citizens with suspected liver disease had FL as compared to 35% of those without suspected liver disease [8]. The estimates made by the Bagnacavallo Study and by the Dionysos Nutrition & Liver Study are unfortunately not comparable because of the different operational definitions of ALE and suspected liver disease. The criteria for suspected liver disease adopted by the Dionysos Nutrition & Liver Study did in fact include an altered GGT (> 35 U/l), did not consider AST, and did consider an ALT > 30 U/l as altered [8]. The Bagnacavallo Study confirms nonetheless, as firstly shown by the Dionysos Nutrition & Liver Study in a general population [8], that FL is quite common (35%) among subjects with normal liver enzymes.

The analysis of the potential risk factors for FL yielded two very interesting findings. The first finding is that ethanol intake was not an independent predictor of FL in the general population. The Dionysos Nutrition & Liver Study reported the same finding even if a direct comparison of the Dionysos Nutrition & Liver Study and the Bagnacavallo Study is not possible because of

the different instruments used to measure alcohol intake [9]. The second finding is that all the components of the MS were associated to FL independently of ALE, gender, age and alcohol intake. The dichotomization implicit in the concept of MS has been criticized by research methodologists on the basis of both clinical and statistical grounds [5, 37]. The findings of the present study offer a further empirical argument for preferring the use of the single components of the MS instead of the whole MS for the study of the association of FL as a whole with cardiometabolic risk factors.

Prevalence of and risks factors for non-alcoholic fatty liver disease and alcoholic fatty liver disease

Although the present study focused on FL as a whole considering ethanol intake as a potential predictor, we performed an analysis of the prevalence of and the risk factors for NAFLD to allow a comparison with the available studies [10].

In the present study, the prevalence of NAFLD was 46% among ALE+ and 22% among ALE- citizens. The corresponding figures for citizens with and without suspected liver disease in the Dionysos Nutrition & Liver Study were 25 and 20% [8]. The Bagnacavallo Study and Dionysos Nutrition & Liver Study estimates are unfortunately not comparable not only because of the different operational definitions of ALE and suspected liver disease as discussed above, but also because the Dionysos Nutrition & Liver Study employed a different cut-point of alcohol intake to diagnose NAFLD in men (≤ 20 g/day) and used a different instrument (7-day prospective diary) to measure ethanol intake [8]. We have, indeed, previously shown that small errors in the estimation of ethanol intake may lead to a substantial difference in the estimated prevalence of NAFLD vs. AFLD [5, 8].

The analysis of the potential risk factors for NAFLD yielded a very interesting finding. All potential risk factors were associated with a lower odds of normal liver vs. NAFLD in all models, which were able to satisfactorily discriminate NAFLD from normal liver. However, the same models were not able to discriminate AFLD from NAFLD. There are several, not mutually exclusive, explanations for this finding. First, the dichotomization of ethanol intake, central to the separation of NAFLD from AFLD [38], could have introduced substantial bias into the inference [37]. Second, we have not cross-validated the recall method used to assess ethanol intake in the present study against an accepted reference method, e.g. the 7-day prospective diary used the Dionysos Nutrition & Liver Study [8]. Thus, we ignore the measurement error of the method used to assess ethanol intake [39]. This is unfortunately the rule in the literature on FL and is especially troublesome because the separation of NAFLD from AFLD is based entirely on the dichotomization of alcohol intake [38]. Third, it is possible that the separation between NAFLD and AFLD is not relevant at the population level because most of the risk factors for FL as whole are not associated with its separation into NAFLD and AFLD. However, without accurate measurements of ethanol intake, this hypothesis remains highly speculative. In view of the fact that ethanol is a well-known hepatotoxic agent, our data should not be taken as evidence that ethanol intake is not an individual risk factor for fatty liver but simply that with conventional instruments used to detect fatty liver and measure ethanol intake, this relationship was not evident at the population level in Bagnacavallo in 2005/2009.

Conclusions

In conclusion, FL was highly prevalent in a Northern Italy town in 2005/9 and was more common among ALE individuals. It had no association with alcohol intake but was strongly associated with anthropometry and all the MS components. NAFLD was more common than AFLD but, while anthropometry and all the MS components were able to discriminate normal liver from NAFLD, they did not discriminate AFLD from NAFLD. The cross-sectional data presented in this paper will inform the ongoing and future analyses of the Bagnacavallo cohort, which we hope will offer new and relevant information on the burden of FL in the general population.

Additional files

Additional file 1: Table S1. Comparison of the citizens with and without liver ultrasonography among those with altered liver enzymes. In this table we compared the 349 citizens with altered liver enzymes (ALE +) and with liver ultrasonography (LUS) to the 28 ALE+ citizens without LUS.

Additional file 2: Table S2. Comparison of the citizens with and without liver ultrasonography among those with normal liver enzymes. In this table we compared the 1810 citizens without altered liver enzymes (ALE-) and with liver ultrasonography (LUS) to the 1692 ALE- citizens without LUS.

Abbreviations

AFLD: Alcoholic fatty liver disease; AIC: Akaike information criterion; ALE: Altered liver enzymes; ALT: Alanine transaminase; anti-HCV: Antibodies against hepatitis C virus; AST: Aspartate transaminase; BIC: Bayesian information criterion; BMI: Body mass index; FL: Fatty liver; GGT: Gamma-glutamyl-transferase; HBsAg: Hepatitis B surface antigen; HDL: High-density lipoprotein; LDL: Low-density lipoprotein; LUS: Liver ultrasonography; MS: Metabolic syndrome; NAFLD: Non-alcoholic fatty liver disease; ROC-AUC: Area the under the receiver-operating characteristic curve; WC: Waist circumference

Acknowledgements
Not applicable.

Funding
The authors state that this work has not received any funding.

Authors' contributions
FGF, PG and GFS made substantial contributions to conception and design and were the study coordinators. MD, ACDA, FD, AL, FC, SS and GS were involved in generation and collection of data. GB performed statistical analysis. GB, MB, PA, AG, ACG, CT, SB were involved in drafting the manuscript or revising it critically. All authors gave final approval of the version to be published.

Consent for publication
Not applicable.

Competing interests
Stefano Bellantani is an Editorial Board Member for BMC Gastroenterology.

Author details
[1]Department of Internal Medicine, Ospedale di Faenza, AUSL Romagna, Faenza, Italy. [2]Liver Research Center, Italian Liver Foundation, Basovizza, Trieste, Italy. [3]Department of Medical and Surgical Sciences, University of Bologna, Via Massarenti 9, 40138 Bologna, Italy. [4]Department of Internal Medicine, Ospedale di Lugo, AUSL Romagna, Locarno, Italy. [5]Research Center for the Study of Hepatitis, Department of Medical and Surgical Sciences, University of Bologna, Bologna, Italy. [6]Institute of Clinical Physiology, National Research Council, Pisa, Italy. [7]Department of Medical Oncology, Istituto Scientifico Romagnolo per lo studio e la cura dei tumori (IRST) IRCCS, Meldola, Italy. [8]Gastroenterology and Hepatology Service, Clinica Santa Chiara, Locarno, Switzerland.

References

1. Chalasani N, Younossi Z, Lavine JE, et al. The diagnosis and management of nonalcoholic fatty liver disease: Practice guidance from the American Association for the Study of Liver Diseases. Hepatology. 2018;67:328–57.
2. EASL-EASD-EASO. EASL-EASD-EASO Clinical Practice Guidelines for the management of non-alcoholic fatty liver disease. J Hepatol. 2016;64:1388–402.
3. Bellentani S, Saccoccio G, Masutti F, et al. Prevalence of and risk factors for hepatic steatosis in Northern Italy. Ann Intern Med. 2000;132:112–7.
4. Hart CL, Morrison DS, Batty GD, Mitchell RJ, Davey Smith G. Effect of body mass index and alcohol consumption on liver disease: analysis of data from two prospective cohort studies. BMJ. 2010;340:c1240.
5. Bedogni G, Nobili V, Tiribelli C. Epidemiology of fatty liver: an update. World J Gastroenterol. 2014;20:9050–4.
6. Smits MM, Ioannou GN, Boyko EJ, Utzschneider KM. Non-alcoholic fatty liver disease as an independent manifestation of the metabolic syndrome: results of a US national survey in three ethnic groups. J Gastroenterol Hepatol. 2013;28:664–70.
7. Lonardo A, Ballestri S, Marchesini G, Angulo P, Loria P. Nonalcoholic fatty liver disease: a precursor of the metabolic syndrome. Dig Liver Dis. 2015;47:181–90.
8. Bedogni G, Miglioli L, Masutti F, Tiribelli C, Marchesini G, Bellantani S. Prevalence of and risk factors for nonalcoholic fatty liver disease: the Dionysos nutrition and liver study. Hepatology. 2005;42:44–52.
9. Bedogni G, Bellantani S, Miglioli L, et al. The Fatty Liver Index: a simple and accurate predictor of hepatic steatosis in the general population. BMC Gastroenterol. 2006;6:33.
10. Younossi ZM, Koenig AB, Abdelatif D, Fazel Y, Henry L, Wymer M. Global epidemiology of nonalcoholic fatty liver disease-Meta-analytic assessment of prevalence, incidence, and outcomes. Hepatology. 2016;64:73–84.
11. Suomela E, Oikonen M, Virtanen J, et al. Prevalence and determinants of fatty liver in normal-weight and overweight young adults. The Cardiovascular Risk in Young Finns Study. Ann Med. 2015;47:40–6.
12. van der Voort EA, Koehler EM, Dowlatshahi EA, et al. Psoriasis is independently associated with nonalcoholic fatty liver disease in patients 55 years old or older: Results from a population-based study. J Am Acad Dermatol. 2014;70:517–24.
13. Volzke H, Robinson DM, Kleine V, et al. Hepatic steatosis is associated with an increased risk of carotid atherosclerosis. World J Gastroenterol. 2005;11:1848–53.
14. Green LA, Fryer GE, Yawn BP, Lanier D, Dovey SM. The ecology of medical care revisited. N Engl J Med. 2001;344:2021–5.

15. Murray CJ, Lopez AD. Measuring the global burden of disease. N Engl J Med. 2013;369:448–57.
16. Parker R, Hodson J, Rowe IAC. Systematic review: Current evidence in non-alcoholic fatty liver disease lacks relevance to patients with advanced fibrosis. J Gastroenterol Hepatol. 2017;32:950–6.
17. Keogh RH, Cox DR. Case-control studies. Cambridge: Cambridge University Press; 2014.
18. Bellentani S, Tiribelli C, Saccoccio G, et al. Prevalence of chronic liver disease in the general population of northern Italy: the Dionysos Study. Hepatology. 1994;20:1442–9.
19. MacDonald I. Health issues related to alcohol consumption. Oxford: Blackwell Science; 1999.
20. Lohman TG, Roche AF, Martorell R. Anthropometric standardization reference manual. Champaign. Illinois: Human Kinetics Books; 1991.
21. Clinical Guidelines on the Identification, Evaluation, and Treatment of Overweight and Obesity in Adults. The Evidence Report. National Institutes of Health. Obes Res. 1998;6(Suppl 2):51S–209S.
22. Bedogni G, Kahn HS, Bellentani S, Tiribelli C. A simple index of lipid overaccumulation is a good marker of liver steatosis. BMC Gastroenterol. 2010;10:98.
23. Alberti KG, Eckel RH, Grundy SM, et al. Harmonizing the metabolic syndrome: a joint interim statement of the International Diabetes Federation Task Force on Epidemiology and Prevention; National Heart, Lung, and Blood Institute; American Heart Association; World Heart Federation; International Atherosclerosis Society; and International Association for the Study of Obesity. Circulation. 2009;120:1640–5.
24. Sanyal AJ. AGA technical review on nonalcoholic fatty liver disease. Gastroenterology. 2002;123:1705–25.
25. Machado JAF, Parente PMDC, Santos Silva JMC. QREG2: Stata module to perform quantile regression with robust and clustered standard errors. Statistical Software Components, Boston College Department of Economics S457369. 2011; https://ideas.repec.org/c/boc/bocode/s457369.html.
26. Hosmer D, Lemeshow L, Sturdivant R. Applied Logistic Regression. Hoboken: Wiley; 2013.
27. Long JS, Freese J. Regression models for categorical dependent variables using Stata. College Station: Stata Press; 2014.
28. Royston P, Cox NJ. A multivariable scatterplot smoother. Stata J. 2005;5:405–12.
29. Royston P, Sauerbrei W. Multivariable model-building: a pragmatic approach to regression analysis based on fractional polynomials for modelling continuous variables. Chichester: John Wiley; 2008.
30. Harrell F. Regression modeling strategies. Switzerland: Springer International Publishing; 2015.
31. Belsley DA, Kuh E, Welsch RE. Regression diagnostics: identifying influential data and sources of collinearity. New York: Wiley; 1980.
32. Williams R. Using the margins command to estimate and interpret adjusted predictions and marginal effects. Stata J. 2012;12:308–31.
33. Wasserstein R. The ASA's statement on p-values: context, process, and purpose. Am Stat. 2016;70:129–33.
34. Bedogni G, Miglioli L, Masutti F, et al. Incidence and natural course of fatty liver in the general population: the Dionysos study. Hepatology. 2007;46:1387–91.
35. Morton SM, Bandara DK, Robinson EM, Carr PE. In the 21st Century, what is an acceptable response rate. Aust N Z J Public Health. 2012;36:106–8.
36. Hernaez R, Lazo M, Bonekamp S, et al. Diagnostic accuracy and reliability of ultrasonography for the detection of fatty liver: A meta-analysis. Hepatology. 2011;54:1082–90.
37. Greenland S. Invited Commentary: The Need for Cognitive Science in Methodology. Am J Epidemiol. 2017;186:639–45.
38. Kleiner DE, Makhlouf HR. Histology of Nonalcoholic Fatty Liver Disease and Nonalcoholic Steatohepatitis in Adults and Children. Clin Liver Dis. 2016;20:293–312.
39. Jurek AM, Maldonado G, Greenland S, Church TR. Exposure-measurement error is frequently ignored when interpreting epidemiologic study results. Eur J Epidemiol. 2006;21:871–6.

17

Diagnostic value of alpha-fetoprotein combined with neutrophil-to-lymphocyte ratio for hepatocellular carcinoma

Jian Hu[1†], Nianyue Wang[2†], Yongfeng Yang[2], Li Ma[2], Ruilin Han[3], Wei Zhang[4], Cunling Yan[3*], Yijie Zheng[5*] and Xiaoqin Wang[1*]

Abstract

Background: To investigate the diagnostic performance of alpha-fetoprotein (AFP) and neutrophil-to-lymphocyte ratio (NLR) as well as their combinations with other markers.

Methods: Serum aspartate aminotransferase (AST), alanine aminotransferase (ALT), AFP and levels as well as the numbers of neutrophils and lymphocytes of all enrolled patients were collected. The NLR was calculated by dividing the number of neutrophils by the number of lymphocytes. Receiver operating characteristic (ROC) curve analysis was conducted to determine the ability of each marker and combination of markers to distinguish HCC and liver disease patients.

Results: In total, 545 patients were included in this study. The area under the ROC curve (AUC) values for AFP, ALT, AST, and NLR were 0.775 (0.738–0.810), 0.504 (0.461–0.547), 0.660 (0.618–0.699), and 0.738 (0.699–0.774) with optimal cut-off values of 24.6 ng/mL, 111 IU/mL, 27 IU/mL, and 2.979, respectively. Of the four biomarkers, AFP and NLR showed comparable specificity (0.881 and 0.858) and sensitivity (0.561 and 0.539). The combination of AFP and NLR showed the highest AUC (0.769) with a significantly higher sensitivity (0.767) and a lower specificity (0.773) compared to AFP or NLR alone, and it had the highest sum of sensitivity and specificity (1.54) among all combinations. In patients with AFP < 20 ng/mL, the NLR showed the highest AUC and combination with other markers did not improve the diagnostic accuracy.

Conclusions: Our data indicate that the combination of AFP and NLR offers better diagnostic performance than either marker alone for differentiating HCC from liver disease, which may benefit clinical screening.

Keywords: Alpha-fetoprotein, Neutrophil-granulocyte ratio, Hepatocellular carcinoma

Background

Liver cancer is the sixth most common cancer and the third leading cause of cancer-related death worldwide [1, 2]. Hepatocellular carcinoma (HCC), which accounts for 70–85% of liver cancer cases, is always diagnosed in an advanced stage and is associated with a poor prognosis, with a 5-year overall survival rate of less than 15% [3, 4]. At present, treatments such as surgery and liver transplantation for early-stage HCC result in better outcomes with a 5-year overall survival rate of more than 70% [5–7]. Therefore, diagnosis of HCC during an early stage is pivotal for improving the clinical outcomes of patients.

Alpha-fetoprotein (AFP) is the most widely used serum marker for screening and initial diagnosis of HCC in clinical practice. However, the sensitivity of AFP is only about 60% at a cut-off value of 20 ng/mL, and the specificity is low [8–10]. Moreover, AFP levels remain normal in 15–30% of patients with advanced stage disease and increase in some patients with chronic hepatitis, liver cirrhosis, and

* Correspondence: yancunling@163.com; yijiezheng2015@163.com; 1493722680@qq.com
†Jian Hu and Nianyue Wang contributed equally to this work.
³Department of Clinical Laboratory, Peking University First Hospital, Beijing 100000, China
⁵Medical Scientific Affairs, Abbott Diagnostics Division, Abbott Laboratories, Shanghai 200032, China
¹Department of Clinical Laboratory, The First Affiliated Hospital of Xi'an Jiaotong University, 277 West Yanta Road, Xi'an 710061, People's Republic of China
Full list of author information is available at the end of the article

other liver diseases [4, 11], leading to high negative and false-positive rates. Therefore, novel markers that complement the limitations of AFP are needed to for screening and more accurate diagnosis of HCC.

Crosstalk between cancer cells and their inflammatory microenvironment plays critical roles in the initiation and progression of cancer, including the promotion of angiogenesis, proliferation, and metastasis [12–14]. Inflammatory infiltrates in the tumor microenvironment largely influence the biological behavior of HCC [15–18]. The neutrophil-to-lymphocyte ratio (NLR) is one parameter reflecting the presence of a systemic inflammatory response and can be readily determined at low cost through routine blood examination. The baseline NLR has been reported to be a valuable predictor in many cancers, including colorectal cancer [19], renal cancer [20], diffuse large B-cell lymphoma [21, 22], and HCC [23]. The NLR also has been reported to be diagnostic marker for peptic ulcer perforation [24], acute mesenteric ischemia [25], and lung cancer [26, 27].

Thus, we questioned whether the NLR can be used as a supplementary diagnostic marker with AFP. This study aimed to evaluate the diagnostic value of AFP in combination with the NLR for HCC. To better investigate the relative diagnostic value of serum biomarkers, two common serum biomarkers for liver function, aspartate aminotransferase (AST) and alanine aminotransferase (ALT), also were analyzed in the present study.

Methods
Patients
Patients diagnosed with HCC and liver disease were enrolled at the three centers (Peking University 1st Hospital, Xi'an Jiaotong University 1st Hospital and The Second Hospital of Nanjing, Affiliated to Medical School of Southeast University) between July 2013 and July 2016. HCC was diagnosed according to the Asian Pacific Association for the Study of the Liver (APASL) consensus recommendations on HCC [28]. Only newly diagnosed

and treatment-naïve patients with HCC were enrolled in the present study. Liver disease samples were mainly from patients infected with hepatitis B virus (HBV) or hepatitis C virus (HCV) and include samples from patients with hepatitis and cirrhosis, which were diagnosed according to APASL guideline.

This study was conducted according to the Declaration of Helsinki and approved by the Ethics of Committee.

Data collection
Serum AST and ALT concentrations and the numbers of neutrophils and lymphocytes were recorded from routine clinical testing. Serum AFP was measured using the Abbott ARCHITECT hepatitis B surface antigen chemiluminescent microparticle immunoassay (Abbott Diagnostics, Abbott Park, IL, USA). The NLR was calculated by dividing the number of neutrophils by the number of lymphocytes.

Statistical analysis
All statistical analyses were performed using SPSS (version 21; IBM, Armonk, NY, USA). Data are presented as mean ± standard derivation for normally distributed continuous data, as median (interquartile range, Q25–Q75) for abnormally distributed continuous data, or as actual values for categorical data. Comparisons between two groups were performed using t test, Wilcoxon test, or chi-square test. Receiver operation characteristic (ROC) curves were used to compare the diagnostic performance of each biomarker. The area under the ROC curve (AUC) for each biomarker for distinguishing HCC and liver disease patients as well as the optimal cut-off value, sensitivity, specificity, positive predictive value (PPV), and negative predictive value (NPV) were calculated using MedCalc. Combinations of markers were analyzed, and the related parameters were calculated with the online statistical software OpenEpi (http://www.openepi.com/Menu/OE_Menu.htm). A P value < 0.05 was considered to indicate a statistically significant difference.

Table 1 Clinical characteristics of the patients

	Liver disease ($n = 176$)	HCC ($n = 369$)	P value
Age (y)	46.34 ± 11.71	56.91 ± 10.04	< 0.001
Gender (M/F)	124/52	318/51	< 0.001
Neutrophils ($\times 10^9$/L)	5.705 (2.97–58.20)	0.674 (0.57–0.78)	< 0.001
Lymphocytes ($\times 10^9$/L)	3.01 (1.65–30.85)	0.209 (0.12–0.295)	< 0.001
NLR	1.851 (1.43–2.53)	3.23 (1.91–6.62)	< 0.001
ALT (IU/mL)	38.5 (26.00–66.50)	38.9 (23.75–73.93)	0.739
AST (IU/mL)	29 (21.00–52.00)	44 (29.78–85.65)	< 0.001
AFP (ng/mL)	3.67 (2.43–10.36)	41.16 (5.59–1030.03)	< 0.001

HCC, hepatocellular carcinoma; M, male; F, female; NLR, neutrophil-granulocyte ratio; ALT, alanine aminotransferase; AST, aspartate aminotransferase; AFP, alpha-fetoprotein
Data are presented as mean ± standard derivation for age, actual values for gender, and median (interquartile range, Q25-Q75) for other parameters
Comparisons between two groups were performed using t test for age, chi-square test for gender, or Wilcoxon test for other parameters

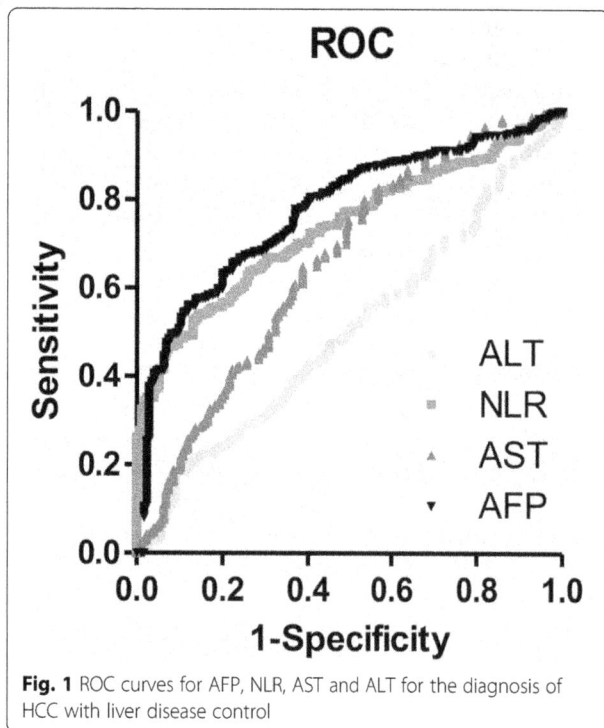

Fig. 1 ROC curves for AFP, NLR, AST and ALT for the diagnosis of HCC with liver disease control

Results
Clinical characteristics of the participants
In total, 545 patients, 369 with HCC and 176 with liver disease (21 cases of cirrhosis, 130 cases of hepatitis, and 25 cases of other diseases including autoimmune liver disease and alcoholic liver disease) were included in this study. The clinical characteristics of all participants are shown in Table 1. While ALT levels did not differ significantly, HCC patients were older, more likely to be male, had fewer neutrophils and lymphocytes, had a higher NLR, and had higher AST and AFP levels than liver disease patients (all $P < 0.001$).

Diagnostic accuracy of serum biomarkers for detecting HCC
The ROC curves for serum biomarkers (AFP, ALT, AST, and NLR) for diagnosing HCC are shown in Fig. 1. The AUC values for AFP, ALT, AST, and NLR were 0.775 (0.738–0.810), 0.504 (0.461–0.547), 0.660 (0.618–0.699), and 0.738 (0.699–0.774) with optimal cut-off values of 24.6 ng/mL, 111 IU/mL, 27 IU/mL, and 2.979, respectively. When applying the common cutoff value of 20 ng/mL for AFP, the AUC was 0.664 (0.6224–0.703) (Table 2). Of the four biomarkers, ALT showed the highest specificity (0.909) with the lowest sensitivity (0.184), and AFP and NLR individually showed both higher specificity (0.881 and 0.858) and higher sensitivity (0.561 and 0.539) compared to AST (Table 2).

Because both AFP and NLR showed low sensitivity values, the diagnostic value of biomarker combinations was evaluated. The AUC, sensitivity, specificity, PPV, and NPV as well as optimal cut-off values for each marker and different combinations of biomarkers are summarized in Table 3. As diagnostic biomarkers for HCC, among all combinations of two biomarkers, the combination of AFP and NLR showed the highest AUC (0.769) with a significantly higher sensitivity (0.767) and a lower specificity (0.773) compared to AFP or NLR alone. In addition, this combination had the highest sum of sensitivity and specificity (1.54) among all the two-marker combinations. However, the combination of NLR and AST was the most sensitive (0.892) with a specificity of 0.409. Among all combinations with three biomarkers, the combination of AFP, NLR, and AST was the most sensitive (0.927) with a specificity of 0.409 and showed the same accuracy as the combination of all four biomarkers (Table 2). The combination of AFP, NLR, and ALT showed the highest AUC (0.773) with the highest sum of sensitivity and specificity (1.524) among all the three-marker combinations.

Table 2 Diagnostic performances of four serum biomarkers for differentiating HCC from liver disease

Marker	Cutoff value	AUC	Sensitivity (Sn)	Specificity (Sp)	Sn + Sp	PPV	NPV
ALT	111	0.504 (0.461–0.547)	0.184 (0.146–0.228)	0.909 (0.857–0.947)	1.093	0.810 (0.709–0.887)	0.347 (0.304–0.392)
AST	27	0.660 (0.618–0.699)	0.802 (0.758–0.842)	0.466 (0.391–0.542)	1.268	0.759 (0.713–0.801)	0.529 (0.447–0.610)
AFP	24.64	0.775 (0.738–0.810)	0.561 (0.509–0.612)	0.881 (0.823–0.925)	1.442	0.908 (0.863–0.942)	0.489 (0.433–0.545)
	20	0.664 (0.624–0.703)	0.577 (0.525–0.628)	0.852 (0.791–0.901)	1.429	0.891 (0.845–0.928)	0.490 (0.433–0.548)
	40	0.633 (0.592–0.672)	0.501 (0.449–0.554)	0.903 (0.850–0.943)	1.404	0.916 (0.869–0.950)	0.464 (0.410–0.518)
	100	0.514 (0.467–0.560)	0.442 (0.390–0.494)	0.938 (0.891–0.968)	1.38	0.937 (0.890–0.968)	0.445 (0.393–0.497)
	200	0.580 (0.538–0.621)	0.396 (0.345–0.448)	0.960 (0.920–0.984)	1.356	0.954 (0.908–0.981)	0.431 (0.382–0.482)
	188.4	0.585 (0.544–0.626)	0.409 (0.359–0.461)	0.955 (0.912–0.980)	1.364	0.950 (0.903–0.978)	0.435 (0.385–0.486)
NLR	2.979	0.738 (0.699–0.774)	0.539 (0.487–0.591)	0.858 (0.797–0.906)	1.397	0.888 (0.840–0.926)	0.470 (0.415–0.527)

HCC, hepatocellular carcinoma; ALT, alanine aminotransferase; AST, aspartate aminotransferase; AFP, alpha-fetoprotein; NLR, neutrophil-granulocyte ratio; AUC, area under the receiver operation characteristics curve

Table 3 Diagnostic performances of combinations of four serum biomarkers for differentiating HCC from liver disease

Markers	AUC	Sensitivity (Sn)	Specificity (Sp)	Sn + Sp	PPV	NPV
AFP + NLR	0.769 (0.732–0.802)	0.767 (0.721–0.807)	0.773 (0.705–0.828)	1.54	0.876 (0.836–0.908)	0.613 (0.547–0.674)
AFP + ALT	0.697 (0.657–0.734)	0.639 (0.578–0.677)	0.841 (0.780–0.888)	1.48	0.892 (0.849–0.924)	0.519 (0.461–0.577)
AFP + AST	0.749 (0.711–0.783)	0.884 (0.847–0.912)	0.466 (0.394–0.540)	1.35	0.776 (0.734–0.813)	0.656 (0.569–0.734)
ALT+AST	0.694 (0.654–0.731)	0.802 (0.759–0.840)	0.470 (0.394–0.540)	1.272	0.759 (0.714–0.799)	0.529 (0.451–0.606)
NLR + ALT	0.653 (0.612–0.692)	0.596 (0.545–0.645)	0.773 (0.705–0.828)	1.369	0.846 (0.797–0.885)	0.477 (0.420–0.535)
NLR + AST	0.736 (0.697–0.771)	0.892 (0.856–0.919)	0.409 (0.339–0.483)	1.301	0.760 (0.717–0.798)	0.643 (0.551–0.726)
AFP + AST + ALT	0.749 (0.711–0.783)	0.884 (0.847–0.912)	0.466 (0.394–0.540)	1.35	0.776 (0.734–0.813)	0.656 (0.569–0.734)
NLR + AST + ALT	0.736 (0.697–0.771)	0.892 (0.856–0.919)	0.409 (0.339–0.483)	1.301	0.760 (0.717–0.798)	0.643 (0.551–0.726)
AFP + NLR + ALT	0.773 (0.735–0.806)	0.791 (0.747–0.830)	0.733 (0.663–0.793)	1.524	0.861 (0.821–0.894)	0.626 (0.558–0.689)
AFP + NLR + AST	0.760 (0.722–0.796)	0.927 (0.896–0.949)	0.409 (0.339–0.483)	1.336	0.767 (0.725–0.804)	0.727 (0.632–0.805)
AFP + AST + ALT+NLR	0.760 (0.722–0.796)	0.927 (0.896–0.949)	0.409 (0.339–0.483)	1.336	0.767 (0.725–0.804)	0.727 (0.632–0.805)

HCC, hepatocellular carcinoma; ALT, alanine aminotransferase; AST, aspartate aminotransferase; AFP, alpha-fetoprotein; NLR, neutrophil-granulocyte ratio; AUC, area under the receiver operating characteristic curve

For combinations of markers, similar results were obtained when applying the common cutoff value of 20 ng/mL AFP or the optimal cutoff value of 24.6 ng/mL AFP (Table 4). When used in combination, AFP and NLR showed the highest sum of sensitivity and specificity (1.511).

Diagnostic accuracy of AFP with different cut-off value as well as in combination with three other biomarkers

Next, the sensitivity, specificity, PPV, and NPV for AFP at different cutoff values were analyzed. As shown in Table 2, with the increase in cutoff value, AFP showed decreased sensitivity (from 0.577 at 20 ng/mL to 0.396 at 200 ng/mL) and increased specificity (from 0.852 at 20 ng/mL to 0.955 at 200 ng/mL), with the highest AUC of 0.775 at 24.64 ng/mL. Then we used the cutoff value of AFP with 95% specificity, which was 188.40 ng/mL, in combination with other

markers. If the sensitivity was as high as 90%, the cut-off values for AST, ALT, and NLR were 26.4–26.6, 20.8, and 1.7, respectively, and the cutoff values for AST and ALT were 29.6 IU/mL and 23.5 IU/mL.

Diagnostic accuracy of NLR in patients with low AFP (< 20 ng/mL)

In the present study, 156 (42.3%) HCC patients and 149 (85.1%) liver disease patients had an AFP level less than 20 ng/mL. We also evaluated the diagnostic accuracy of these biomarkers for HCC in these patients. As shown in Fig. 2 and Table 5, among all three biomarkers, the NLR showed the highest AUC (0.685). ALT and AST showed the same AUC and cutoff values as in the whole population, whereas the NLR had a lower AUC (0.685 vs 0.738) and a higher cutoff value (3.355 vs 2.979) with an increased specificity (0.926 vs 0.858) in patients with a low

Table 4 Diagnostic performances of combinations of four serum biomarkers for differentiating HCC from liver disease using AFP = 20 ng/mL as cutoff value

Markers	AUC	Sensitivity (Sn)	Specificity (Sp)	Sn + Sp	PPV	NPV
AFP + NLR	0.762 (0.724–0.795)	0.772 (0.727–0.812)	0.739 (0.669–0.798)	1.511	0.861 (0.820–0.894)	0.608 (0.541–0.671)
AFP + ALT	0.697 (0.657–0.734)	0.694 (0.654–0.731)	0.807 (0.742–0.858)	1.501	0.874 (0.829–0.909)	0.516 (0.4458–0.575)
AFP + AST	0.749 (0.711–0.783)	0.889 (0.853–0.917)	0.470 (0.394–0.540)	1.359	0.777 (0.735–0.813)	0.667 (0.579–0.744)
ALT+AST	0.694 (0.654–0.731)	0.802 (0.759–0.840)	0.470 (0.394–0.540)	1.272	0.759 (0.714–0.799)	0.529 (0.451–0.606)
NLR + ALT	0.653 (0.612–0.692)	0.596 (0.545–0.645)	0.773 (0.705–0.828)	1.369	0.846 (0.797–0.885)	0.477 (0.420–0.535)
NLR + AST	0.736 (0.697–0.771)	0.892 (0.856–0.919)	0.409 (0.339–0.483)	1.301	0.760 (0.717–0.798)	0.643 (0.551–0.726)
AFP + AST + ALT	0.749 (0.711–0.783)	0.889 (0.853–0.917)	0.470 (0.394–0.540)	1.359	0.777 (0.735–0.813)	0.667 (0.579–0.744)
NLR + AST + ALT	0.736 (0.697–0.771)	0.892 (0.856–0.919)	0.409 (0.339–0.483)	1.301	0.760 (0.717–0.798)	0.643 (0.551–0.726)
AFP + NLR + ALT	0.765 (0.728–0.799)	0.799 (0.759–0.835)	0.699 (0.627–0.762)	1.498	0.847 (0.806–0.881)	0.621 (0.552–0.686)
AFP + NLR + AST	0.762 (0.724–0.795)	0.930 (0.899–0.952)	0.409 (0.339–0.484)	1.339	0.767 (0.73–0.804)	0.736 (0.640–0.812)
AFP + AST + ALT+NLR	0.762 (0.724–0.795)	0.930 (0.8998–0.952)	0.409 (0.339–0.484)	1.339	0.767 (0.73–0.804)	0.736 (0.640–0.812)

HCC, hepatocellular carcinoma; ALT, alanine aminotransferase; AST, aspartate aminotransferase; AFP, alpha-fetoprotein; NLR, neutrophil-granulocyte ratio; AUC, area under the receiver operating characteristic curve

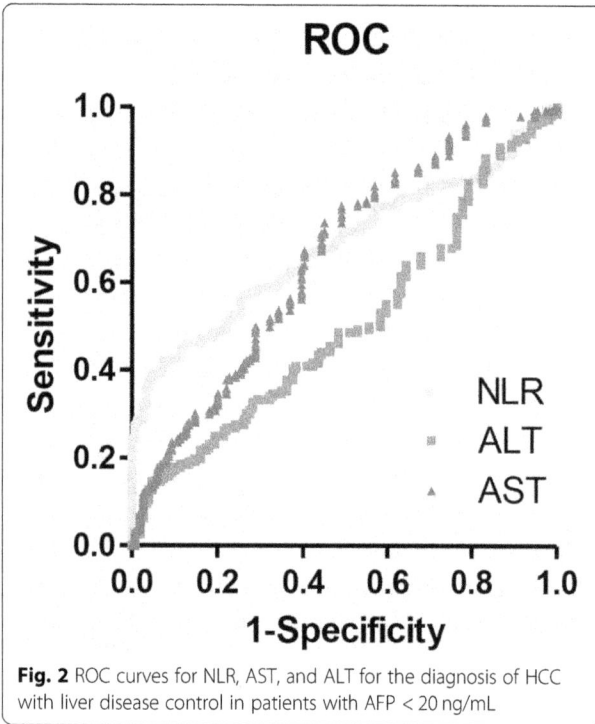

Fig. 2 ROC curves for NLR, AST, and ALT for the diagnosis of HCC with liver disease control in patients with AFP < 20 ng/mL

AFP level. Among biomarker combinations, NLR and ALT together showed the highest AUC (0.682) with the highest sum of sensitivity and specificity (1.423; Table 6).

Discussion

In the present study, the diagnostic values of AFP, NLR, AST, and ALT as well as their combinations were evaluated and compared. The data showed that AFP remained the best single marker, and the NLR was a comparable single marker to AFP. The combination of AFP and NLR had the best diagnostic performance (with a sum of sensitivity and specificity of 1.54) compared to all other combinations, even in patients with AFP < 20 ng/mL. Combination of three or four markers did not improve the diagnostic performance compared to the combination of AFP and NLR. In patients with AFP < 20 ng/mL, the NLR showed the best AUC as a single marker, and the combination of NLR and ALT showed the best AUC as a combination marker.

At present, early diagnosis of HCC is still a challenge. Although AFP is a well-known and widely used clinical

marker for screening, diagnosing and monitoring HCC, the low sensitivity restricts its clinical application [4, 10]. Researchers are looking for new efficient diagnosis markers. microRNAs, osteopontin, glypican-3, and Cavin-2 are several biomarkers reported to be potential diagnostic indicators of HCC [4, 11, 29–31]. However, these biomarkers show limited improvement or even no improvement in HCC diagnosis compared to AFP, and they are not competitive candidates. Several studies also have investigated the combination of AFP with other biomarkers such as osteopontin, Dickkopf-1(DKK-1), protein induced by vitamin K absence (PIVKA-II) and *Lens culinaris* agglutinin-reactive fraction of AFP (AFP-L3) [10, 32]. However, the conclusions from different studies are controversial. Lim et al. found that PIVK A-II was the most accurate diagnostic marker and diagnostic accuracy was improved by combining the AFP, PIVKA-II, and AFP-L3 markers compared to each marker alone for HCC diagnosis [32]. Jang et al. found that AFP was still the most useful single biomarker and diagnostic accuracy was improved by combining AFP and DKK-1 but not other biomarkers [10]. Moreover, these added biomarkers are not common clinically measured parameters. Considering the limited diagnostic accuracy improved by combination, it is not cost-effective to introduce such new biomarkers in routine clinical detection. The diagnostic accuracy of AFP combined with some more common and available markers from routine examinations should be investigated.

The NLR is a simple biomarker of inflammation and clinically available through routine examination. It has been proposed to be of prognostic value in HCC. The NLR can predict HCC recurrence after liver transplantation or in recurrent HCC patients following thermal ablation [33, 34], and an elevated NLR indicates a poor prognosis for HCC patients [23]. All these data indicate that the NLR may reflect the disease status of the patients and may be used for screening.

In the present study, we investigated the diagnostic values of AFP, NLR, AST, and ALT alone as well as their combinations. Our data indicate that AFP is still the most effective single diagnostic marker for HCC, although the NLR is comparable to AFP. The AUC for AFP at the optimal cutoff value of 24.64 ng/mL was 0.775, which is consistent with previous reports [10, 32].

Table 5 Diagnostic performances of three serum biomarkers for differentiating HCC from liver disease in patients with AFP < 20 ng/mL

Marker	Cutoff value	AUC	Sensitivity (Sn)	Specificity (Sp)	Sn + Sp	PPV	NPV
ALT	111	0.507 (0.449–0.564)	0.147 (0.096–0.213)	0.953 (0.906–0.981)	1.1	0.767 (0.577–0.901)	0.516 (0.456–0.577)
AST	27	0.660 (0.603–0.713)	0.981 (0.945–0.996)	0.168 (0.112–0.238)	1.149	0.552 (0.492–0.612)	0.893 (0.718–0.977)
NLR	3.355	0.685 (0.629–0.737)	0.423 (0.344–0.505)	0.926 (0.872–0.963)	1.349	0.857 (0.759–0.926)	0.605 (0.539–0.669)

HCC, hepatocellular carcinoma; ALT, alanine aminotransferase; AST, aspartate aminotransferase; AFP, alpha-fetoprotein; NLR, neutrophil-granulocyte ratio; AUC, area under the receiver operating characteristic curve

Table 6 Diagnostic performances of combinations of four serum biomarkers for differentiating HCC from liver disease in patients with AFP < 20 ng/mL

Markers	AUC	Sensitivity (Sn)	Specificity (Sp)	Sn + Sp	PPV	NPV
ALT+AST	0.646 (0.591–0.698)	0.737 (0.66–0.800)	0.550 (0.470–0628)	1.287	0.632 (0.560–0.699)	0.667 (0.5794–0.744)
NLR + ALT	0.682 (0.628–0.732)	0.500 (0.423–0.578)	0.873 (0.809–0.917)	1.423	0.804 (0.714–0.871)	0.645 (0.558–0.688)
NLR + AST	0.666 (0.611–0.716)	0.821 (0.753–0.873)	0.503 (0.424–0.583)	1.324	0.634 (0.565–0.697)	0.728 (0.635–0.805)
NLR + AST + ALT	0.666 (0.611–0.716)	0.821 (0.753–0.873)	0.503 (0.424–0.583)	1.324	0.634 (0.565–0.697)	0.728 (0.635–0.805)

HCC, hepatocellular carcinoma; ALT, alanine aminotransferase; AST, aspartate aminotransferase; AFP, alpha-fetoprotein; NLR, neutrophil-granulocyte ratio; AUC, area under the receiver operating characteristic curve

However, when applying the most common cutoff value of AFP (20 ng/mL), the AUC was only 0.664, indicating that in our study population, 20 ng/mL is not an optimal cutoff value. The AUC for the NLR in the present study was 0.738, suggesting the NLR is a promising diagnostic marker for HCC.

Further evaluation of biomarker combinations showed that the combination of AFP and NLR had the highest diagnostic accuracy, and the AUC for this combination was 0.769 with a sensitivity of 0.767 and specificity of 0.773, which showed a comparable diagnostic accuracy to the combination of AFP and DKK-1 or AFP, PICKA-II, and AFP-L3 as previously reported [10, 32]. Our data indicate that combination of AFP and NLR is a promising diagnostic marker for HCC.

When we evaluated the diagnostic value of NLR in patients with AFP < 20 ng/mL, we found that compared to AST and ALT, the NLR still showed a relative high AUC (0.685) with a sensitivity of 0.423 and specificity of 0.926, and the PPV was 0.857, indicating its possible application in this population. Further analysis of combinations of biomarkers showed that addition of other biomarkers did not improve diagnostic accuracy beyond that of NLR alone.

There are a few limitations in the present study. First, this was a retrospective study, and thus, selection bias could not be avoided. Second, only patients with liver disease caused by HBV or HCV infection were enrolled as the control group, and thus, the influencing factors may not be complex enough to reflect the whole liver disease population. Therefore, the conclusions should be further confirmed. Third, we did not collect enough data for HCC stage, and thus, the association between the screening value of AFP and HCC stage cannot be evaluated. Fourth, due to a lack of follow-up data, the impact of AFP/NLR on the development and progression of HCC over time cannot be evaluated. We will evaluate the longitudinal significance of AFP/NLR in a future study.

Conclusions

In conclusion, a combination of AFP and NLR showed better accuracy than either marker alone for differentiating HCC from liver disease. Because the NLR is a readily measurable marker on routine examination, this study provides further insight into their clinical applications.

Abbreviations

AFP: Alpha-fetoprotein; ALT: Alanine aminotransferase; AST: Aspartate aminotransferase; HCC: Hepatocellular carcinoma; NLR: Neutrophil-to-lymphocyte ratio; NPV: Negative predictive value; PPV: Positive predictive value; ROC: Receiver operation characteristic

Acknowledgments

None.

Funding

This study received reagents support from Abbott Laboratories. The authors declare that they have no financial relationship with the organization that sponsored the research, and the funding body was not involved in study design, data collection, analysis and writing of the study.

Authors' contributions

JH, NW, YZ and XW designed the study. JH, NW, YY, LM, RH and CY contributed samples collection and testing. WZ, JH and YZ contributed to data analysis. JH, CY, XW and YZ drafted and wrote the manuscript. All authors read and approved the final manuscript.

Consent for publication

All data published here are under the consent for publication.

Competing interests

Yijie Zheng is employee of Abbott Laboratories. The other authors declare that they have no competing interests.

Author details

[1]Department of Clinical Laboratory, The First Affiliated Hospital of Xi'an Jiaotong University, 277 West Yanta Road, Xi'an 710061, People's Republic of China. [2]Department of Clinical Laboratory and Liver Diseases, The Second Hospital of Nanjing, Affiliated to Medical School of Southeast University, Nanjing 210000, China. [3]Department of Clinical Laboratory, Peking University First Hospital, Beijing 100000, China. [4]Department of Mathematics & Statistics, University of Arkansas at Little Rock, Little Rock, AR 72204, USA. [5]Medical Scientific Affairs, Abbott Diagnostics Division, Abbott Laboratories, Shanghai 200032, China.

References

1. Global Burden of Disease Cancer C, Fitzmaurice C, Dicker D, Pain A, Hamavid H, Moradi-Lakeh M, et al. The global burden of Cancer 2013. JAMA Oncol. 2015;1:505–27.
2. Ferlay J, Soerjomataram I, Dikshit R, Eser S, Mathers C, Rebelo M, et al. Cancer incidence and mortality worldwide: sources, methods and major patterns in GLOBOCAN 2012. Int J Cancer. 2015;136:E359–86.
3. Perz JF, Armstrong GL, Farrington LA, Hutin YJ, Bell BP. The contributions of hepatitis B virus and hepatitis C virus infections to cirrhosis and primary liver cancer worldwide. J Hepatol. 2006;45:529–38.
4. Jia X, Liu J, Gao Y, Huang Y, Du Z. Diagnosis accuracy of serum glypican-3 in patients with hepatocellular carcinoma: a systematic review with meta-analysis. Arch Med Res. 2014;45:580–8.
5. Llovet JM, Bruix J. Early diagnosis and treatment of hepatocellular carcinoma. Baillieres Best Pract Res Clin Gastroenterol. 2000;14:991–1008.

6. Huang TS, Shyu YC, Turner R, Chen HY, Chen PJ. Diagnostic performance of alpha-fetoprotein, lens culinaris agglutinin-reactive alpha-fetoprotein, des-gamma carboxyprothrombin, and glypican-3 for the detection of hepatocellular carcinoma: a systematic review and meta-analysis protocol. Syst Rev. 2013;2:37.

7. Ioannou GN, Perkins JD, Carithers RL Jr. Liver transplantation for hepatocellular carcinoma: impact of the MELD allocation system and predictors of survival. Gastroenterology. 2008;134:1342–51.

8. Bruix J, Sherman M. American Association for the Study of liver D. management of hepatocellular carcinoma: an update. Hepatology. 2011;53: 1020–2.

9. Marrero JA, Feng Z, Wang Y, Nguyen MH, Befeler AS, Roberts LR, et al. Alpha-fetoprotein, des-gamma carboxyprothrombin, and lectin-bound alpha-fetoprotein in early hepatocellular carcinoma. Gastroenterology. 2009; 137:110–8.

10. Jang ES, Jeong SH, Kim JW, Choi YS, Leissner P, Brechot C. Diagnostic performance of alpha-fetoprotein, protein induced by vitamin K absence, Osteopontin, Dickkopf-1 and its combinations for hepatocellular carcinoma. PLoS One. 2016;11:e0151069.

11. Jing W, Luo P, Zhu M, Ai Q, Chai H, Tu J. Prognostic and diagnostic significance of SDPR-Cavin-2 in hepatocellular carcinoma. Cell Physiol Biochem. 2016;39:950–60.

12. Balkwill F, Mantovani A. Inflammation and cancer: back to Virchow? Lancet. 2001;357:539–45.

13. Coussens LM, Werb Z. Inflammation and cancer. Nature. 2002;420:860–7.

14. Grivennikov SI, Greten FR, Karin M. Immunity, inflammation, and cancer. Cell. 2010;140:883–99.

15. Allavena P, Sica A, Solinas G, Porta C, Mantovani A. The inflammatory micro-environment in tumor progression: the role of tumor-associated macrophages. Crit Rev Oncol Hematol. 2008;66:1–9.

16. Unitt E, Marshall A, Gelson W, Rushbrook SM, Davies S, Vowler SL, et al. Tumour lymphocytic infiltrate and recurrence of hepatocellular carcinoma following liver transplantation. J Hepatol. 2006;45:246–53.

17. Gao Q, Qiu SJ, Fan J, Zhou J, Wang XY, Xiao YS, et al. Intratumoral balance of regulatory and cytotoxic T cells is associated with prognosis of hepatocellular carcinoma after resection. J Clin Oncol. 2007;25:2586–93.

18. Chen KJ, Zhou L, Xie HY, Ahmed TE, Feng XW, Zheng SS. Intratumoral regulatory T cells alone or in combination with cytotoxic T cells predict prognosis of hepatocellular carcinoma after resection. Med Oncol. 2012;29: 1817–26.

19. Li MX, Liu XM, Zhang XF, Zhang JF, Wang WL, Zhu Y, et al. Prognostic role of neutrophil-to-lymphocyte ratio in colorectal cancer: a systematic review and meta-analysis. Int J Cancer. 2014;134:2403–13.

20. Hu K, Lou L, Ye J, Zhang S. Prognostic role of the neutrophil-lymphocyte ratio in renal cell carcinoma: a meta-analysis. BMJ Open. 2015;5:e006404.

21. Sun HL, Pan YQ, He BS, Nie ZL, Lin K, Peng HX, et al. Prognostic performance of lymphocyte-to-monocyte ratio in diffuse large B-cell lymphoma: an updated meta-analysis of eleven reports. Onco Targets Ther. 2016;9:3017–23.

22. Zhou D, Liang J, Xu LI, He F, Zhou Z, Zhang Y, et al. Derived neutrophil to lymphocyte ratio predicts prognosis for patients with HBV-associated hepatocellular carcinoma following transarterial chemoembolization. Oncol Lett. 2016;11:2987–94.

23. Xiao WK, Chen D, Li SQ, Fu SJ, Peng BG, Liang LJ. Prognostic significance of neutrophil-lymphocyte ratio in hepatocellular carcinoma: a meta-analysis. BMC Cancer. 2014;14:117.

24. Tanrikulu Y, Sen Tanrikulu C, Sabuncuoglu MZ, Kokturk F, Temi V, Bicakci E. Is the neutrophil-to-lymphocyte ratio a potential diagnostic marker for peptic ulcer perforation? A retrospective cohort study. Am J Emerg Med. 2016;34:403–6.

25. Aktimur R, Cetinkunar S, Yildirim K, Aktimur SH, Ugurlucan M, Ozlem N. Neutrophil-to-lymphocyte ratio as a diagnostic biomarker for the diagnosis of acute mesenteric ischemia. Eur J Trauma Emerg Surg. 2016;42:363–8.

26. Kemal Y, Yucel I, Ekiz K, Demirag G, Yilmaz B, Teker F, et al. Elevated serum neutrophil to lymphocyte and platelet to lymphocyte ratios could be useful in lung cancer diagnosis. Asian Pac J Cancer Prev. 2014;15:2651–4.

27. Nikolic I, Kukulj S, Samarzija M, Jelec V, Zarak M, Orehovec B, et al. Neutrophil-to-lymphocyte and platelet-to-lymphocyte ratio help identify patients with lung cancer, but do not differentiate between lung cancer subtypes. Croat Med J. 2016;57:287–92.

28. Omata M, Lesmana LA, Tateishi R, Chen PJ, Lin SM, Yoshida H, et al. Asian Pacific Association for the Study of the liver consensus recommendations on hepatocellular carcinoma. Hepatol Int. 2010;4:439–74.

29. Jiang L, Cheng Q, Zhang BH, Zhang MZ. Circulating microRNAs as biomarkers in hepatocellular carcinoma screening: a validation set from China. Medicine (Baltimore). 2015;94:e603.

30. Li G, Shen Q, Li C, Li D, Chen J, He M. Identification of circulating MicroRNAs as novel potential biomarkers for hepatocellular carcinoma detection: a systematic review and meta-analysis. Clin Transl Oncol. 2015;17: 684–93.

31. Wan HG, Xu H, Gu YM, Wang H, Xu W, Zu MH. Comparison osteopontin vs AFP for the diagnosis of HCC: a meta-analysis. Clin Res Hepatol Gastroenterol. 2014;38:706–14.

32. Lim TS, Kim do Y, Han KH, Kim HS, Shin SH, Jung KS, et al. Combined use of AFP, PIVKA-II, and AFP-L3 as tumor markers enhances diagnostic accuracy for hepatocellular carcinoma in cirrhotic patients. Scand J Gastroenterol. 2016;51:344–53.

33. Xiao GQ, Liu C, Liu DL, Yang JY, Yan LN. Neutrophil-lymphocyte ratio predicts the prognosis of patients with hepatocellular carcinoma after liver transplantation. World J Gastroenterol. 2013;19:8398–407.

34. Li X, Han Z, Cheng Z, Yu J, Liu S, Yu X, et al. Preoperative neutrophil-to-lymphocyte ratio is a predictor of recurrence following thermal ablation for recurrent hepatocellular carcinoma: a retrospective analysis. PLoS One. 2014; 9:e110546.

18

Prevalence of medication discrepancies in patients with cirrhosis

Kelly L. Hayward[1,2], Patricia C. Valery[3], W. Neil Cottrell[4], Katharine M. Irvine[5], Leigh U. Horsfall[5], Caroline J. Tallis[6], Veronique S. Chachay[7], Brittany J Ruffin[5], Jennifer H. Martin[8†] and Elizabeth E. Powell[5,6*†]

Abstract

Background: Cirrhosis patients are prescribed multiple medications for their liver disease and comorbidities. Discrepancies between medicines consumed by patients and those documented in the medical record may contribute to patient harm and impair disease management. The aim of the present study was to assess the magnitude and types of discrepancies among patient-reported and medical record-documented medications in patients with cirrhosis, and examine factors associated with such discrepancies.

Methods: Fifty patients who attended a hospital hepatology outpatient clinic were interviewed using a questionnaire composed of mixed short-response and multiple-choice questions. Patients' reported medication use was compared with documentation in the hospital medical records and pharmacy database. Medication adherence was assessed using the 8-question ©Morisky Medication Adherence Scale (MMAS-8). The multivariate logistic regression model was constructed using clinically relevant and/or statistically significant variables as determined by univariate analysis. All p-values were 2-sided ($\alpha = 0.05$).

Results: Twenty-seven patients (54.0 %) had ≥1 discrepancy between reported and documented medicines. Patients with ≥1 discrepancy were older ($p = 0.04$) and multivariate analysis identified taking ≥5 conventional medicines or having a 'low' or 'medium' adherence ranking as independent predictors of discrepancy (adjusted OR 11.0 (95 % CI 1.8–67.4), 20.7 (95 % CI 1.3–337.7) and 49.0 (95 % CI 3.3–718.5) respectively). Concordance was highest for liver disease medicines (71.9 %) and lowest for complementary and alternative medicines (14.5 %) and respiratory medicines (0 %).

Conclusion: There is significant discrepancy between sources of patient medication information within the hepatology clinic. Medication reconciliation and medicines-management intervention may address the complex relationship between medication discrepancies, number of medications and patient adherence identified in this study.

Keywords: Medication reconciliation, Medication adherence, Liver cirrhosis, Complementary therapies, Ambulatory care

Background

Liver disease is gaining global recognition as an important chronic health disorder, due to increasing prevalence of non-alcoholic fatty liver disease (NAFLD), hazardous alcohol intake and viral hepatitis [1]. Regardless of aetiology, morbidity and mortality occurs predominantly among patients with cirrhosis, a late stage of progressive fibrosis with liver vascular and architectural alterations. Clinically, cirrhosis is defined as "compensated", a latency period with median survival times of more than 12 years, or "decompensated", a rapidly progressive phase marked by complications of portal hypertension or liver insufficiency and median survival times of less than 2 years [2].

The morbidity and health care costs associated with the complications of decompensated cirrhosis are substantial, as people require complex medical care and have very high use of hospital services [3, 4]. With the growing prevalence of liver cirrhosis worldwide, it is becoming increasingly important to identify potentially-modifiable factors that may contribute to disease burden.

* Correspondence: e.powell@uq.edu.au
†Equal contributors
5Centre for Liver Disease Research, The University of Queensland, Brisbane, Australia
6Department of Gastroenterology and Hepatology, Princess Alexandra Hospital, Woolloongabba 4102, Brisbane, Queensland, Australia
Full list of author information is available at the end of the article

People with cirrhosis are often prescribed multiple medications for therapeutic or prophylactic use [3] and the number of medications prescribed on hospital discharge is a risk factor for early readmission [5]. Although the precise reason for this has not been established, and increased medication use is common in people with more severe illness, medication misuse and non-adherence may have contributed. Polypharmacy is strongly related to poor adherence and both factors have also been associated with medication misuse and a higher prevalence of discrepancies between patient-reported and clinician-documented medications [6, 7]. Discrepancies between the type and frequency of medications prescribed by clinicians and the drugs actually consumed by patients may contribute to patient harm or reduce the efficacy of therapy. Unresolved medication discrepancies have been correlated with increased length of hospital stay, readmission within 30 days and adverse events post-discharge [8–10].

In contrast to other chronic diseases, the prevalence of medication discrepancies has not been examined in patients with cirrhosis. Examination of the types and magnitude of discrepancies that are present and the potential harms associated with them is important to improve clinician recognition of this potential barrier to care, especially with the growing push for treatment and follow-up of chronic liver disease (CLD) patients in community settings.

Aims

To assess the magnitude and types of discrepancies between reported and documented medications in patients with cirrhosis seen in a hospital hepatology clinic, and examine factors associated with such discrepancies.

Methods

Patients and clinical data

A convenience sample of 50 English-speaking patients with cirrhosis were invited to participate when they attended the hepatology outpatient clinic at the Princess Alexandra Hospital (Brisbane, Australia) from August to December 2014.

Participants (and carers/family members if present) were interviewed by the research co-ordinator using a questionnaire composed of mixed short-response and multiple-choice questions designed to elicit demographic information, patient knowledge of their medications and liver disease and related lifestyle factors. Self-reported adherence to cirrhosis medications was evaluated using the eight-item Morisky Medication Adherence Scale© (MMAS-8) with approval from the developer [11–13]. The MMAS-8 is a previously validated questionnaire used to estimate self-reported adherence to treatment and is widely used in chronic diseases. It consists of

seven questions with "yes" or "no" alternatives, and one item featuring a 5-point Likert scale. The MMAS-8 scores range from 0–8, with levels of adherence classified as: high adherence (score 8); medium adherence (score 6–7.75); and low adherence (score <6).

Patients' medical records, standard biochemical and serological assays and liver imaging were used to confirm the diagnosis of liver disease and cirrhosis. In addition, Fibroscan®, gastroscopy and histological assessment of a liver biopsy were also used, if performed. The severity of liver disease was evaluated using the Child-Turcotte-Pugh classification.

Patient reported medications

Subjects were asked to list the dose, frequency and indication for each of their medicines and specifically prompted for over-the-counter (OTC) and complementary medicines (CAMs). Qualitative questions were also asked throughout the interview to elicit individual medication-taking behaviour. Medications were not actively verified with other sources such as the GP or local pharmacy, as medication reconciliation was not standard practice within the clinic at the time this study was conducted.

Documented medications

Medications were considered current if documented less than 3 months prior to patient interview, without subsequent documentation of cessation or modification. Each patient's medical record and the pharmacy database 'ELMs' (Enterprise-wide Liaison Medication System) were interrogated to determine documented medications and compare to patient responses. ELMs is a state-wide hospital pharmacy database that is routinely updated by hospital pharmacists at the point of admission and/or discharge from hospital. Within the outpatient hepatology clinic there was no assigned clinician or assistant who routinely verified and updated the patient's medication list. Consequently, medications were not consistently recorded within the outpatient section of the medical record, and thus correspondence letters from GPs, other specialists and admission notes were also used to determine documented medications.

Data analysis

'Medication discrepancy' was defined as a difference between what was reported by the patient and what was documented in the medical record or in ELMs. Documented medications in the ELMs database which were annotated or classified as 'temporary' by the study clinicians (antibiotic courses, post-operative analgesia, some PRN medications, medicines with a documented cessation date) were not included in the discrepancy analysis.

Correlation between reported and documented medicine name, dose, frequency and indication was attempted, but due to patient ambiguity and limited chart documentation of dosage, only the name of medications could be analysed for this study. The clinical significance of discrepancies was determined by a panel of clinicians experienced in treating cirrhosis patients (pharmacist, hepatologist and nurse). A significant discrepancy was defined as one which may lead to potential harm within 7 days if the patient was administered, or not administered, a drug due to misdocumentation or misreporting. Medications which were in agreement between 2 sources were considered 'concordant'.

Medications were categorised as 'conventional medications' (including prescription medicines, OTCs, vitamins and protein supplements prescribed for the treatment of cirrhosis-related complications and other comorbidities) or 'CAMs'. Medications were grouped into 12 drug-disease categories: liver, gastrointestinal-luminal, cardiovascular, diabetes, psychomodulators, analgesia, CAMs, respiratory and 'others'. Proton-pump inhibitors (PPIs) were classified as a 'liver' medication in patients with gastric and/or oesophageal varices or a 'gastro-luminal' medication when prescribed for gastro-oesophageal reflux disease. Liver disease medications were further analysed by drug name and/or indication.

Statistical analysis

Data analysis was conducted using SPSS Inc. version 20.0 (College Station TX: StatCorp LP; 2013). Participant characteristics are presented as means and standard deviation (normally distributed data), and proportions. Univariate analysis was performed using Pearson's Chi-squared analysis or Fisher's Exact test for categorical data (proportions), and t-test for normally-distributed data (means). The association between medication discrepancy and demographic and clinical variables was determined by calculating the odds ratios (OR) and 95 % confidence interval (CI). The multivariate logistic regression analysis model was constructed by testing variables of clinical relevance and/or statistical significance as determined by univariate analysis. The Hosmer-Lemeshow test was performed on selected models to assess goodness-of-fit. The final model was used to assess associations after adjustment for the total number of conventional medications taken by patients (excluding CAMs), and MMAS ranking. Interactions between individual variables (age, gender, regular general practitioner (GP), comorbidities, number of conventional medications and MMAS ranking) were not found to be statistically significant. All p values were 2-sided and statistical significance was set at alpha = 0.05.

Results

Patient characteristics

Fifty-three cirrhotic patients who attended the hepatology clinic at the Princess Alexandra Hospital were invited to participate; 50 (94.0 %) were interviewed, and three declined to participate. Overall, the mean age of participants was 58.5 (±10.2) years; 39 patients (78.0 %) were men and 43 (86.0 %) were Caucasian. Primary liver disease aetiology was Hepatitis C in 26 patients; non-alcoholic steatohepatitis in 11; alcoholic liver disease in 10; Hepatitis B in one; primary biliary cirrhosis in one; cryptogenic in one. Twenty patients (40.0 %) had decompensated cirrhosis at the time of interview, including five with a history of hepatic encephalopathy, 14 with ascites and 15 with oesophageal/gastric varices.

A total of 307 medications were identified from all sources; 244 were classified as 'conventional', 63 as CAMs, and the drug-disease classes comprised liver-related (22.8 %), CAM (20.5 %), cardiovascular (15.6 %), diabetes (8.8 %), "other" (8.5 %), psychomodulators (8.1 %), analgesia (7.2 %), gastro-luminal (4.9 %) and respiratory (3.6 %) medications. Seven patients (14.0 %) stated that they took no medications, however two disclosed OTC/CAMs when prompted and one had salbutamol 'when required' documented within their medical record. Twenty-seven patients (54.0 %) had ≥5 conventional medications identified from all sources.

Medication discrepancies

Significant discrepancies between patient-reported conventional medications (including prescribed CAMs) and the medical record were present in 27 patients (54.0 %). All 27 patients reported conventional medications which were not recorded in the medical record and 16 patients also did not report conventional medications that were documented in the medical record. Twenty-four percent of patients had three or more discrepancies among conventional medicines identified (Fig. 1).

Sixteen patients had medications recorded in the ELMs database. Of these 16 patients, discrepancies in conventional medicines were present in 11 patients (68.8 %); five reported conventional medications which

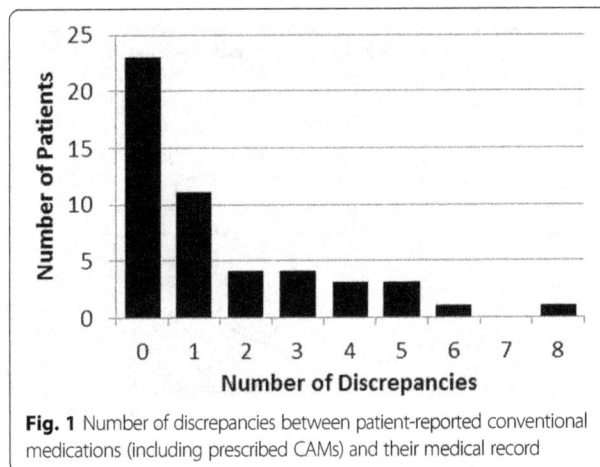

Fig. 1 Number of discrepancies between patient-reported conventional medications (including prescribed CAMs) and their medical record

were not recorded in ELMs, and nine had medications recorded in ELMs which they did not report.

Figure 2 describes the overall concordance and discordance between medications reported by patients and documented in their medical records and the ELMs database. A total of 246 medications (including CAMs) were reported by the cohort of 50 patients and 160 were documented in their medical records. Overall, 125 of 281 medications (44.5 %) were concordant between the patient and their medical record. Twenty-six medications documented in ELMs were not reported by patients or documented in their medical record; these included records of insulin, liver, cardiovascular and respiratory medicines. A large proportion of patient-reported medications that were not documented in the medical record were CAMs.

The distribution of medication discrepancies by drug-disease class between patients and their medical records, and between the medical record and ELMs is presented in Fig. 3a and 3b respectively. Discrepancies in medications prescribed for the management of liver disease and cirrhosis-related complications are summarised in Table 1. Propranolol and anti-viral therapies were 100 % concordant between the patient and the medical record. Only two of the five patients who were recorded as taking lactulose for hepatic encephalopathy reported using it. The one patient who reported taking trimethoprim-sulfamethoxazole for spontaneous bacterial peritonitis (SBP) prophylaxis did not have this medication documented within their medical record.

Qualitative analysis of medication discrepancies identified three patients using benzodiazepines and five patients who were taking opiates or non-steroidal anti-inflammatory analgesics not documented in their medical record. One patient took moclobemide, a monoamine-oxidase inhibitor (MAOI) which was not documented, and two patients had angiotensin II receptor antagonists documented in the chart, but not reported by the patient. Five patients had discrepancies involving insulin. Only

two of the six patients with documented inhalers reported using them.

Factors associated with medication discrepancy

The demographic and clinical characteristics of patients according to the presence or absence of medication discrepancies between the patient and medical record is summarised in Table 2. Patients with ≥ 1 medication discrepancy were older ($p = 0.04$), more likely to be taking ≥ 5 conventional medications ($p = 0.01$), had a regular GP ($p = 0.04$), comorbidities ($p = 0.02$) and a lower adherence ranking ($p < 0.01$). Multivariate analysis identified the total number of conventional medications and the MMAS ranking as the most significant predictors of discrepancy (Table 3). Patients taking ≥ 5 conventional medications were 11.0 (95 % CI 1.8–67.4) times more likely to have at least one discrepancy; those with a 'low' or 'medium' adherence ranking were 20.7 (95 % CI 1.3–337.7) and 49.0 (95 % CI 3.3–718.5) times more likely to have at least one medication discrepancy compared to those with a 'high' MMAS ranking.

Of the 20 participants who had decompensated cirrhosis, five had a history of hepatic encephalopathy. Encephalopathy was not associated with medication discrepancies in the whole group ($n = 50$, $p = 0.36$), nor in the subset of decompensated patients ($n = 20$, $p = 0.60$) although this finding may be limited by sample size.

Over-the-counter (OTC), complementary and alternative medications (CAMs)

When initially asked to list their medications, only 31.8 % of over-the-counter, complementary and alternative medications were volunteered by patients. Further specific questioning about OTC products and CAMs were required to elicit these medicines. In total, twenty-seven patients reported taking CAMs, including two patients who stated that they took no medications at all. Only 14.5 % of CAMs reported by

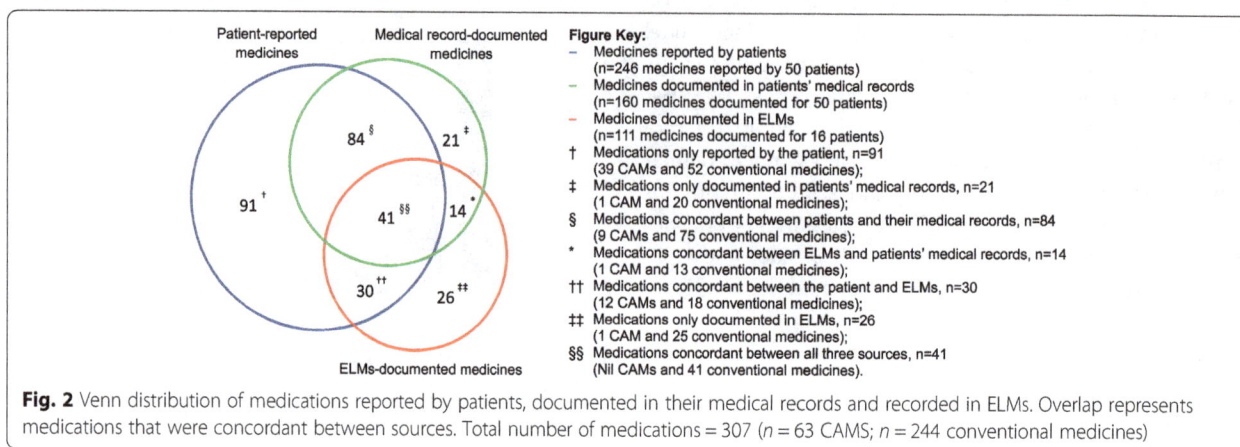

Patient-reported medicines   Medical record-documented medicines

Figure Key:
– Medicines reported by patients
  (n=246 medicines reported by 50 patients)
– Medicines documented in patients' medical records
  (n=160 medicines documented for 50 patients)
– Medicines documented in ELMs
  (n=111 medicines documented for 16 patients)
† Medications only reported by the patient, n=91
  (39 CAMs and 52 conventional medicines);
‡ Medications only documented in patients' medical records, n=21
  (1 CAM and 20 conventional medicines);
§ Medications concordant between patients and their medical records, n=84
  (9 CAMs and 75 conventional medicines);
* Medications concordant between ELMs and patients' medical records, n=14
  (1 CAM and 13 conventional medicines);
†† Medications concordant between the patient and ELMs, n=30
  (12 CAMs and 18 conventional medicines);
‡‡ Medications only documented in ELMs, n=26
  (1 CAM and 25 conventional medicines);
§§ Medications concordant between all three sources, n=41
  (Nil CAMs and 41 conventional medicines).

84 §   21 ‡
91 †
41 §§   14 *
30 ††   26 ‡‡
ELMs-documented medicines

Fig. 2 Venn distribution of medications reported by patients, documented in their medical records and recorded in ELMs. Overlap represents medications that were concordant between sources. Total number of medications = 307 ($n = 63$ CAMS; $n = 244$ conventional medicines)

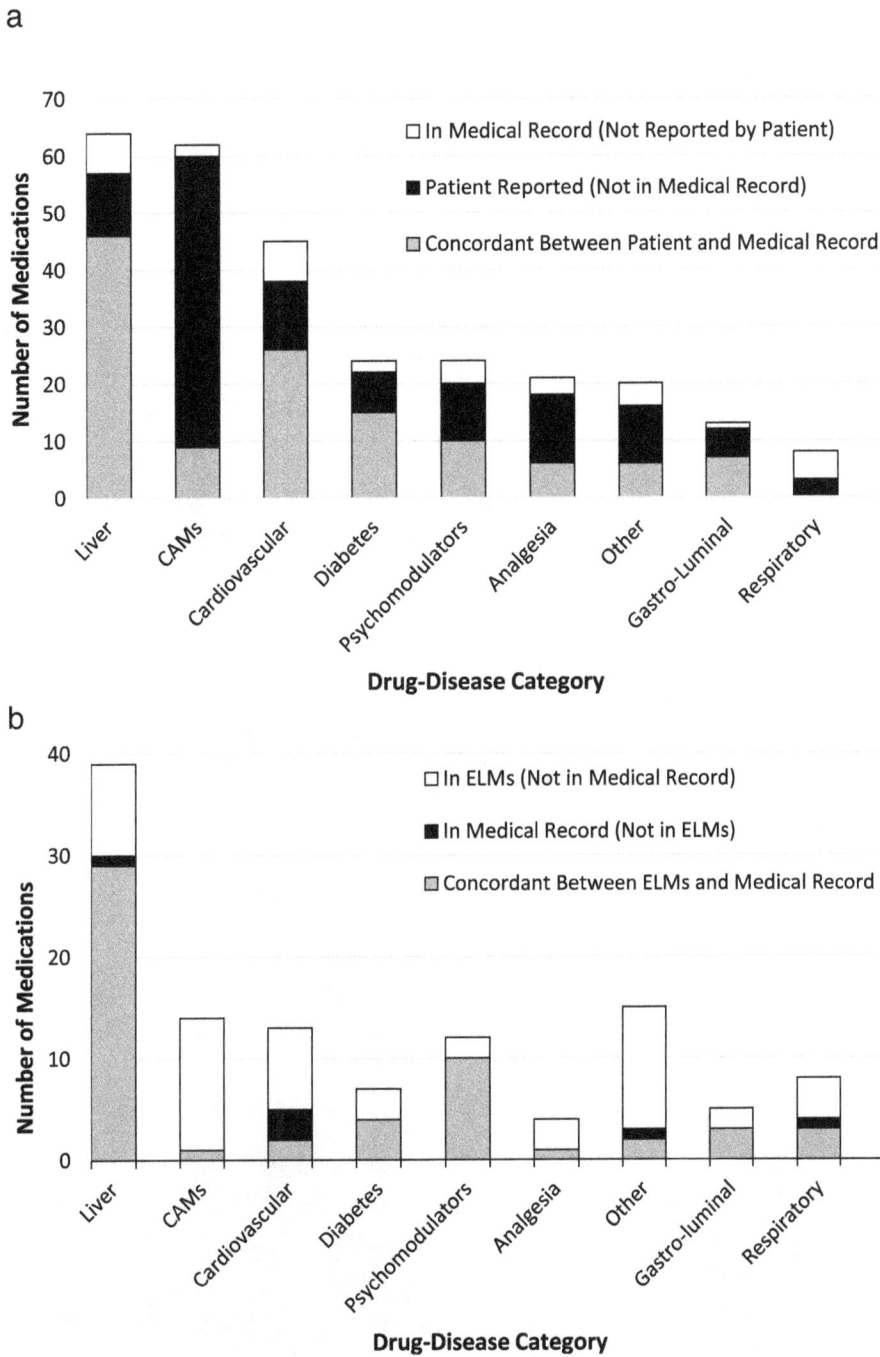

Fig. 3 a. Concordance between medications reported by the patient and documented in their medical record with respect to drug-disease category. Patients (*n* = 50) taking ≥1 medication in drug-disease class: liver *n* = 28; CAMs *n* = 28; cardiovascular *n* = 22; diabetes *n* = 14; psychomodulators *n* = 13; analgesia *n* = 17; other *n* = 14; gastro-luminal *n* = 10; respiratory *n* = 5. **b**. Concordance between medications recorded in ELMs and documented in the medical record with respect to drug-disease category. Patients (*n* = 16) taking ≥1 medication in drug-disease class: liver *n* = 11; CAMs *n* = 10; cardiovascular *n* = 7; diabetes *n* = 5; psychomodulators *n* = 3; analgesia *n* = 5; other *n* = 5; gastro-luminal *n* = 5; respiratory *n* = 4

all patients were recorded in the medical record, whereas ELMs had a 60.0 % concordance rate within the group of 16 patients who had records in this database.

Barriers to knowledge and adherence

Of the 43 patients who reported taking medications, only 24 patients (56.0 %) recalled being told how to take them. Eighty-five percent of decompensated patients

Table 1 Discrepancies between reported and documented medications prescribed for the management of liver-related complications

Number of liver medications[a]	Patient reported but not documented in medical record	Documented in medical record but not reported by patient	Concordant medications	Proportion (%) discordant records within drug-disease category
Diuretics $n = 16$	1	2	13	18.8 %
Propranolol $n = 9$	0	0	9	0.0 %
Cholecalciferol $n = 8$	4	0	4	50.0 %
PPIs $n = 7$	2	1	4	42.9 %
Thiamine $n = 6$	1	0	5	16.7 %
Lactulose $n = 5$	0	3	2	60.0 %
Antivirals $n = 4$	0	0	4	0.0 %
Other $n = 9^b$	3	1	5	44.4 %

[a]Excluding 6 liver medications which were only documented in ELMs ($n = 1$ for thiamine, rifaximin, PPI, lactulose, cholecalciferol, spironolactone)
[b]Rifaximin, spontaneous bacterial peritonitis prophylaxis, ursodeoxecholic acid, other vitamins and protein supplements prescribed for complications of cirrhosis

reported being told to maintain a low salt diet compared to 40 % of compensated cirrhotics ($p < 0.01$), which is consistent with disease management of ascites. Decompensated patients were also more likely to be taking diuretics ($p < 0.01$), but less than one-third knew to keep a record of weight and blood pressure which can both be variably affected by disease and pharmacotherapy.

Fourteen patients (33.0 %) stated that they could not afford their medications, though this was not found to be related to employment status, polypharmacy or disease severity ($p > 0.05$). Of the 40 patients who completed the adherence tool, only 7 were categorised as having 'high' adherence.

Discussion

In this sample of patients with cirrhosis, over half had at least one discrepancy between their reported medicines and those documented in their medical records. Overall

Table 2 Demographic and clinical characteristics for patients with and without medication discrepancies between the patient and their medical record

		≥1 Medication Discrepancy $n = 27$	Medication Discrepancy Absent $n = 23$	P
Age, mean (±SD)		61 ± 8	55 ± 11	0.04
Male, no (%)		20 (74.1 %)	19 (82.6 %)	0.52
Years attending clinic, median (range)		2.6 (0.0 – 19.4)	2.9 (0.1 - 13.4)	0.86
Liver disease severity	Compensated	55.6 %	65.2 %	0.49
	Decompensated	44.4 %	34.8 %	
Patient has a regular GP		96.3 %	73.9 %	0.04
Comorbidities present[a]		85.2 %	52.2 %	0.02
Level of Education	Primary/High School	66.7 %	73.9 %	0.58
	Higher Education[b]	33.3 %	26.1 %	
Currently employed		25.9 %	43.5 %	0.19
Patient reported being 'told how to take your medications'[c]		59.3 %	50.0 %	0.56
Patient reported being able to afford medications[c]		59.3 %	81.2 %	0.19
No. of conventional medicines[c]	1-4	22.2 %	62.5 %	<0.01
	≥5	77.8 %	37.5 %	
Adherence ranking (MMAS-8)[d]	High	4.2 %	37.5 %	<0.01
	Medium	70.8 %	31.2 %	
	Low	25.0 %	31.2 %	

[a]Comorbidities included cardiovascular disease, hypertension, diabetes, gastro-oesophageal reflux disease, hypothyroidism, benign prostatic hyperplasia, osteoporosis, rheumatoid arthritis, depression, anxiety, schizophrenia, asthma, chronic obstructive pulmonary disease, and neuropathic pain
[b]Trade, technical certificate, diploma
[c]Excluding 4 patients who took no medications, 2 patients who only took CAMs and 1 patient who did not answer the question (total $n = 43$ patients; ≥1 significant discrepancy $n = 27$; no significant discrepancy $n = 16$). Conventional medicines included vitamins and protein supplements prescribed for the management of cirrhosis or other medical conditions (including: vitamin B1, vitamin D, vitamin A, ferrous sulphate in 1 patient with chronic anaemia, magnesium for 2 patients with symptomatic hypomagnesemia due to diuretic use, and calcium in 1 patient with osteoporosis)
[d]Excluding 10 patients who did not complete this section of the questionnaire (total $n = 40$; ≥1 medication discrepancy $n = 24$; No medication discrepancy $n = 16$)

Table 3 Crude and multivariate predictors of medication discrepancies

		Crude OR (95 % CI)	Adjusted OR[a] (95 % CI)
Age ≥60		1.5 (0.5 – 4.7)	0.9 (0.2 – 4.7)
Male gender		0.6 (0.2 – 2.4)	1.0 (0.1 – 6.6)
Regular GP		9.2 (1.0 – 83.1)	-
≥1 Comorbidity		5.3 (1.4 – 20.1)	2.8 (0.3 – 23.9)
≥5 Conventional Medicines		5.8 (1.5 – 22.7)	11.0 (1.8 – 67.4)
MMAS ranking	Low	7.2 (0.6 – 81.5)	20.7 (1.3 – 337.7)
	Medium	20.4 (2.00 – 211.89)	49.0 (3.3 – 718.5)

[a]Odds ratio adjusted for number of conventional medicines and the MMAS score. Analysis excludes 10 patients who did not complete the MMAS section of the questionnaire

concordance between patients and their medical records was under 50 %. Those patients with a discrepancy were more likely to be taking ≥5 medicines and have a medium to low medication adherence ranking.

Discrepancies among CAMs were not unexpected as miscommunication between patients and prescribers on this subject is known to be extensive [14]. However, much like conventional medicines, CAMs are not without potential harm. Adverse reactions are not uncommon [15], and a number of herbal remedies and dietary supplements have been linked to drug-induced liver injury, including traditional Chinese medicines (xiao-chai-hu-tang, rheum palmatum (rhubarb), shou-wu pian), green tea extract, greater celandine, and chaparral [16, 17]. A number of these CAMs are purported to have benefits for patients with pre-existing liver disease, therefore cirrhosis patients who are dissatisfied with conventional medicine may seek out these agents. Hepatologists should be aware of this and actively ask patients about their alternative medication use.

A number of discrepancies among conventional medications had potential for patient harm, such as the misdocumentation or misreporting of insulin, analgesics, benzodiazepines and a MAOI. Errors involving insulin can lead to hospitalisation, MAOIs have potential for severe drug-drug interactions, opioids have reduced clearance in cirrhosis and increased risk of constipation and hepatic encephalopathy, and NSAIDs may contribute to renal impairment and hepatorenal syndrome. Discrepancies involving SBP prophylaxis, diuretics and lactulose among patients with decompensated cirrhosis are also cause for concern, as failure to appropriately manage or monitor these medicines may contribute to hospitalisation with life-threatening decompensation events.

Patients with decompensated cirrhosis average two to three hospital admissions per year [3, 5, 18]. Upon hospitalisation many patients are too unwell to discuss their current medications and may therefore be administered a regimen according to the documented list, which contains discrepancies. Unresolved medication discrepancies have been linked to prolonged hospital stay in people with other chronic diseases [8]. With recurrent hospitalisation, additional pharmacotherapy is often prescribed to manage complications of cirrhosis [3]. With an increase in pharmacotherapy there is a greater chance for patient-clinician miscommunication about medications and thus patients prescribed complex and frequently changing medication regimens are often reported to have poorer adherence [19]. These factors may be further compounded by varying degrees of encephalopathy in people with advanced cirrhosis; only 7 participants in the present study were ranked as having 'high' levels of adherence, which is lower than other chronic diseases [12, 20, 21]. Increasing polypharmacy, intentional and unintentional non-adherence, and discrepancies that arise from patient-clinician miscommunication may contribute to re-hospitalisation.

Among decompensated cirrhotics, the number of medications prescribed at discharge has been found to predict hospitalization rate and time to first hospital readmission, independently of the Model for End-stage Liver Disease (MELD) score and serum sodium which also predict poor outcomes [5]. Volk and colleagues estimated that 22 % of 30-day readmissions among patients with decompensated cirrhosis were possibly preventable with improved patient understanding of their medications or more frequent outpatient monitoring [5]. Improved patient understanding may partially be achieved by simplification of the prescribed regimen, which may further improve reporting and adherence due to ease of memory, reduction in side effects and general patient satisfaction [22–24]. However this is difficult to achieve without knowledge of the patient's entire medication regimen. Routine medication reconciliation within the hepatology clinic may improve this.

In existing outpatient models of collaborative practice, pharmacists have a designated role in medication education and reconciliation, with a number of studies concluding pharmacist intervention reduced hospital admissions, increased adherence to therapy and improved patient outcomes [25–27]. Enhancing the level of disease education in patients of a low educational background has been shown to improve medication adherence [28–31], and use of multiple sources to construct an accurate medication record and identify medication-related problems reduces patient harm [32, 33]. Implementation of a pharmacist within this hepatology practice whose role is to focus on medication reconciliation and management may improve patient outcomes.

Strengths and limitations

The use of face-to-face interviews conducted by a data collector who had experience with chronic liver disease and was familiar with the patient group allowed for directed qualitative expansion of some patient responses. In addition, a pharmacist conducted the ELMs reviews, assisted with the construction of medication-related questions and discrepancy analysis. Whilst interviewer administration accommodated for potential literacy problems, all patients who completed this survey spoke and read English. Therefore cirrhotic patients requiring an interpreter during the consultation were excluded from assessment. Furthermore, the study relied heavily on patient recall as most patients did not bring their medicines or a list of them to clinic. Some patients with cirrhosis have a carer or family member who assists with managing their medications; this person was not always present at the time of the interview. Decompensated patients may also have had low-grade encephalopathy, affecting medication recall. However these factors reflect the clinic scenario existing in reality, which is what this study aimed to investigate.

Conclusion

This study demonstrates that there is significant discrepancy between medication sources within the hepatology clinic with potential for harm or impaired disease management. While the aforementioned limitations and single-centre nature of the study may impact on applicability of findings to other sites, we have identified an important potential barrier to care, which may present in similar general hepatology models of care globally. There is much room for improvement in medication reconciliation within the clinic, and our patients may benefit from targeted medication-management intervention.

Abbreviations

NAFLD: Non-alcoholic fatty liver disease; CLD: Chronic liver disease; CAMs: Complementary and alternative medicines; OTC: Over-the-counter; MMAS: Morisky Medication Adherence Scale; ELMs: Enterprise-wide Liaison Medication System; GP: General practitioner; PPI: Proton pump inhibitor; CI: Confidence interval; OR: Odds ratio; SBP: Spontaneous bacterial peritonitis; MAOI: Monoamine oxidase inhibitor; MELD: Model for End-stage Liver Disease

Acknowledgements

The authors would like to acknowledge and extend their appreciation Nursing staff, Dina Fetahagic, Sheree Brown, Kate Choi and Karl Dew along with A/Prof. Graeme Macdonald and Dr Paul Clark at the Princess Alexandra Hospital who assisted with recruitment.
Use of the ©MMAS is protected by US copyright laws. Permission for use is required. A license agreement is available from: Donald E. Morisky, ScD, ScM, MSPH, Professor, Department of Community Health Sciences, UCLA School of Public Health, 650 Charles E. Young Drive South, Los Angeles, CA 90095-1772.

Funding

PV was supported by the Australian National Health and Medical Research Council (Career Development Fellowship #1083090).
EP was supported the National Health and Medical Research Council (Practitioner Fellowship #1004242) and the Queensland Government (Health Research Fellowship).

Authors' contributions

KH: Development of survey questionnaire, ELMs review, medication discrepancy review, data synthesis and analysis, interpretation of results, manuscript preparation, revision and submission. PV: Study concept and design, development of survey questionnaire, data synthesis and analysis, interpretation of results, manuscript preparation and revision. NC: Clinical advice, data analysis, interpretation of results, manuscript preparation and revision. KI: Data analysis, interpretation of results and manuscript revision. LH: Study coordination, development of survey questionnaire, conducted patient interviews, medical record reviews and data collection. CT: Clinical advice, manuscript preparation and revision. VC: Development of survey questionnaire, clinical advice, manuscript preparation and revision. BR: Conducted patient interviews, medical record reviews and data collection. JM: Study concept and design, development of survey questionnaire, clinical advice, medication discrepancy review, data analysis, interpretation of results, manuscript preparation and revision. EP: Study concept and design, development of survey questionnaire, clinical advice, medication discrepancy review, data analysis, interpretation of results, manuscript preparation and revision.

Authors' information

KH PhD candidate, School of Medicine, The University of Queensland, Brisbane, Australia.
Clinical Pharmacist, Pharmacy Department, Princess Alexandra Hospital, Brisbane, Australia.
PV Team Head, Cancer and Chronic Disease Research Group, QIMR Berghofer Medical Research Institute, Brisbane, Australia.
NC Associate Professor, School of Pharmacy, University of Queensland, Brisbane, Australia.
KI Laboratory Head, Centre for Liver Disease Research, University of Queensland, Brisbane, Australia.
LH Research Coordinator, Centre for Liver Disease Research, University of Queensland, Brisbane, Australia.
CT Gastroenterologist and Hepatologist, Department of Gastroenterology and Hepatology, Princess Alexandra Hospital, Brisbane, Australia.
VC Lecturer, Accredited Practicing Dietitian, School of Human Movement and Nutrition Sciences, University of Queensland, Brisbane, Australia.
BR Nursing Student, Centre for Liver Disease Research, University of Queensland, Brisbane, Australia.
JM Chair of Clinical Pharmacology, School of Medicine and Public Health, University of Newcastle, Newcastle, Australia.
EP Director, Centre for Liver Disease Research, University of Queensland, Brisbane, Australia.
Hepatologist, Department of Gastroenterology and Hepatology, Princess Alexandra Hospital, Brisbane, Australia.

Competing interests

The authors declare no competing interests.

Consent for publication

Not applicable.

Author details

[1]School of Medicine, The University of Queensland, Translational Research Institute, Brisbane, Australia. [2]Pharmacy Department, Princess Alexandra Hospital, Brisbane, Australia. [3]QIMR Berghofer Medical Research Institute, Brisbane, Australia. [4]School of Pharmacy, The University of Queensland, Brisbane, Australia. [5]Centre for Liver Disease Research, The University of Queensland, Brisbane, Australia. [6]Department of Gastroenterology and Hepatology, Princess Alexandra Hospital, Woolloongabba 4102, Brisbane, Queensland, Australia. [7]School of Human Movement and Nutrition Sciences, The University of Queensland, Brisbane, Australia. [8]School of Medicine and Public Health, The University of Newcastle, Newcastle, Australia.

References

1. Mokdad AA, Lopez AD, Shahraz S, Lozano R, Mokdad AH, Stanaway J, et al. Liver cirrhosis mortality in 187 countries between 1980 and 2010: a systematic analysis. BMC Med. 2014;12:145.
2. Zipprich A, Garcia-Tsao G, Rogowski S, Fleig W, Seufferlein T, Dollinger M. Prognostic indicators of survival in patients with compensated and decompensated cirrhosis. Liver Int. 2012;32:1407–14.
3. Fagan KJ, Zhao EY, Horsfall LU, Ruffin BJ, Kruger MS, McPhail SM, et al. Burden of decompensated cirrhosis and ascites on hospital services in a tertiary care facility: time for change? Intern Med J. 2014;44:865–72.
4. Deloitte Access Economics. The economic cost and health burden of liver diseases in Australia. Kingston: The Gastroenterological Society of Australia/ Australian Liver Association; 2013.
5. Volk ML, Tocco RS, Bazick J, Rakoski MO, Lok AS. Hospital readmissions among patients with decompensated cirrhosis. Am J Gastroenterol. 2012; 107:247–52.
6. Coletti DJ, Stephanou H, Mazzola N, Conigliaro J, Gottridge J, Kane JM. Patterns and predictors of medication discrepancies in primary care. J Eval Clin Pract. 2015;21:831–9.
7. Mulhem E, Lick D, Varughese J, Barton E, Ripley T, Haveman J. Adherence to medications after hospital discharge in the elderly. Int J Family Med. 2013; 2013:901845.
8. Tompson AJ, Peterson GM, Jackson SL, Hughes JD, Raymond K. Utilizing community pharmacy dispensing records to disclose errors in hospital admission drug charts. Int J Clin Pharmacol Ther. 2012;50:639–46.
9. Stowasser D, Collins D, Stowasser M. A randomised controlled trial of medication liaison services - patient outcomes. J Pharm Pract Res. 2002;32:133–40.
10. Coleman EA, Smith JD, Raha D, Min SJ. Posthospital medication discrepancies: prevalence and contributing factors. Arch Intern Med. 2005;165:1842–7.
11. Morisky DE, Ang A, Krousel-Wood M, Ward HJ. Predictive validity of a medication adherence measure in an outpatient setting. J Clin Hypertens (Greenwich). 2008;10:348–54.
12. Krousel-Wood M, Islam T, Webber LS, Re RN, Morisky DE, Muntner P. New medication adherence scale versus pharmacy fill rates in seniors with hypertension. Am J Manag Care. 2009;15:59–66.
13. Morisky DE, DiMatteo MR. Improving the measurement of self-reported medication nonadherence: response to authors. J Clin Epidemiol. 2011;64:255–7.
14. Ventola CL. Current Issues Regarding Complementary and Alternative Medicine (CAM) in the United States: Part 1: The Widespread Use of CAM and the Need for Better-Informed Health Care Professionals to Provide Patient Counseling. P T. 2010;35:461–8.
15. Braun LA, Tiralongo E, Wilkinson JM, Poole S, Spitzer O, Bailey M, et al. Adverse reactions to complementary medicines: the Australian pharmacy experience. Int J Pharm Pract. 2010;18:242–4.
16. Calitz C, du Plessis L, Gouws C, Steyn D, Steenekamp J, Muller C, et al. Herbal hepatotoxicity: current status, examples, and challenges. Expert Opin Drug Metab Toxicol. 2015;11:1551–65.
17. Stickel F, Shouval D. Hepatotoxicity of herbal and dietary supplements: an update. Arch Toxicol. 2015;89:851–65.
18. Ganesh S, Rogal SS, Yadav D, Humar A, Behari J. Risk factors for frequent readmissions and barriers to transplantation in patients with cirrhosis. PLoS One. 2013;8, e55140.
19. Witticke D, Seidling HM, Lohmann K, Send AF, Haefeli WE. Opportunities to reduce medication regimen complexity: a retrospective analysis of patients discharged from a university hospital in Germany. Drug Saf. 2013;36:31–41.
20. Trindade AJ, Ehrlich A, Kornbluth Asher, Ullman TA. Are your patients taking their medicine? Validation of a new adherence scale in patients with inflammatory bowel disease and comparison with physician perception of adherence. Inflamm Bowel Dis. 2011;17:599–604.
21. Cohen HW, Shmukler C, Ullman R, Rivera CM, Walker EA. Measurements of medication adherence in diabetic patients with poorly controlled HbA1c. Diabet Med. 2010;27:2–6.
22. Murray MD, Kroenke K. Polypharmacy and medication adherence: small steps on a long road. J Gen Intern Med. 2001;16:137–9.
23. Hilmer SN. The dilemma of polypharmacy. Aust Prescr. 2008;31:2–3.
24. Pasina L, Brucato AL, Falcone C, Cucchi E, Bresciani A, Sottocorno M, et al. Medication non-adherence among elderly patients newly discharged and receiving polypharmacy. Drugs Aging. 2014;31:283–9.
25. Wang HY, Chan AL, Chen MT, Liao CH, Tian YF. Effects of pharmaceutical care intervention by clinical pharmacists in renal transplant clinics. Transplant Proc. 2008;40:2319–23.
26. Koshman SL, Charrois TL, Simpson SH, McAlister FA, Tsuyuki RT. Pharmacist care of patients with heart failure: a systematic review of randomized trials. Arch Intern Med. 2008;168:687–94.
27. Chisholm MA, Mulloy LL, Jagadeesan M, DiPiro JT. Impact of clinical pharmacy services on renal transplant patients' compliance with immunosuppressive medications. Clin Transplant. 2001;15:330–6.
28. Dash D, Sebastian TM, Aggarwal M, Tripathi M. Impact of health education on drug adherence and self-care in people with epilepsy with low education. Epilepsy Behav. 2015;44:213–7.
29. Cani CG, Lopes Lda S, Queiroz M, Nery M. Improvement in medication adherence and self-management of diabetes with a clinical pharmacy program: a randomized controlled trial in patients with type 2 diabetes undergoing insulin therapy at a teaching hospital. Clinics (Sao Paulo). 2015;70:102–6.
30. Kuntz JL, Safford MM, Singh JA, Phansalkar S, Slight SP, Her QL, et al. Patient-centered interventions to improve medication management and adherence: a qualitative review of research findings. Patient Educ Couns. 2014;97:310–26.
31. Spence MM, Makarem AF, Reyes SL, Rosa LL, Nguyen C, Oyekan EA, et al. Evaluation of an outpatient pharmacy clinical services program on adherence and clinical outcomes among patients with diabetes and/or coronary artery disease. J Manag Care Spec Pharm. 2014;20:1036–45.
32. Milone AS, Philbrick AM, Harris IM, Fallert CJ. Medication reconciliation by clinical pharmacists in an outpatient family medicine clinic. J Am Pharm Assoc (2003). 2014;54:181–7.
33. Kheir N, Awaisu A, Sharfi A, Kida M, Adam A. Drug-related problems identified by pharmacists conducting medication use reviews at a primary health center in Qatar. Int J Clin Pharm. 2014;36:702–6.

19

Portal hypertensive gastropathy as a prognostic index in patients with liver cirrhosis

Chang Seok Bang[1†], Hyo Sun Kim[1†], Ki Tae Suk[1], Sung Eun Kim[1], Ji Won Park[1], Seung Ha Park[2], Hyoung Su Kim[1], Myoung Kuk Jang[1], Sang Hoon Park[1], Myung Seok Lee[1], Choong Kee Park[1] and Dong Joon Kim[1*]

Abstract

Background: Portal hypertensive gastropathy (PHG) is a frequently overlooked complication of liver cirrhosis (LC). The clinical implications of PHG as a prognostic factor of LC or a predictive factor for the development of hepatocellular carcinoma (HCC) have not been established. The aim of this study was to assess the clinical significance of PHG in patients with LC.

Methods: Patients with LC were prospectively enrolled and followed in a single tertiary hospital in the Republic of Korea. Baseline hepatic vein pressure gradient (HVPG) was measured, and esophagogastroduodenoscopy (EGD) was performed. The associations of PHG with HVPG, survival and the development of HCC were evaluated.

Results: A total of 587 patients were enrolled. The mortality rate was 20.3 % ($n = 119$), and HCC developed in 9.2 % ($n = 54$) during the follow-up period (32.6 ± 27.8 months). The grade of PHG was well correlated with HVPG (no PGH: median 9.2 [IQR: 7.2–16.7], mild PHG: 14.6 [10.1–19.3], and severe PHG: 17.3 [12.3–21.5], $P < 0.001$), as well as with Child-Pugh class, MELD score or survival. However, it was not associated with the development of HCC. The grade of PHG (HR 3.29, 95 % CI: 1.12–9.63, severe vs. no PHG) and Child-Pugh class (HR 3.53, 95 % CI: 1.79–6.97, Child C vs A) showed significant associations with mortality.

Conclusion: PHG was well correlated with portal hypertension and could be used as a prognostic factor for LC but not for the prediction of HCC.

Keywords: Cirrhosis, Portal hypertension, Portal hypertensive gastropathy, Hepatocellular carcinoma

Background

Portal hypertension is a complication of liver cirrhosis (LC) and the main pathophysiologic mechanism that potentiates various adverse gastrointestinal consequences, including esophageal or gastric varices, gastropathy, and enteropathy [1, 2].

Portal hypertensive gastropathy (PHG) is a frequently overlooked complication in patients with LC. More attention has been focused on the detection or evaluation of esophageal or gastric varices by endoscopists. This complex secondary change in the gastric mucosa resulting from portal hypertension is a potential cause of acute or chronic hemorrhage [3]. It can also be severe and fatal, although less frequently than variceal hemorrhage [4].

In addition to the potential hemorrhagic focus, the clinical implications of PHG have not been well established. Previous studies have also shown conflicting results regarding the correlation between PHG and the severity of liver disease [5–13]. The aim of this study was to evaluate the clinical implications of PHG as a prognostic factor of LC or a predictive factor for the development of hepatocellular carcinoma (HCC) in patients with LC.

Methods
Patients

Patients with chronic liver disease were prospectively enrolled and followed in a single tertiary hospital in the Republic of Korea. Baseline hepatic vein pressure gradient

* Correspondence: djkim@hallym.ac.kr
†Equal contributors
[1]Department of Internal Medicine, Hallym University College of Medicine, Chuncheon, Gangwon-do 24253, South Korea
Full list of author information is available at the end of the article

(HVPG) was measured, and esophagogastroduodenoscopy (EGD) was performed in all consecutive patients for the detection or evaluation of the severity of PHG. Both procedures were performed consecutively and the time interval between 2 procedures was minimal. Patients without LC or with incomplete data were excluded from this study. The clinical and endoscopic characteristics of patients with LC were reviewed and analyzed. Data were recorded for the following variables: sex, age, the etiology of LC, endoscopic findings, laboratory findings, and HVPG. Laboratory findings including Child-Pugh classification and Model for End-stage Liver disease (MELD) score were assessed based on hospitalization day.

Differentiation of etiology

The differentiation between LC and chronic hepatitis relied on clinical, laboratory, radiologic and histologic information. The final determination of LC was made by two hepatologists (K.T.S and D.J.K).

In terms of the etiology, chronic hepatitis B was defined as positive for hepatitis B surface antigen (HBsAg) with abnormal levels of aspartate transaminase (AST) / alanine transaminase (ALT) for a period longer than 6 months. Chronic hepatitis C was defined as positivity for hepatitis C antibodies (Anti-HCV) and serum RNA (HCV-RNA) with abnormal levels of AST/ALT for a period longer than 6 months. Determination of alcoholic hepatitis used history of alcohol abuse (>40 g/day for men, >20 g/day for women) [14, 15], physical findings (delirium tremens or alcohol withdrawal seizure), laboratory tests (AST/ALT >2, elevated level of gamma glutamyl transpeptidase, or enlarged mean corpuscular volume), or liver biopsy (steatosis, hepatocyte ballooning, Mallory-Denk bodies, megamitochondria, canalicular and/or lobular

bilirubinostasis, or polymorphonuclear neutrophil infiltration), after excluding other potential etiologies. The determination of non-alcoholic steatohepatitis relied on history (exclusion of significant alcohol consumption), laboratory tests (AST or ALT elevation), imaging modalities (hepatic steatosis), or liver biopsy (macrovesicular fatty changes, hepatocyte ballooning, or inflammatory cell infiltrate), after excluding other potential etiologies.

Endoscopy and HVPG measurement

PHG was evaluated by EGD performed by 6 experienced endoscopists (>6000 cases of endoscopy). The diagnosis and determination of degree were based on the Baveno III scoring system [16]. To minimize the inter-observer variability, all of the endoscopic data and diagnoses were reviewed by 6 experienced endoscopists. Cases of disagreement were discussed and resolved by consensus, according to the Baveno III scoring system. To exclude single gastric antral vascular ectasia cases, not relevant to portal hypertension, authors categorized enrolled population according to the presence of PHG or not (binary criteria), in addition to the Baveno III scoring system for PHG, and six experienced endoscopists made decisions by consensus.

HVPG was measured with transjugular access under fluoroscopic guidance by 2 experienced hepatologists (K.T.S and S.H.P >300 cases of HVPG measurements). A catheter was placed into one of the hepatic vein branches, and the pressure was measured three times using the ballooning and deballooning method of the hepatic vein. The average number was recorded and decided upon as the patient's HVPG. Informed consent was obtained. Vital signs were continuously monitored,

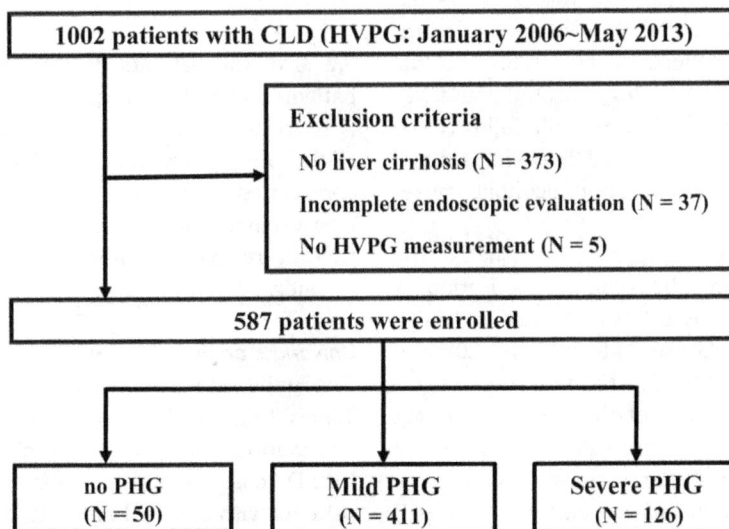

Fig. 1 Flow diagram of study design

and the patients were observed carefully to detect the development of serious complications during and after the measurement of HVPG.

Statistical analysis

Continuous variables are expressed as the medians and interquartile ranges (IQRs) because they were not normally distributed. Categorical variables are expressed as numbers and percentages. The Mann-Whitney test and Fisher's exact test were used to compare two variables. The Kruskal-Wallis test and Fisher's exact test were used to evaluate the three study arms. Post hoc analysis was performed using Bonferroni's correction. Survival analysis, including the development of HCC, was performed using the Kaplan-Meier method and the log rank test. The Cox proportional hazard model was applied for the detection of associated factors for survival and the development of HCC. A P value < 0.05 (2-tailed) was adopted as the threshold of statistical significance for all of the tests. The analysis was performed using SPSS software, version 21.0 (SPSS Inc., Chicago, IL, USA). All of the authors had access to the study data and reviewed and approved the final manuscript.

Results

Characteristic of patients

Between January 2006 and May 2013, 1002 patients were initially enrolled. Patients without LC or with incomplete data were excluded from this study. The number of excluded cases from each category was as follows: no LC ($n = 373$), incomplete endoscopic evaluation ($n = 37$), and incomplete HVPG measurement ($n = 5$). Finally, 587 patients were included in the analysis of this study (Fig. 1).

The clinical characteristics of these patients are summarized in Table 1. The median age was 51 years old (IQR: 45–59) in the total population. Male predominance was observed in the collected data for 78.7 % of the total patients. In terms of the etiology, alcohol abuse was the most frequent cause of LC (69.8 %), followed by hepatitis B virus (HBV) infection (24.2 %), hepatitis C virus (HCV) infection (5.8 %), and non-alcoholic causes (0.2 %).

Regarding the severity of LC, approximately half of the patients were included in Child-Pugh classification A (48.2 %), followed in order by B (39.9 %) and C (11.9 %). The median value of HVPG was 14.8 (IQR: 10–20), and the MELD score was 9.3 (IQR: 5.7–13.0).

PHG was detected in 91.5 % of the patients. Among the patients with PHG, the severe category constituted 21.5 %, and 70 % of the patients showed mild PHG. Patients with only gastric antral vascular ectasia was 3 (0.51 %). During the follow-up period (32.59 ± 27.77 months), the overall survival rate was 79.7 %, and

Table 1 Clinical characteristics of total patients

Characteristics, N (%)	Total (N = 587)
Age (years), Median (Interquartile range)	51 (45–59)
Sex	
Male	462 (78.7 %)
Female	125 (21.3 %)
Etiology	
Alcohol	410 (69.8 %)
HBV	142 (24.2 %)
HCV	34 (5.8 %)
Non-alcoholic	1 (0.2 %)
PHG	
No PHG	50 (8.5 %)
Mild PHG	411 (70 %)
Severe PHG	126 (21.5 %)
Child-Pugh classification	
Class A	283 (48.2 %)
Class B	234 (39.9 %)
Class C	70 (11.9 %)
HVPG (mmHg), Median (Interquartile range)	14.8 (10–20)
MELD score	9.3 (6.0–13.0)
Albumin (g/dL)	3.3 (2.8–3.8)
Total bilirubin (mg/dL)	1.4 (0.8–2.7)
Platelet count (x 10^3/mL)	105 (74–160)
Prothrombin time (INR)	1.26 (1.11–1.44)
Follow-up duration (months), Mean ± SD	32.59 ± 27.77
Survival	468 (79.7 %)
HCC	54 (9.2 %)

N number, HBV hepatitis B virus, HCV hepatitis C virus, PHG portal hypertensive gastropathy, HVPG hepatic vein pressure gradient, MELD model for end-stage liver disease, INR international normalized ratio, SD standard deviation, HCC hepatocellular carcinoma

9.2 % of the patients developed HCC. The proportion patients lost to follow-up was 12.8 % ($n = 75$).

There were no serious complications during or after HVPG measurements. Transient ventricular premature contraction was frequently noted when the tip of the measurement catheter passed the right atrium. Cardiac rhythm recovered without any treatment after a few seconds.

Univariate analysis for PHG

The univariate analyses for PHG in LC are listed in Tables 2 and 3. There were significant differences in the distributions of Child-Pugh classification, HVPG, and MELD score, as well as laboratory parameters, between patients with and without PHG (Table 2). In the analysis stratified by the severity of PHG (no PHG vs mild PHG vs severe PHG), this finding was consistent (Table 3).

Table 2 Univariable analysis for PHG in patients with liver cirrhosis

Variables, N (%)	No PHG	PHG	P value
	N = 50 (8.5 %)	N = 537 (91.5 %)	
Age (years), Median (Interquartile range)	52 (43–60.25)	51 (45–59)	0.64
Sex			0.002
Male	30 (60 %)	432 (80.4 %)	
Female	20 (40 %)	105 (19.6 %)	
Etiology			<0.001
Alcohol	20 (40 %)	390 (72.6 %)	
HBV	26 (52 %)	116 (21.6 %)	
HCV	4 (8 %)	30 (5.6 %)	
Non-alcoholic	0 (0 %)	1 (0.2 %)	
Child-Pugh classification			<0.001
Class A	37 (74 %)	246 (45.8 %)	
Class B	12 (24 %)	222 (41.3 %)	
Class C	1 (2 %)	69 (12.8 %)	
HVPG (mmHg), Median (Interquartile range)	9.2 (7.23–16.73)	15 (11–20)	<0.001
MELD score	6.00 (6.00–8.07)	9.83 (6.00–13.58)	<0.001
Albumin (g/dL)	3.7 (3.0–4.1)	3.2 (2.8–3.7)	0.001
Total bilirubin (mg/dL)	0.9 (0.6–1.2)	1.5 (0.9–2.9)	<0.001
Platelet count (x 10^3/mL)	141.5 (94.8–214.3)	104 (71–157)	0.001
Prothrombin time (INR)	1.12 (1.04–1.32)	1.28 (1.12–1.45)	<0.001
Survival	46 (92 %)	422 (78.6 %)	0.004
HCC	5 (10 %)	49 (9.1 %)	0.33

N number, HBV hepatitis B virus, HCV hepatitis C virus, PHG portal hypertensive gastropathy, HVPG hepatic vein pressure gradient, MELD model for end-stage liver disease, INR international normalized ratio, SD standard deviation, HCC hepatocellular carcinoma

In the analysis of survival, patients without PHG showed a higher survival rate than patients with PHG (92 % vs 78.6 %, 95.33 ± 3.78 vs 74.53 ± 2.21 months, $P = 0.004$) (Table 2 and Fig. 2a). This finding was also consistent with the analysis stratified by the severity of PHG (severe PHG vs mild PHG, $P = 0.008$; severe PHG vs no PHG, $P < 0.001$; mild PHG vs no PHG, $P = 0.008$) (Table 3, Fig. 2b). The detailed survival months and survival rates are reported in Table 4.

For the development of HCC, there was no significant difference between patients with or without PHG (9.1 % vs 10 %, $P = 0.33$) (Table 2). This finding was also consistent with the analysis stratified by the severity of PHG (severe PHG vs mild PHG: $P = 0.63$; severe PHG vs no PHG: $P = 0.34$; mild PHG vs no PHG: $P = 0.32$) (Table 3).

The distribution of sex and etiology of LC was different between patients with PHG and without PHG. However, the survival rate was not different between men and women ($P = 0.44$, log-rank test). In terms of the etiology of LC, the survival rate was only different between patients with CHB-associated LC and those with alcoholic LC ($P = 0.03$) (Fig. 3). The development of HCC was not significantly different between men and women ($P = 0.66$, log-rank test). In terms of the etiology of LC, the survival rate was not also different according to the etiology (Additional file 1: Figure S1).

Multivariate analysis for the prediction of survival in patients with LC

In the multivariate analysis of independent risk factors for survival, PHG (severe PHG vs no PHG, HR: 3.29, 95 % CI: 1.12–9.63, $P = 0.03$) and Child-Pugh classification (Child C vs A, HR: 3.53, 95 % CI: 1.79–6.97, $P < 0.001$) (Child B vs A, HR: 2.15, 95 % CI: 1.35–3.44, $P = 0.001$) showed statistically significant associations with survival in patients with LC. Age (HR 1.03, 95 % CI: 1.01–1.06, $P = 0.001$) and HVPG (HR 1.06, 95 % CI: 1.03–1.08, $P < 0.001$) showed marginal statistical significance (Table 5). This analysis was controlled for age, sex, etiology of LC, and MELD score.

Discussion

Blood flow congestion secondary to portal hypertension is considered the primary cause of PHG [17]. Imbalances between mucosal protective mechanisms and injury factors resulting from mucosal hemodynamic alterations are believed to induce PHG [18]. Although portal hypertension is the prerequisite for the development of PHG,

Table 3 Univariable analysis for PHG in patients with liver cirrhosis

Variables, N (%)	No PHG N = 50 (8.5 %)	Mild PHG N = 411 (70 %)	Severe PHG N = 126 (21.5 %)	P value
Age (years), Median (Interquartile range)	52 (43–60.25)	52 (46–60)	51 (45–56)	0.24
Sex				0.001
Male	30 (60 %)	324 (78.8 %)	108 (85.7 %)	
Female	20 (40 %)	87 (21.2 %)	18 (14.3 %)	
Etiology				<0.001
Alcohol	20 (40 %)	284 (69.1 %)	106 (84.1 %)	
HBV	26 (52 %)	99 (24.1 %)	17 (13.5 %)	
HCV	4 (8 %)	27 (6.6 %)	3 (2.4 %)	
Non-alcoholic	0 (0 %)	1 (0.2 %)	1 (0 %)	
Child-Pugh classification				<0.001
Class A	37 (74 %)	197 (47.9 %)	49 (38.9 %)	
Class B	12 (24 %)	169 (41.1 %)	53 (42.1 %)	
Class C	1 (2 %)	45 (10.9 %)	24 (19 %)	
HVPG (mmHg), Median (Interquartile range)	9.2 (7.2–16.7)	14.6 (10.1–19.3)	17.3 (12.3–21.5)	<0.001
MELD score	6.00 (6.00–8.07)	9.41 (6.00–12.85)	10.64 (6.94–14.73)	<0.001
Albumin (g/dL)	3.7 (3.0–4.1)	3.3 (2.8–3.8)	3.2 (2.8–3.6)	0.001
Total bilirubin (mg/dL)	0.9 (0.6–1.2)	1.4 (0.8–2.5)	1.9 (1.0–4.3)	<0.001
Platelet count (x 10^3/mL)	141.5 (94.8–214.3)	103 (75–156)	104 (66.8–167)	0.004
Prothrombin time (INR)	1.12 (1.04–1.32)	1.26 (1.11–1.44)	1.29 (1.15–1.49)	<0.001
Survival	46 (92 %)	327 (79.6 %)	95 (75.4 %)	
HCC	5 (10 %)	43 (10.5 %)	6 (4.8 %)	

HVPG, Severe PHG vs Mild PHG: $P = 0.001$, Severe PHG vs No PHG: $P < 0.001$, Mild PHG vs No PHG: $P < 0.001$
MELD score, Severe PHG vs Mild PHG: $P = 0.015$, Severe PHG vs No PHG: $P < 0.001$, Mild PHG vs No PHG: $P < 0.001$
Albumin, Severe PHG vs Mild PHG: $P = 0.18$, Severe PHG vs No PHG: $P < 0.001$, Mild PHG vs No PHG: $P = 0.002$
Total bilirubin, Severe PHG vs Mild PHG: $P < 0.001$, Severe PHG vs No PHG: $P < 0.001$, Mild PHG vs No PHG: $P < 0.001$
Platelet, Severe PHG vs Mild PHG: $P = 0.49$, Severe PHG vs No PHG: $P = 0.004$, Mild PHG vs No PHG: $P = 0.001$
INR, Severe PHG vs Mild PHG: $P = 0.14$, Severe PHG vs No PHG: $P < 0.001$, Mild PHG vs No PHG: $P < 0.001$
Survival, Severe PHG vs Mild PHG: $P = 0.08$, Severe PHG vs No PHG: $P < 0.001$, Mild PHG vs No PHG: $P = 0.008$
HCC, severe PHG vs Mild PHG: $P = 0.63$, Severe PHG vs No PHG: $P = 0.34$, Mild PHG vs No PHG: $P = 0.32$
N number, HBV hepatitis B virus, HCV hepatitis C virus, PHG portal hypertensive gastropathy, HVPG hepatic vein pressure gradient, MELD model for end-stage liver disease, INR international normalized ratio, SD standard deviation, HCC hepatocellular carcinoma

various other factors, such as inflammatory response, local vascular tone, hepatic function, gastric mucosal perfusion, endotoxin, and gastric sucrose permeability, are suspected to influence the development of PHG [19–22]. Reversible mucosal changes in the stomach have suggested that PHG is a dynamic condition [23, 24]. Several studies have evaluated the correlation of PHG with the severity of liver disease or portal hypertension [5–13]. However, most of these studies have included small populations, and the association remains unclear. Our study included the largest population (n = 587) and evaluated the association of PHG with the development of HCC, as well as with portal hypertension and survival.

PHG was detected in 91.5 % of the total population in our study. This result was consistent with several previous studies (90.1 % in the study by Kim et al. and 93.4 % in the study by Curvêlo et al.) [7, 8]. The reported prevalence of PHG has shown great variation (7–98 %) [25, 26].

Selection bias in the studies, inconsistent endoscopic diagnosis criteria, and the lack of interobserver reliability are suspected causes of variation [27]. A recent study of the reliability of endoscopic diagnosis in PHG showed unsatisfactory results regarding the currently available diagnostic criteria (Baveno, McCormack, and NIEC classification) [27]. Binary criteria, such as the presence or absence of a mosaic-like pattern, red-point lesions and cherry-red spots, showed high inter-observer agreement and high specificity [27]. To minimize bias, our study adopted an analysis of group created according to the presence of PHG or not (binary criteria), in addition to the Baveno III scoring system for PHG, and six experienced endoscopists made decisions by consensus.

In the analysis of the correlation between PHG and the severity of liver disease, PHG showed correlations with Child-Pugh classification, HVPG, and MELD score, as well as laboratory parameters (Table 2). These correlations

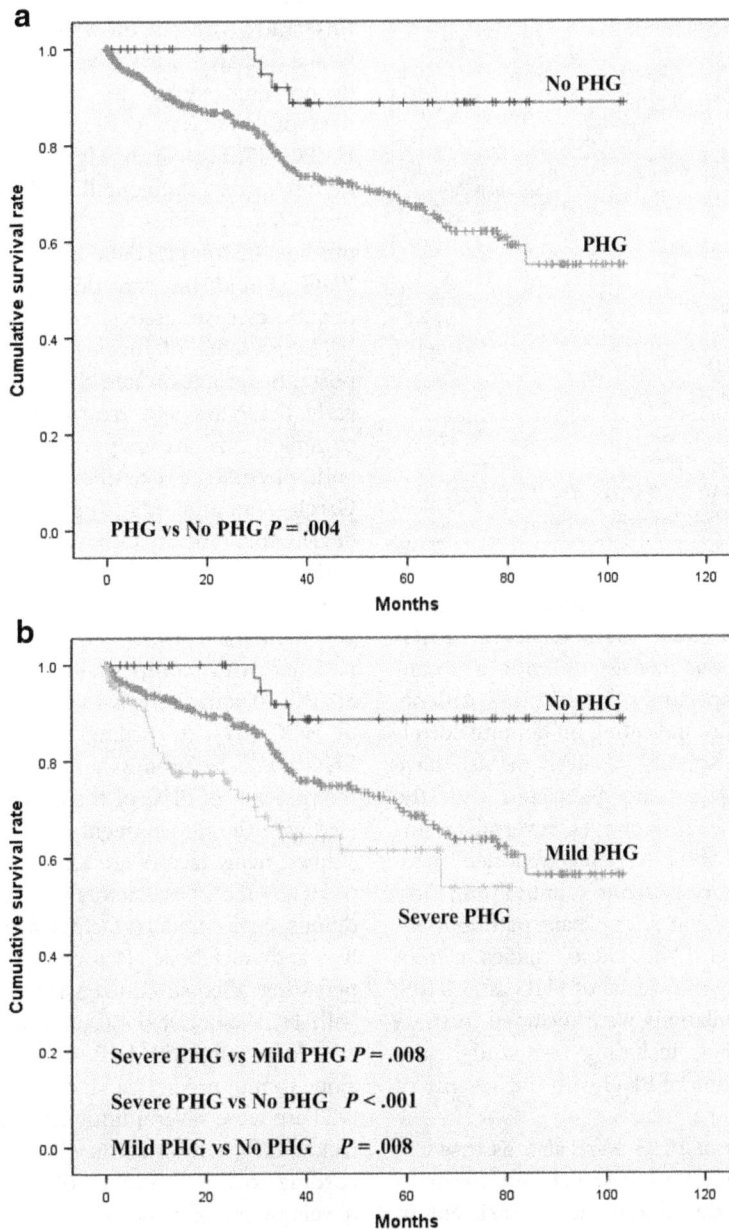

Fig. 2 Survival curve according to the presence of PHG (**a**) and PHG grade (**b**). PHG, portal hypertensive gastropathy

Table 4 Survival rate according to the PHG grade

PHG grade	Mean survival (months), Mean ± SD	Survival rate			Overall mortality (%)
		1 year (%)	3 years (%)	7 years (%)	
No PHG	95.33 ± 3.78	100	88.6	88.6	8
Overall PHG	74.53 ± 2.21	89.9	75.5	54.9	21.4
Mild PHG	76.68 ± 2.40	92.8	78.5	56.4	20.4
Severe PHG	55.48 ± 2.05	79.7	64.3	53.8 (5 years)	24.6

N number, *PHG* portal hypertensive gastropathy, *SD* standard deviation

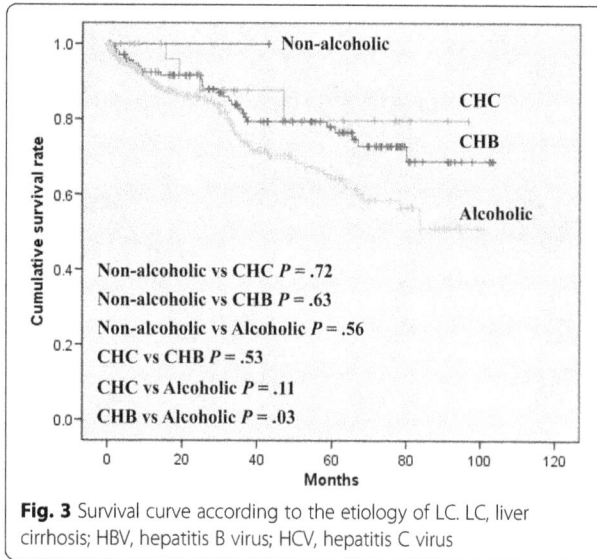

Fig. 3 Survival curve according to the etiology of LC. LC, liver cirrhosis; HBV, hepatitis B virus; HCV, hepatitis C virus

were also consistent in the analysis according to the severity of PHG (no PHG vs mild PHG vs severe PHG) (Table 3). This finding was consistent with a recent Korean study, which prospectively enrolled 331 patients with LC [8]. Previous studies indicating no definite correlation of PHG with the severity of liver disease have suggested that various factors are associated with the development of PHG [11, 12]. However, reversal or improvement of PHG was observed after treatment with transjugular intrahepatic portosystemic shunt (TIPS), indicating that portal hypertension is the main pathophysiologic mechanism of PHG [24]. These studies cannot definitely explain the cause of reversal of PHG after TIPS. Moreover, only small populations were included in these studies. Large scale studies, including our study, have shown a common association of PHG with the severity of liver disease [8].

Prognostic implications of PHG were also assessed in our study. The survival rates were statistically lower in patients with PHG, and this finding was consistent in the stratified analysis based on the severity of PHG (Tables 2 and 3; Fig. 2). Another large-scale study by Kim et al [8]. also showed consistent results. There was a report indicating an association of HVPG with

mortality in patients with decompensated LC [28]. In this study, the cut-off value of HVPG of 18 mm Hg was associated with 2-year mortality in patients with decompensated LC [28]. This value was similar to our data of HVPG in patients with severe PHG (median HVPG 17.3 of mm Hg). Without definite mucosal hemorrhage, incidentally detected PHG is easily neglected by endoscopists. Although this study cannot provide histologic data about the liver, patients with PHG should be considered to have more advanced hepatic disease, associated with a poorer prognosis.

The presence of advanced hepatic fibrosis is related to portal hypertension and the development of HCC. Thus, early detection and treatment of liver fibrosis and its complications are important. After the suggestion of pathophysiologic classification of LC using HVPG by Garcia-Tsao et al. [29], the association of HVPG and the development of HCC have been studied. In a study of patients with decompensated alcoholic LC, the cut-off value for HVPG of 15 mm Hg was associated with the development of HCC [30]. However, in another study of patients with compensated LC, the cut-off value of HVPG 10 mm Hg was associated with the development of HCC [31]. According to our data, the presence of PHG could be used as an index of prognosis. However, the presence of PHG or the degree of PHG was not associated with the development of HCC. As shown in previous studies, many factors are associated with the development of HCC [32]. These factors include viral predisposing conditions, environmental factors, age, sex, genetic susceptibility, and metabolic factors [32]. Considering the risk persisting after sustained virological response in patients with HCV-associated LC or even after HBsAg seroclearance in patients with HBV infection, hemodynamic staging alone cannot predict the development of HCC [33–35].

There were several limitations of our study. This study lacked information about changes in PHG or HVPG according to the treatment of LC. The association of the development of PHG with esophageal or gastric varices could not be assessed because various treatments or even non-treated cases of varices were included in the total population. Despite these limitations, our study included the largest population, and long-term observation

Table 5 Multivariable analysis for the prediction of survival in patients with LC

Variables, n (%)	HR (95 % CI)	P value
PHG	3.29 (1.12–9.63) (Severe PHG vs No PHG)	$P = 0.03$
Age	1.03 (1.01–1.06)	$P = 0.001$
Child-Pugh classification	3.53 (1.79–6.97) (Child C vs A)	$P < 0.001$
	2.15 (1.35–3.44) (Child B vs A)	$P = 0.001$
HVPG	1.06 (1.03–1.08)	$P < 0.001$

Controlled for age, sex, etiology, and MELD score

N number, HVPG hepatic vein pressure gradient, PUD peptic ulcer disease, NSAIDs non-steroid anti-inflammatory drugs, LC liver cirrhosis, OR Odds ratio

was undertaken for the evaluation of prognosis and the development of HCC.

Conclusion

In conclusion, PHG was well correlated with portal hypertension. It could be used as a prognostic factor for LC but not for the prediction of HCC.

Abbreviations
ALT, alanine transaminase; AST, aspartate transaminase; CI, confidence interval; EGD, esophagogastroduodenoscopy; HCC, hepatocellular carcinoma; HCV, hepatitis C virus; HR, hazard ratio; HVPG, hepatic vein pressure gradient; IQR, interquartile ranges; LC, liver cirrhosis; MELD score, The Model for End-stage Liver disease score; n, number; HBV, hepatitis B virus; PHG, portal hypertensive gastropathy

Acknowledgements
Not applicable.

Funding
This research was supported by Hallym University Research Fund 2014 (HURF-2014-20).

Authors' contributions
CSB participated data analysis and interpretation, and article drafting. HSK participated data analysis and interpretation, and article drafting. KTS participated to data analysis and interpretation. SEK participated to data analysis and interpretation. JWP participated to data analysis and interpretation. SHP participated to data analysis and interpretation. HSK participated to data analysis and interpretation. MKJ participated to data analysis and interpretation. SHP participated to data analysis and interpretation. MSL participated to data analysis and interpretation. CKP participated to data analysis and interpretation and revising it critically for important intellectual content. DJK participated to study design, data analysis and interpretation, and gave final approval for publication. All authors read and approved the final manuscript.

Competing interests
The authors declare that they have no competing interests.

Consent for publication
Voluntary participation was encouraged and informed consent to participate in the study was obtained from each patient. Patient records or information was anonymized and de-identified prior to analysis. Consent to publish of each patient data was obtained.

Author details
[1]Department of Internal Medicine, Hallym University College of Medicine, Chuncheon, Gangwon-do 24253, South Korea. [2]Department of Internal Medicine, Inje University Haeundae-Paik Hospital, Busan, South Korea.

References
1. de Franchis R. Evolving consensus in portal hypertension. Report of the Baveno IV consensus workshop on methodology of diagnosis and therapy in portal hypertension. J Hepatol. 2005;43(1):167–76.
2. De Palma GD, Rega M, Masone S, Persico F, Siciliano S, Patrone F, Matantuono L, Persico G. Mucosal abnormalities of the small bowel in patients with cirrhosis and portal hypertension: a capsule endoscopy study. Gastrointest Endosc. 2005;62(4):529–34.
3. Westerhoff M, Tretiakova M, Hovan L, Miller J, Noffsinger A, Hart J. CD61, CD31, and CD34 improve diagnostic accuracy in gastric antral vascular ectasia and portal hypertensive gastropathy: An immunohistochemical and digital morphometric study. Am J Surg Pathol. 2010;34(4):494–501.
4. Schepis F, Camma C, Niceforo D, Magnano A, Pallio S, Cinquegrani M, D'amico G, Pasta L, Craxì A, Saitta A, et al. Which patients with cirrhosis should undergo endoscopic screening for esophageal varices detection? Hepatology. 2001;33(2):333–8.
5. Panes J, Bordas JM, Pique JM, Bosch J, García-Pagán JC, Feu F, Casadevall M, Terés J, Rodés J. Increased gastric mucosal perfusion in cirrhotic patients with portal hypertensive gastropathy. Gastroenterology. 1992;103(6):1875–82.
6. Merkel C, Schipilliti M, Bighin R, Bellini B, Angeli P, Bolognesi M, Vescovi F, Gatta A. Portal hypertension and portal hypertensive gastropathy in patients with liver cirrhosis: a haemodynamic study. Dig Liver Dis. 2003;35(4):269–74.
7. Curvelo LA, Brabosa W, Rhor R, Lanzoni V, Parise ER, Ferrari AP, Kondo M. Underlying mechanism of portal hypertensive gastropathy in cirrhosis: a hemodynamic and morphological approach. J Gastroenterol Hepatol. 2009; 24(9):1541–6.
8. Kim MY, Choi H, Baik SK, Yea CJ, Won CS, Byun JW, Park SY, Kwon YH, Kim JW, Kim HS, et al. Portal hypertensive gastropathy: correlation with portal hypertension and prognosis in cirrhosis. Dig Dis Sci. 2010;55(12):3561–7.
9. Iwao T, Toyonaga A, Sumino M, Takagi K, Oho K, Nishizono M, Ohkubo K, Inoue R, Sasaki E, Tanikawa K. Portal hypertensive gastropathy in patients with cirrhosis. Gastroenterology. 1992;102(6):2060–5.
10. Ohta M, Hashizume M, Higashi H, Ueno K, Tomikawa M, Kishihara F, Kawanaka H, Tanoue K, Sugimachi K. Portal and gastric mucosal hemodynamics in cirrhotic patients with portal-hypertensive gastropathy. Hepatology. 1994;20(6):1432–6.
11. Bellis L, Nicodemo S, Galossi A, Guarisco R, Spilabotti L, Durola L, Dell'Unto O, Puoti C. Hepatic venous pressure gradient does not correlate with the presence and the severity of portal hypertensive gastropathy in patients with liver cirrhosis. J Gastrointestin Liver Dis. 2007;16(3):273–7.
12. Quintero E, Pique JM, Bombi JA, Bordas JM, Sentis J, Elena M, Bosch J, Rodes J. Gastric mucosal vascular ectasias causing bleeding in cirrhosis. A distinct entity associated with hypergastrinemia and low serum levels of pepsinogen I. Gastroenterology. 1987;93(5):1054–61.
13. Sarin SK, Sreenivas DV, Lahoti D, Saraya A. Factors influencing development of portal hypertensive gastropathy in patients with portal hypertension. Gastroenterology. 1992;102(3):994–9.
14. Becker U, Deis A, Sorensen TI, Grønbaek M, Borch-Johnsen K, Müller CF, Schnohr P, Jensen G. Prediction of risk of liver disease by alcohol intake, sex, and age: a prospective population study. Hepatology. 1996;23(5):1025–9.
15. McQuade WH, Levy SM, Yanek LR, Davis SW, Liepman MR. Detecting symptoms of alcohol abuse in primary care settings. Arch Fam Med. 2000; 9(9):814–21.
16. de Franchis R. Updating consensus in portal hypertension: report of the Baveno III Consensus Workshop on definitions, methodology and therapeutic strategies in portal hypertension. J Hepatol. 2000;33(5):846–52.
17. Ripoll C, Garcia-Tsao G. Management of gastropathy and gastric vascular ectasia in portal hypertension. Clin Liver Dis. 2010;14(2):281–95.
18. Perini RF, Camara PR, Ferraz JG. Pathogenesis of portal hypertensive gastropathy: translating basic research into clinical practice. Nat Clin Pract Gastroenterol Hepatol. 2009;6(3):150–8.
19. Abbasi A, Bhutto AR, Butt N, Munir SM, Dhillo AK. Frequency of portal hypertensive gastropathy and its relationship with biochemical, haematological and endoscopic features in cirrhosis. J Coll Physicians Surg Pak. 2011;21(12):723–6.
20. Giofre MR, Meduri G, Pallio S, Calandra S, Magnano A, Niceforo D, Cinquegrani M, di Leo V, Mazzon E, Sturniolo GC, et al. Gastric permeability to sucrose is increased in portal hypertensive gastropathy. Eur J Gastroenterol Hepatol. 2000;12(5):529–33.
21. Panes J, Bordas JM, Pique JM, García-Pagán JC, Feu F, Terés J, Bosch J, Rodés J. Effects of propranolol on gastric mucosal perfusion in cirrhotic patients with portal hypertensive gastropathy. Hepatology. 1993;17(2):213–8.
22. Lan C, Sun X, Dong L, Huang B, Yuan S, Wu K. The role of endotoxin in the pathogenesis of gastric mucosal damage in cirrhotic rats with portal hypertensive gastropathy. Asian Pac J Trop Med. 2011;4(3):212–4.
23. Primignani M, Carpinelli L, Preatoni P, Battaglia G, Carta A, Prada A, Cestari R, Angeli P, Gatta A, Rossi A, et al. Natural history of portal hypertensive gastropathy in patients with liver cirrhosis. The New Italian Endoscopic Club for the study and treatment of esophageal varices (NIEC). Gastroenterology. 2000;119(1):181–7.
24. Kamath PS, Lacerda M, Ahlquist DA, McKusick MA, Andrews JC, Nagorney

25. McCormack TT, Sims J, Eyre-Brook I, Kennedy H, Goepel J, Johnson AG, Triger DR. Gastric lesions in portal hypertension: inflammatory gastritis or congestive gastropathy? Gut. 1985;26(11):1226–32.

26. Vigneri S, Termini R, Piraino A, Scialabba A, Pisciotta G, Fontana N. The stomach in liver cirrhosis. Endoscopic, morphological, and clinical correlations. Gastroenterology. 1991;101(2):472–8.

27. de Macedo GF, Ferreira FG, Ribeiro MA, Szutan LA, Assef MS, Rossini LG. Reliability in endoscopic diagnosis of portal hypertensive gastropathy. World J Gastrointest Endosc. 2013;5(7):323–31.

28. Suk KT, Kim CH, Park SH, Sung HT, Choi JY, Han KH, Hong SH, Kim DY, Yoon JH, Kim YS, et al. Comparison of hepatic venous pressure gradient and two models of end-stage liver disease for predicting the survival in patients with decompensated liver cirrhosis. J Clin Gastroenterol. 2012;46(10):880–6.

29. Garcia-Tsao G, Friedman S, Iredale J, Pinzani M. Now there are many (stages) where before there was one: In search of a pathophysiological classification of cirrhosis. Hepatology. 2010;51(4):1445–9.

30. Kim MY, Baik SK, Yea CJ, Lee IY, Kim HJ, Park KW, Kim HK, Suk KT, Kim JW, Kim HS, et al. Hepatic venous pressure gradient can predict the development of hepatocellular carcinoma and hyponatremia in decompensated alcoholic cirrhosis. Eur J Gastroenterol Hepatol. 2009;21(11):1241–6.

31. Ripoll C, Groszmann RJ, Garcia-Tsao G, Bosch J, Grace N, Burroughs A, Planas R, Escorsell A, Garcia-Pagan JC, Makuch R, et al. Hepatic venous pressure gradient predicts development of hepatocellular carcinoma independently of severity of cirrhosis. J Hepatol. 2009;50(5):923–8.

32. Herbst DA, Reddy KR. Risk factors for hepatocellular carcinoma. Clinical Liver Disease. 2012;1(6):180–2.

33. Pinzone MR, Zanghì AM, Rapisarda L, D'Agata V, Benanti F, Spartà D, Nunnari G, Cacopardo B. Cirrhotic patients are still at risk of developing hepatocellular carcinoma despite Interferon-induced sustained virological response. Eur Rev Med Pharmacol Sci. 2014;18(2 Suppl):11–5.

34. Aleman S, Rahbin N, Weiland O, Davidsdottir L, Hedenstierna M, Rose N, Verbaan H, Stål P, Carlsson T, Norrgren H, et al. A risk for hepatocellular carcinoma persists long-term after sustained virologic response in patients with hepatitis C-associated liver cirrhosis. Clin Infect Dis. 2013;57(2):230–6.

35. Simonetti J, Bulkow L, McMahon BJ, Homan C, Snowball M, Negus S, Williams J, Livingston SE. Clearance of hepatitis B surface antigen and risk of hepatocellular carcinoma in a cohort chronically infected with hepatitis B virus. Hepatology. 2010;51(5):1531–7.

20

Prognostic significance of synergistic hexokinase-2 and beta2-adrenergic receptor expression in human hepatocelluar carcinoma after curative resection

Zhi-Feng Zhang[1†], Xiao-Sha Feng[1†], He Chen[1†], Zhi-Jun Duan[1*], Li-Xia Wang[1], Dong Yang[1], Pi-Xu Liu[2], Qiu-Ping Zhang[3], Yan-Ling Jin[3], Zhi-Gang Sun[3] and Han Liu[2]

Abstract

Background: Hexokinase-2 (HK2) and Beta2-adrenergic receptor (Beta2AR) are overexpressed in hepatocellular carcinoma (HCC) tissues and associated with poor prognosis. However, the synergistic effect of HK2 and Beta2AR in HCC prognosis is not elucidated. The present study aims to investigate the association between HK2 and Beta2AR expressions in HCC tissues, and to evaluate the synergistic effect of HK2 and Beta2AR in HCC prognosis.

Methods: Immunohistochemistry of HK2 and Beta2AR was performed on 155 paraffin embedded HCC samples retrieved from the archives of pathology department. Corresponding clinical data and prognostic data were collected through searching medical record systems, death registration systems and interviews with patient families. Spearman correlation test was performed to evaluate the association between HK2 and Beta2AR expression. Kaplan-Meier survival curves and Cox regressions were employed to evaluate HK2 and Beta2AR expression in HCC prognosis, respectively and synergistically.

Results: 109 of 155 HCC patients reached the death point, the survival time of HCC patients was 46.23 ± 31.01 months after curative surgical resections of HCC. Kaplan-Meier survival analysis showed that large tumor size (more than 5 cm) (hazard ratio (HR) = 8.42, 95 % confidence interval (CI) = 3.81–18.59, $P < 0.0001$), advanced TNM stage (III and IV stages) (HR = 2.09, 95%CI = 1.21–3.62, $P < 0.001$) and AFP more than 20 μg/L (HR = 1.49, 95%CI = 1.02–2.18, $P = 0.0302$) were predictors for poor prognosis. HK2 and Beta2AR positive expression was detected in 66 (42.58) and 122 (78.71 %) HCC samples respectively. In univariate analysis, HK2(+) (HR = 2.70, 95%CI = 1.76–4.15, $P < 0.0001$) and Beta2AR(+) (HR = 4.61, 96%CI = 3.14–6.76, $P < 0.0001$) were associated with poor prognosis. In multivariate analysis, HK2(+) ($P < 0.0001$) and Beta2AR(+) ($P < 0.0001$) were also associated with poor prognosis. HK2(+)/Beta2AR(+) in HCC samples had poorer prognosis compared with HK2(−)/Beta2AR(−) in both univariate analysis (HR = 4.69, 95%CI = 2.91–7.57, $P < 0.0001$) and multivariate analysis ($P < 0.0001$). HK2(+)/Beta2AR(+) in HCC samples had poorer prognosis compared with HK2(−)/Beta2AR(+) in both univariate analysis (HR = 1.76, 95%CI = 1.17–2.64, $P = 0.003$) and multivariate analysis ($P = 0.004$).

(Continued on next page)

* Correspondence: cathydoctor@sina.com
†Equal contributors
[1]Department of Gastroenterology, The First Affiliated Hospital of Dalian Medical University, 116000 Dalian, Liaoning Province, China
Full list of author information is available at the end of the article

(Continued from previous page)

Conclusion: HK2 and Beta2AR play important roles in HCC progression. HK2 and Beta2AR expression in HCC is correlated positively. Beta2AR may increase HCC invasion and metastasis in collaboration with HK2. HK2 and Beta2AR can predict HCC prognosis both independently and synergistically.

Keywords: Hepatocellular carcinoma, Hexokinase-2, Beta2-adrenergic receptor, Prognosis, Immunohistochemistry

Background

Hepatocellular carcinoma (HCC) is the fifth most common cancer in men and seventh most common cancer in women worldwide [1]. HCC is also the third most common cause of death from carcinomas worldwide [1, 2]. Although new treatment modalities for HCC have been developed in recent years, improvement of the five-year survival rates mainly relies on diagnosis at early stages of HCC. Early stage HCC can be treated with curative surgical resections, radiofrequency ablation, percutaneous ethanol injection and transarterial chemoembolization [2]. Moreover, only curative surgical resection has the possibility to cure HCC. As for the advanced stage HCC, although tyrosine kinase inhibitors, such as Sorafenib and Linifanib have been developed to improve survival rates, the cure of advanced stage HCC is rarely achieved [3, 4]. Therefore, how to choose the optimal therapy for the individual patient in order to maximize the survival time is of great importance to both clinicians and patients. Another issue of importance to clinicians and patients is to predict prognosis of HCC especially for the patients underwent curative HCC resections and for the patients with advanced stage HCC. Proper prediction of prognosis can guide clinicians to choose the right therapies and help patients to arrange the remaining life appropriately. To date, no individual biomarker can predict prognosis of HCC accurately. The combination of two or more correlated biomarkers for HCC prognosis may improve the power of prognosis predictions of HCC.

Beta2-adrenergic receptor (Beta2AR) is a transmembrane G protein-coupled receptor (GPCR), which can regulate cell proliferation via cyclic adenosine monophosphate and protein kinase A pathways [5]. Beta2AR are overexpressed in multiple cancers especially in gastrointestinal cancers and HCC [6–8]. It has been proved that Beta2AR agonist can promote DNA synthesis and beta-blockers can block DNA synthesis in pancreatic ductal carcinoma cell lines [7]. Selective Beta2AR blockage can also suppress colorectal cancer growth via EGFR-Akt/ERK signaling, G1-phase arrest and apoptosis [9]. Through increasing DNA synthesis, accelerating cell cycle and decreasing apoptosis, activation of Beta2AR promotes cancer growth, invasion and metastasis. High expression of Beta2AR may play a role in the canceration of injured hepatocytes, and may represent high grade of malignancy of HCC. So high expression of Beta2AR in HCC tissues is proposed be a biomarker for poor prognosis, which is supported by a previous survival study of HCC with immunohistochemistry [10].

Besides increased DNA synthesis, accelerated cell cycle and decreased apoptosis, another feature of cancer is the energy shift to aerobic glycolysis called Warburg effect, even in adequate oxygen environments [11]. Accelerated aerobic glycolysis is of importance to cancer cell survival, growth and metastasis [11]. Hexokinase (HK) is a key enzyme in glycolysis, to date, four HK isoforms were identified in mammals [12]. It is shown that HK2 is overexpressed in HCC tissues [13, 14]. Overexpression of HK2 may also represent high grade of malignancy. Two survival studies proved this hypothesis, and showed that high level expression of HK2 was an independent poor prognostic biomarker for HCC [13, 14].

Moreover, HK2 and Beta2AR are not independent, they are related in HCC development. Recently, one study indicates that activation of Beta2AR can promote HK2 expression, and inhibition of Beta2AR can decrease HK2 expressions in breast cancer cell lines [15]. It is deduced that Beta2AR might increase the grade of malignancy of cancers via promoting HK2 expression. However, the relationship between Beta2AR and HK2 expression in HCC tissues is not fully elucidated. We postulate that Beta2AR and HK2 expression in HCC tissues correlates positively; overexpression of HK2 and beta2AR in HCC can predict prognosis of HCC patients synergistically; Beta2AR may increase the grade of malignancy of HCC via promoting HK2 expression. In the current study, we performed immunohistochemistry assays to prove the above hypotheses.

Methods

HCC patients and tissue samples

This study is a retrospective study. 160 HCC patients underwent curative resections between January 2000 and December 2013 in the First affiliated hospital of Dalian Medical University were included in our study. Surgical treatment selection was mainly based on the Barcelona Clinic Liver Cancer (BCLC) algorithm [16]. Moreover, ten HCC patients with regional metastasis underwent HCC resections and lymph node dissections were also included into our study. Paraffin embedded pathologic samples were retrieved from the archives of the Department of Pathology. All the tissue sections were evaluated by experienced pathologist to confirm the diagnosis of HCC. Cholangiocellular carcinoma and other carcinomas of the liver were excluded during pathology evaluation. HCC patients accompanied with other site carcinomas were also excluded from our study. Because Beta2AR and HK2 were associated with metabolism, HCC patients accompanied with metabolic diseases including diabetes mellitus and thyroid diseases were also excluded from our study. This study was approved by Medical Ethics Committee of First Affiliated Hospital of Dalian Medical University. Consent was obtained from all participants (alive HCC patients or relatives of deceased HCC patients).

Survival data and clinical data collection

Clinical and laboratory data of each included patient during the hospital stay for curative resection were retrieved from the medical record system of the First Affiliated Hospital of Dalian Medical University. The computed tomography (CT) scanning and magnetic resonance images (MRI) of each patient were collected via Picture Archiving and Communication Systems. The records of operational procedures and observations during operations were also collected via medical record system. The CT images, MRI images and observations during operation were used to evaluate the tumor size (maximum diameter of the tumor). The survival data and the death date of each patient were retrieved through telephone interviews with patient families, and confirmed by searching the municipal death registration system of Dalian (the final collection date was 20th March 2014, the data collection period was limited in two weeks). Overall survival was used to evaluate HCC patient survival after surgical curative resections. Paraffin embedded pathologic samples of each patient were reevaluated by experienced pathologist to determine the differentiation grade of HCC according to Edmondson-Steiner histopathologic grading [17]. The HCC staging evaluation before operation was based on American Joint Commission on Cancer 7th edition TNM system [18].

Immunohistochemistry and density scoring

Immunohistochemistry was performed with the MaxVisionTM AP kit (Fuzhou Maixin Biotech. Co., Ltd, Fuzhou, China) according to the manufacture manuals. HK2 expression was evaluated with a rabbit anti-human HK2 monoclonal antibody (Cell Signaling Technology, Inc., Danvers, MA, USA) in accordance with the manufacturer's protocol

with antibody dilution of 1:50. Beta2AR was evaluated using a rabbit anti-human Beta2AR monoclonal antibody (Abcam, Cambridge, MA, USA) in accordance with the manufacturer's protocol with antibody dilution of 1:50. Both the intensity and proportion of stained cells in a HCC section (200×) were inspected and evaluated. Staining intensity was classified with a four grade system: no staining (0), weak (1), moderate (2), strong (3). The percentage of positive stained cells was also classified into a four scale system: <5 % (0), 5–25 % (1), 26–50 % (2), >50 % (3). All the scores were based on the mean scores of ten randomly selected fields of tissue sections. The staining intensity score plus the percentage score made the final score of each sample (the final score ranged from 0 to 6). If the final score is more than 3, the sample was determined to be positive. Otherwise, the sample was determined to be negative.

Statistical analysis

Pearson Chi-square test was used to analyze the associations between protein expression and clinical data. Survival time was shown as mean and standard deviation (SD). One-way ANOVA analysis and least significant difference (LSD) test were employed to determine the difference of live time among different groups. Spearman correlation test was performed to evaluate the association between HK2 and beta2AR expression with the final scores. Kaplan-Meier survival curve was employed to evaluate HK2 expression, Beta2AR expression and clinical data in HCC prognosis, respectively and synergistically. Cox regression analysis was also performed for multivariate analyses (all the selected clinical data was included in Cox regression) for HK2, Beta2AR and clinical data in HCC prognosis. $P < 0.05$ was considered statistically significant. Pearson Chi-square test and One-way ANOVA analysis were performed with the SPSS16.0 statistical software package (SPSS Inc., Chicago, IL, USA). Survival analysis and Cox regression analysis were performed with MedCalc 11.4.2.0 (MedCalc Software bvba, Acacialaan, Ostend, Belgium). Survival curve, Cox regression curve, Spearman correlation diagram and One-way ANOVA diagram were depicted with MedCalc 11.4.2.0 (MedCalc Software bvba, Acacialaan, Ostend, Belgium).

Results

The association between clinical data and survival

160 paraffin embedded HCC samples were retrieved from the archives of pathology department. Complete clinical data and prognostic data were collected through searching medical record systems and taking interviews with patient families. The survival data were confirmed by searching municipal death registration system of Dalian. Survival information of 155 patients was retrieved successfully, the rate of lost to follow-up was 3.13 %. 155 patients were included into final analyses. 109 (70.32 %)

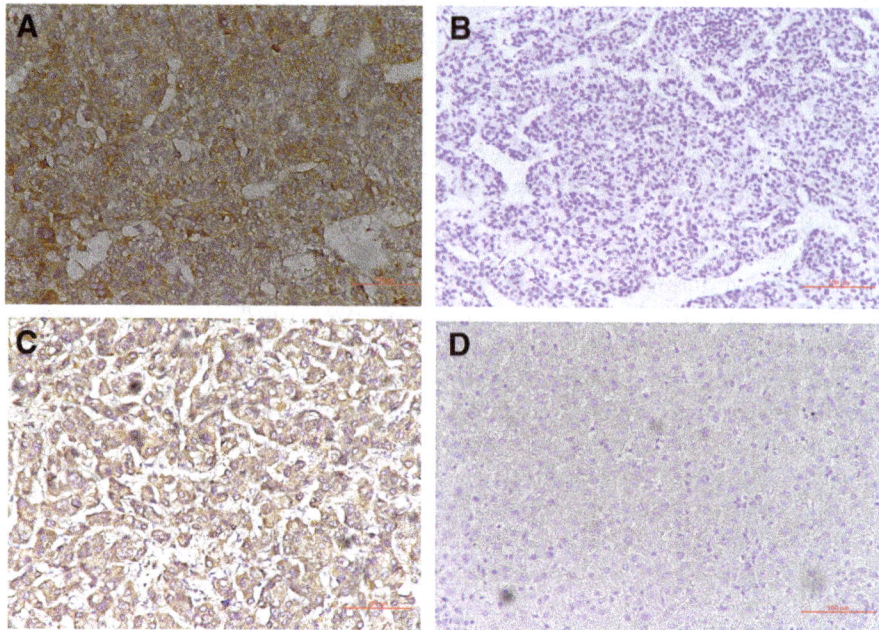

Fig. 1 Immunochemistry of HCC tissues. **a** Representative positive staining of HK2 in HCC tissues. **b** Representative negative staining of HK2 in HCC tissues. **c** Representative positive staining of Beta2AR in HCC tissues. **d** Representative negative staining of Beta2AR in HCC tissues

HCC patients reached the death point, the survival time of HCC patients was 46.23 ± 31.01 months after curative surgical resections of HCC. Kaplan-Meier survival analysis showed that large tumor size (more than 5 cm) (hazard ratio (HR) = 8.42, 95 % confidence interval (CI) = 3.81–18.59, $P < 0.0001$), advanced TNM stage (III and IV stages) (HR = 2.09, 95%CI = 1.21–3.62, $P < 0.001$) and AFP more than 20ug/L (HR = 1.49, 95%CI = 1.02–2.18, $P = 0.0302$) were predictors for poor prognosis. Age, gender, Hepatitis viral infection, tumor number, tumor

differentiation grade and post operational treatment are not associated with prognosis of HCC patients. Cox regression showed that only large tumor size and advanced TNM stage were associated with poor prognosis of HCC patients.

HK2 and Beta2AR are over expressed in HCC
Positive staining of HK2 was detected in the cytoplasm of HCC tissues. And positive staining of Beta2AR was also detected in the membrane and cytoplasm of HCC

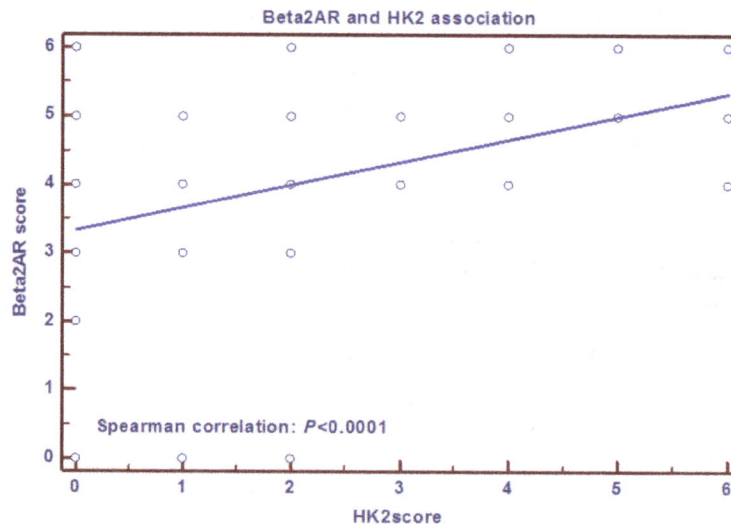

Fig. 2 Spearman correlation between HK2 and Beta2AR. Spearman correlation test shows that HK2 and Beta2AR expression is correlated positively ($P < 0.0001$)

Table 1 The details of association between Beta2AR expression and clinical data

	Beta2AR positive	Beta2AR negative	P value
Age			0.391
≤ 50 year	35	7	
> 50 year	87	26	
Gender			0.848
Male	98	27	
Female	24	6	
Hepatitis virus infection			0.439
HBV	106	29	
HCV	4	2	
HBV + HCV	1	1	
None	11	1	
AFP level			0.685
≤ 20ug/L	58	17	
> 20ug/L	64	16	
Tumor number			0.154
Solitary	118	30	
Multiple	4	3	
Tumor size			0.0001
≤ 5 cm	82	33	
> 5 cm	40	0	
TNM stage			0.795
I	44	12	
II	49	14	
III	22	4	
IV	7	3	
Differentiation			0.328
Well	36	14	
Moderate	58	14	
Poor	28	5	
Post operation treatment			0.483
None	77	23	
TACE	45	10	

Table 2 The details of association between HK2 expression and clinical data

	HK2 positive	HK2 negative	P value
Age			0.062
≤ 50 year	23	19	
> 50 year	43	70	
Gender			0.360
Male	51	74	
Female	15	15	
Hepatitis virus infection			0.594
HBV	57	78	
HCV	3	3	
HBV + HCV	0	2	
None	6	6	
AFP level			0.054
≤ 20ug/L	26	49	
> 20ug/L	40	40	
Tumor number			0.121
Solitary	65	83	
Multiple	1	6	
Tumor size			0.001
≤ 5 cm	40	75	
> 5 cm	26	14	
TNM stage			0.015
I	26	30	
II	18	45	
III	16	10	
IV	6	4	
Differentiation			0.145
Well	19	31	
Moderate	28	44	
Poor	19	14	
Post operation treatment			0.630
None	44	56	
TACE	22	33	

tissues. Representative positive staining and negative staining of HK2 and Beta2AR in HCC tissues are shown in Fig. 1. According to the scores of staining, HK2 and Beta2AR positive expression was detected in 66 (42.58) and 122 (78.71 %) HCC samples, respectively. Spearman correlation test showed that HK2 and Beta2AR expression was correlated positively ($P < 0.0001$), as shown in Fig. 2.

The association between HK2/Beta2AR expression and clinical data

There was no significant difference between HK2 positive staining samples and HK2 negative staining samples in age, gender, Hepatitis viral infection, AFP level, tumor number, tumor differentiation grade and post operational treatment. Only large tumor size and advanced TNM stage were correlated with HK2 positive staining positively. There was also no significant difference between Beta2AR positive staining samples and Beta2AR negative staining samples in age, gender, Hepatitis viral infection, AFP level, tumor number, TNM stage, tumor differentiation grade and post operational treatment. Only large tumor size was correlated with Beta2AR positive staining positively. The details of the association tests between HK2/Beta2AR expression and clinical data are shown in Tables 1 and 2.

Table 3 The details of association between HK2 expression and clinical data in Beta2AR positive samples

| | Beta2AR positive | | |
	HK2 positive	HK2 negative	P value
Age			0.102
≤ 50 year	23	12	
> 50 year	43	44	
Gender			0.357
Male	51	47	
Female	15	9	
Hepatitis virus infection			0.596
HBV	57	49	
HCV	3	1	
HBV + HCV	0	1	
None	6	5	
AFP level			0.050
≤ 20ug/L	26	32	
> 20ug/L	40	24	
Tumor number			0.235
Solitary	65	53	
Multiple	1	3	
Tumor size			0.091
≤ 5 cm	40	42	
> 5 cm	26	14	
TNM stage			0.006
I	26	18	
II	18	31	
III	16	6	
IV	6	1	
Differentiation			0.229
Well	19	17	
Moderate	28	30	
Poor	19	9	
Post operation treatment			0.377
None	44	33	
TACE	22	23	

HK2 and Beta2AR can predict HCC prognosis independently and synergistically

Positive Beta2AR staining was observed in all HK2 positive HCC samples. Moreover, when Beta2AR was negative in the HCC tissues, HK2 was also negative in the corresponding samples. In the Beta2AR positive staining HCC tissues, there was no significant difference between HK2 positive samples and HK2 negative ones in age, gender, Hepatitis viral infection, AFP level, tumor number, tumor differentiation grade and post operational treatment. Only advanced TNM stage was correlated

with HK2 positive staining. The details of the association tests between HK2 expression and clinical data in Beta2AR positive samples are shown in Table 3.

In univariate analysis, HK2(+) (HR = 2.70, 95%CI = 1.76–4.15, $P < 0.0001$) and Beta2AR(+) (HR = 4.61, 96%CI = 3.14–6.76, $P < 0.0001$) were associated with poor prognosis. In multivariate analysis, HK2(+) ($P < 0.0001$) and Beta2AR(+) ($P < 0.0001$) were also associated with poor prognosis. HK2(+)/Beta2AR(+) in HCC samples had poorer prognosis as compared with HK2(–)/Beta2AR(–) in both univariate analysis (HR = 4.69, 95%CI = 2.91–7.57, $P < 0.0001$) and multivariate analysis ($P < 0.0001$). HK2(+)/Beta2AR(+) in HCC samples had the poorer prognosis as compared with HK2(–)/Beta2AR(+) in both univariate analysis (HR = 1.76, 95%CI = 1.17–2.64, $P = 0.003$) and multivariate analysis ($P = 0.004$). The survival analysis curves are shown in Fig. 3.

Regarding patients that reached death point, one-way ANOVA analysis showed that survival time of HK2(–)/Beta2AR(–) patients (106.29 ± 26.68 months) was longer than that of HK2(–)/Beta2AR(+) patients (45.61 ± 19.12 months) ($P < 0.0001$) and HK2(+)/Beta2AR(+) patients (31.13 ± 18.00 months) ($P < 0.0001$) significantly. The survival time of HK2(–)/Beta2AR(+) patients was also longer than that of HK2(+)/Beta2AR(+) patients ($P = 0.001$). The details of one-way ANOVA analysis are shown in Fig. 4.

Discussion

HCC is the third most common cause of death from carcinomas worldwide [1, 2]. Moreover HCC is also one of the main causes of death of liver cirrhosis irrespective of cirrhotic etiology [19]. Due to the increasing incidence of hepatitis C virus (HCV) infections and non-alcoholic fatty liver disease (NAFLD), the incidence of HCC in USA has doubled in the past twenty years. Based on the trend of HCC incidence, it is postulated that HCC is likely to replace breast cancer and colorectal cancer to become the third cause of death from carcinomas in USA [20]. Different from developed countries, the etiology of HCC in developing countries especially southeastern Asian countries is hepatitis B virus (HBV) infection [21, 22]. The high incidence of HBV infection also makes HCC to be a big healthy problem in southeastern Asian countries. Irrespective of the etiology of HCC, the prognosis of HCC mainly relies on diagnosis at early stage and the possibility of curative surgical resections. However, even in USA, the rate of HCC diagnosed at early stage is only 46 % [20]. And only a small portion of HCC patients diagnosed at early stage can receive curative resections [20]. In the developing countries, the rates of HCC diagnosed at early stage and the portions of HCC patients at early stage received curative resections are very low. Although tyrosine kinase

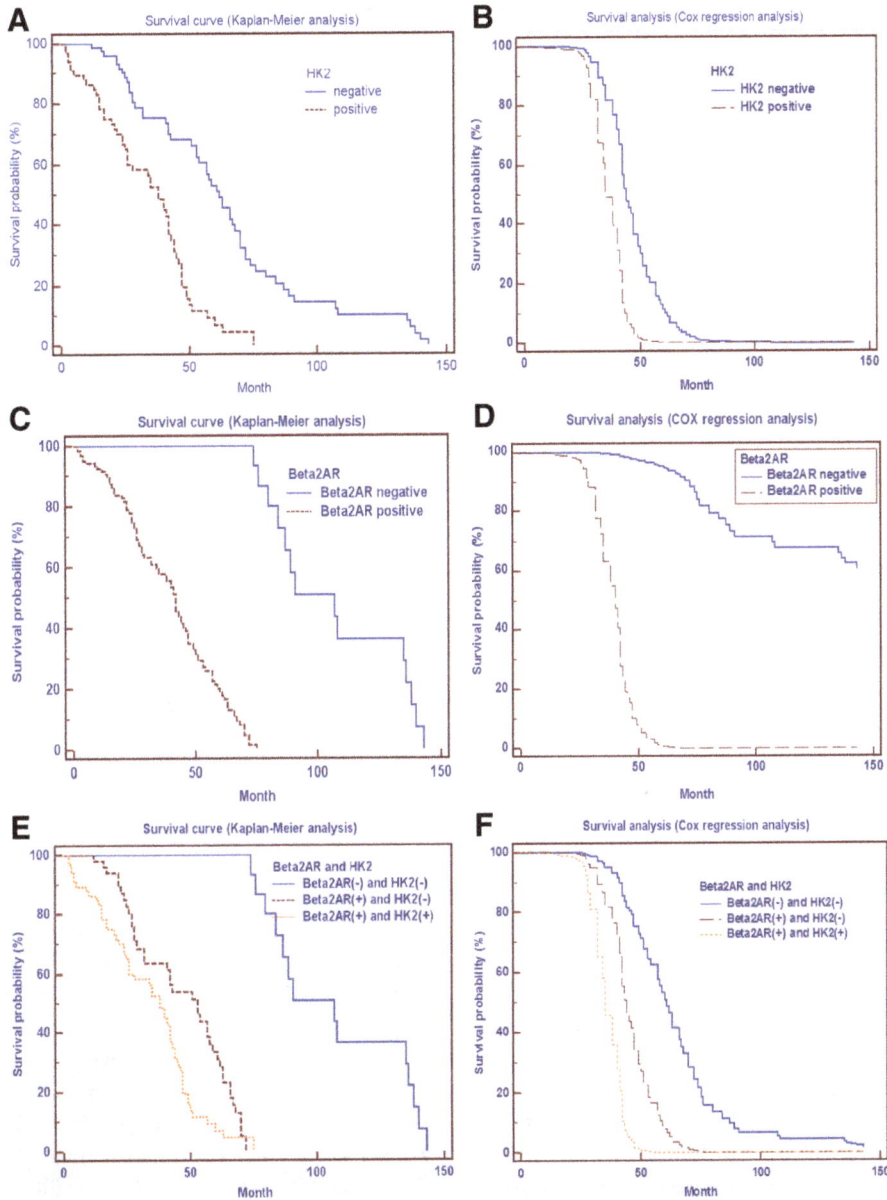

Fig. 3 Survival curve. **a** and **b** HK2(+) is associated with poor prognosis in both univariate analysis (HR = 2.70, 95%CI = 1.76–4.15, $P < 0.0001$) and multivariate analysis ($P < 0.0001$). **c** and **d** Beta2AR(+) is associated with poor prognosis in both univariate analysis (HR = 4.61, 96%CI = 3.14–6.76, $P < 0.0001$) and multivariate analysis ($P < 0.0001$). **e** and **f** HK2(+)/Beta2AR(+) in HCC samples shows poorer prognosis as compared with HK2(−)/Beta2AR(−) in both univariate analysis (HR = 4.69, 95%CI = 2.91–7.57, $P < 0.0001$) and multivariate analysis ($P < 0.0001$). HK2(+)/Beta2AR(+) in HCC samples shows poorer prognosis as compared with HK2(−)/Beta2AR(+) in both univariate analysis (HR = 1.76, 95%CI = 1.17–2.64, $P = 0.003$) and multivariate analysis ($P = 0.004$)

inhibitors (such as Sorafeniband Linifanib) have been developed to treat HCC at advanced stage, the outcome of treatment at advanced stage is not satisfactory [3, 4]. Scientists are still searching for new HCC treatment targets. Exploring the mechanism of HCC development may shed light on developing new therapies. Another realistic issue of importance to clinicians and patients is to predict prognosis of HCC. Proper prediction of prognosis can guide clinicians to

choose the right therapies and help patients to arrange the remaining life appropriately.

Beta2AR regulates cell proliferation via cyclic adenosine monophosphate and protein kinase A pathways [5]. Through increasing DNA synthesis, accelerating cell cycle and decreasing apoptosis, activation of Beta2AR promotes cancer growth, invasion and metastasis. A previous study indicates that high expression of Beta2AR in HCC tissues is a biomarker for poor prognosis [10]. The

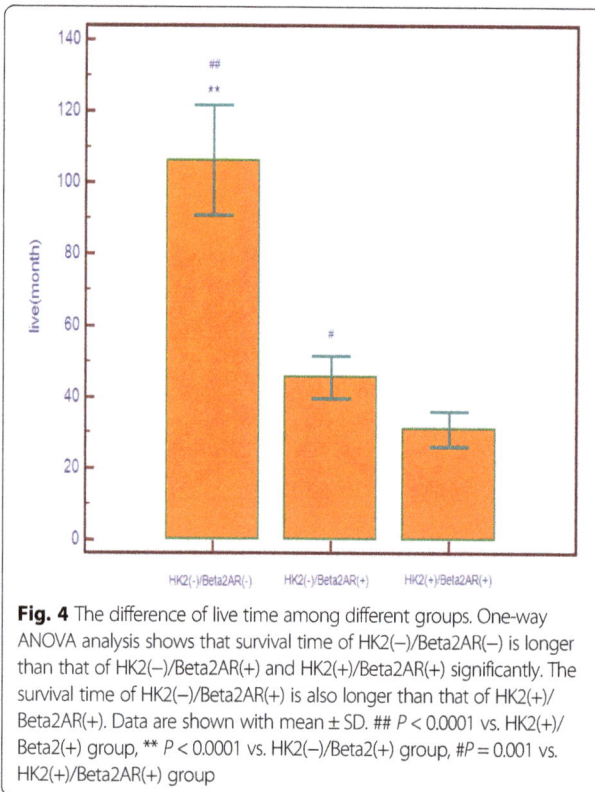

Fig. 4 The difference of live time among different groups. One-way ANOVA analysis shows that survival time of HK2(−)/Beta2AR(−) is longer than that of HK2(−)/Beta2AR(+) and HK2(+)/Beta2AR(+) significantly. The survival time of HK2(−)/Beta2AR(+) is also longer than that of HK2(+)/Beta2AR(+). Data are shown with mean ± SD. ## $P < 0.0001$ vs. HK2(+)/Beta2(+) group, ** $P < 0.0001$ vs. HK2(−)/Beta2(+) group, # $P = 0.001$ vs. HK2(+)/Beta2AR(+) group

Kaplan-Meier survival analysis and Cox regression analysis of our study are in consistence with the findings of this study. Our study also proves that high expression of Beta2AR in HCC is associated with large tumor size, which implies high expression Beta2AR in HCC playing an important role in tumor growth.

Glycolysis is the the key step for cellular energy metabolism, which converts glucose into pyruvate to produce adenosine triphosphate (ATP) [23]. Ten steps and corresponding enzymes participate in this process. Among these enzymes, HK is the first step enzyme converting glucose into glucose 6-phosphate, and pyruvate kinase (PK) is the final step enzyme converting phosphoenolpyruvate into pyruvate [23]. When abundant oxygen is present, pyruvate enters tricarboxylic acid (TCA) cycle to produce ATP in mitochondria. Under hypoxia conditions, pyruvate will be converted into lactate by lactate dehydrogenase (LDH) to produce ATP. Tumor prefers the latter instead of entering the TCA cycle to produce energy, even under sufficient oxygen conditions, which is called Warburg effect [11]. HK and PK play important roles in this energy shift [24]. To date, four HK isoforms and four PK isoforms are identified in mammals [12, 25, 26]. Different from normal liver cells, HCC tissues express HK2 and PKM2 predominantly [13, 14, 27]. This isoform alteration makes cancer cells prefer aerobic glycolysis instead of aerobic oxidation [11]. Accelerated aerobic glycolysis supplies abundant energy to cancer cells

for their survival, growth and metastasis [11]. HK2 participates in tumor initiation and maintenance, and HK2 depletion inhibits the neoplastic phenotype of human lung and breast cancer cells in vitro and in vivo [25]. Previous study showed that 3-bromopyruvate (3-BP), a HK2 inhibitor induced apoptosis of HCC cells via augmenting ER stress and anti-angiogenesis by protein disulfide isomerase inhibition [28]. In another study, Resveratrol (a HK2 inhibitor) also induces apoptosis of HCC cells via inhibiting aerobic glycolysis [29]. All the above evidence indicates that HK2 might be a potential therapeutic target for HCC.

Recently one study also revealed that the levels of HK2 expression in dysplastic cirrhosis and HCC was higher than that of non dysplastic cirrhosis and normal liver, which indicates that high expression of HK2 is associated with high grade of malignancy [30]. Previous studies also showed that high expression of HK2 was an independent poor prognostic biomarker for HCC [13, 14]. The results of our study are in consistence with these two survival studies. Our study also suggests that high expression of HK2 is associated with large tumor size and advanced TNM stages, which indicates that high expression of HK2 in HCC represents high levels of malignancy. High HK2 expression in HCC tissues can also be used as a biomarker for poor HCC prognosis.

Moreover, HK2 and Beta2AR are correlated in HCC development. Previous study indicates that activation of Beta2AR can promote HK2 expression, and inhibition of Beta2AR can decrease HK2 expressions in breast cancer cell lines [15]. Our study also shows positive associations between HK2 and Beta2AR in HCC tissues. Additionally, Beta2AR positive staining in HCC is not associated with TNM stage in our study. However, in Beta2AR positive stained samples, HK2 positive staining is associated with TNM stage. This may imply that Beta2AR increases HCC invasion and metastasis through HK2 activation. Detecting HK2 and Beta2AR simultaneously may help clinicians to evaluate the malignant status of HCC. Combination therapy of targeting HK2 and Beta2AR might be a promising strategy for HCC.

Combination of HK2 and Beta2AR detection also improves the predictive power for prognosis. The Kaplan-Meier survival analysis and Cox regression analysis of our study showed that HK2(+)/Beta2AR(+) HCC patients had poorer prognosis compared with HK2(−)/Beta2AR(+) and HK2(−)/Beta2AR(−) HCC patients. Detecting HK2 and Beta2AR expression in HCC simultaneously has clinical significance in prognosis prediction. However, there are some limitations of our study. Firstly, the sample number of our study is not very large, which could attenuate the statistical power. Secondly, because of the limitations of pathologic samples, only immunohistochemistry was employed in our study, other methods to detect HK2 and Beta2AR (Western blot and quantitative real time PCR) are needed to confirm the results of this study. Moreover, in vitro studies are also required to prove these findings. Thirdly, we were not able to calculate the score of Child Pugh due to incomplete information collection, the effect of liver function reservoir on HCC survival and Cox regression analyses could not be evaluated. Fourthly, we were unable to retrieved the recurrence information of HCC, so we did not evaluate the expression of HK2 and Beta2AR on the recurrence of HCC. Despite of the above limitations, our study will shed new light on HCC treatment and prognosis predictions.

Conclusion

In summary, Beta2AR and HK2 expression in HCC tissues is positively correlated. High expression of HK2 and beta2AR in HCC can predict prognosis of HCC patients independently and synergistically. Beta2AR might increase the grade of malignancy of HCC via promoting HK2 expression. Combined targeting of HK2 and Beta2AR might be a promising therapy for HCC.

Abbreviations
BCLC, Barcelona Clinic Liver Cancer algorithm; Beta2AR, Beta2-adrenergic receptor; CT, computed tomography scanning; GPCR, transmembrane G protein-coupled receptor; HBV, hepatitis B virus; HCC, hepatocellular carcinoma; HCV, hepatitis C virus; HK2, Hexokinase-2; MRI, magnetic resonance images

Acknowledgment
We would like to acknowledge librarian Jiao He of the first affiliated hospital of Dalian Medical University for the retrieving of related articles. All authors declare that there is no fund provided to this research.

Funding
The authors have no support or funding to report.

Authors' contributions
Conceived and designed the experiments: ZFZ, ZJD, PXL and HL. Performed the experiments: ZFZ, XSF, HC, LXW, QPZ, YLJ, ZGS and DY. Analyzed the data and wrote the paper: ZFZ, ZJD, PXL and HL. All authors read and approved the final manuscript as submitted.

Competing interests
The authors declare that they have no competing interests.

Consent for publication
Not applicable.

Author details
[1]Department of Gastroenterology, The First Affiliated Hospital of Dalian Medical University, 116000 Dalian, Liaoning Province, China. [2]Institute of Cancer Stem Cell, Dalian Medical University, 116000 Dalian, Liaoning Province, China. Department of Pathology, The First Affiliated Hospital of Dalian Medical University, 116000 Dalian, Liaoning Province, China.

References
1. Ferlay J, Shin HR, Bray F, Forman D, Mathers C, Parkin DM. Estimates of worldwide burden of cancer in 2008: GLOBOCAN 2008. Int J Cancer. 2010; 127(12):2893–917.
2. Forner A, Llovet JM, Bruix J. Hepatocellular carcinoma. Lancet. 2012;379: 1245–55.
3. Cainap C, Qin S, Huang WT, Chung IJ, Pan H, Cheng Y, Kudo M, Kang YK, Chen PJ, Toh HC, Gorbunova V, Eskens FA, Qian J, McKee MD, Ricker JL, Carlson DM, El-Nowiem S. Linifanib versus Sorafenib in patients with advanced hepatocellular carcinoma: results of a randomized phase III trial. J Clin Oncol. 2015;33(2):172–9.
4. Peng S, Zhao Y, Xu F, Jia C, Xu Y, Dai C. An updated meta-analysis of randomized controlled trials assessing the effect of sorafenib in advanced hepatocellular carcinoma. PLoS One. 2014;9(12):e112530.
5. Maudsley S, Pierce KL, Zamah AM, Miller WE, Ahn S, Daaka Y, Lefkowitz RJ, Luttrell LM. The beta(2)-adrenergic receptor mediates extracellular signal-regulated kinase activation via assembly of a multireceptor complex with the epidermal growth factor receptor. J Biol Chem. 2000;275:9572–80.
6. Masur K, Niggermann B, Zanker KS, Entschladen F. Norepinephrine-induced mi-gration of SW 480 colon carcinoma cells is inhibited by beta-blockers. Cancer Res. 2001;61:2866–9.
7. Weddle DL, Tithof PK, Williams M, Schuller HM. Beta-adrenergic growth regulation of human cancer cell lines derived from pancreatic ductal carcinomas. Carcinogenesis. 2001;22:473–9.
8. Kassahun WT, Guenl B, Ungemach FR, Jonas S, Abraham G. Expression and functional coupling of liver β2-adrenoceptors in the human hepatocellular carcinoma. Pharmacology. 2012;89(5–6):313–20.
9. Chin CC, Li JM, Lee KF, Huang YC, Wang KC, Lai HC, Cheng CC, Kuo YH, Shi CS. Selective β2-AR blockage suppresses colorectal cancer growth through regulation of EGFR-Akt/ERK1/2 signaling, G1-phase arrest, and apoptosis. J Cell Physiol. 2016;231(2):459–72.
10. Chen D, Xing W, Hong J, Wang M, Huang Y, Zhu C, Yuan Y, Zeng W. The beta2- adrenergic receptor is a potential prognostic biomarker for human hepatocellular carcinoma after curative resection. Ann Surg Oncol. 2012; 19(11):3556–65.
11. Vander Heiden MG, Cantley LC, Thompson CB. Understanding the Warburg effect: the metabolic requirements of cell proliferation. Science. 2009;324: 1029–33.
12. Wilson JE. Isozymes of mammalian hexokinase: structure, subcellular localization and metabolic function. J Exp Biol. 2003;206:2049–57.
13. Kwee SA, Hernandez B, Chan O, Wong L. Choline kinase alpha and hexokinase-2 protein expression in hepatocellular carcinoma: association with survival. PLoS One. 2012;7(10):e46591.
14. Peng SY, Lai PL, Pan HW, Hsiao LP, Hsu HC. Aberrant expression of the glycolytic enzymes aldolase B and type II hexokinase in hepatocellular carcinoma are predictive markers for advanced stage, early recurrence and poor prognosis. Oncol Rep. 2008;19(4):1045–53.
15. Kang F, Ma W, Ma X, Shao Y, Yang W, Chen X, Li L, Wang J. Propranolol inhibits glucose metabolism and 18 F-FDG uptake of breast cancer through posttranscriptional downregulation of hexokinase-2. J Nucl Med. 2014;55(3):439–45.
16. Llovet JM, Brú C, Bruix J. Prognosis of hepatocellular carcinoma: the BCLC staging classification. Semin Liver Dis. 1999;19:329–38.
17. Edmondson HA, Steiner PE. Primary carcinoma of the liver: a study of 100 cases among 48,900 necropsies. Cancer. 1954;7(3):462–503.
18. Sobin LH, Compton CC. TNM seventh edition: what's new, what's changed: communication from the International Union against Cancer and the American Joint Committee on Cancer. Cancer. 2010;116:5336–9.
19. El-Serag HB. Hepatocellular carcinoma. N Engl J Med. 2011;365:1118–27.
20. Njei B, Rotman Y, Ditah I, Lim JK. Emerging trends in hepatocellular carcinoma incidence and mortality. Hepatology. 2015;61:191–9.
21. Luo Z, Li L, Ruan B. Impact of the implementation of a vaccination strategy on hepatitis B virus infections in China over a 20-year period. Int J Infect Dis. 2012;16:e82–8.
22. Zacharias T, Wang W, Dao D, Wojciechowski H, Lee WM, Do S, Singal AG. HBV outreach programs significantly increase knowledge and vaccination rates among Asian pacific islanders. J Community Health. 2015;40:619–24.

23. Zwerschke W, Mazurek S, Stöckl P, Hütter E, Eigenbrodt E, Jansen-Dürr P. Metabolic analysis of senescent human fibroblasts reveals a role for AMP in cellular senescence. Biochem J. 2003;376:403–11.

24. Li XB, Gu JD, Zhou QH. Review of aerobic glycolysis and its key enzymes-new targets for lung cancer therapy. Thorac Cancer. 2015;6(1):17–24.

25. Patra KC, Wang Q, Bhaskar PT, Miller L, Wang Z, Wheaton W, Chandel N, Laakso M, Muller WJ, Allen EL, Jha AK, Smolen GA, Clasquin MF, Robey RB, Hay N. Hexokinase 2 is required for tumor initiation and maintenance and its systemic deletion is therapeutic in mouse models of cancer. Cancer Cell. 2013;24(2):213–28.

26. Israelsen WJ, Vander Heiden MG. Pyruvate kinase: function, regulation and role in cancer. Semin Cell Dev Biol. 2015;43:43–51.

27. Chen Z, Lu X, Wang Z, Jin G, Wang Q, Chen D, Chen T, Li J, Fan J, Cong W, Gao Q, He X. Co-expression of PKM2 and TRIM35 predicts survival and recurrence in hepatocellular carcinoma. Oncotarget. 2015;6(4):2538–48.

28. Yu SJ, Yoon JH, Yang JI, Cho EJ, Kwak MS, Jang ES, Lee JH, Kim YJ, Lee HS, Kim CY. Enhancement of hexokinase II inhibitor-induced apoptosis in hepatocellular carcinoma cells via augmenting ER stress and anti-angiogenesis by protein disulfide isomerase inhibition. J Bioenerg Biomembr. 2012;44(1):101–15.

29. Dai W, Wang F, Lu J, Xia Y, He L, Chen K, Li J, Li S, Liu T, Zheng Y, Wang J, Lu W, Zhou Y, Yin Q, Abudumijiti H, Chen R, Zhang R, Zhou L, Zhou Z, Zhu R, Yang J, Wang C, Zhang H, Zhou Y, Xu L, Guo C. By reducing hexokinase 2, resveratrol induces apoptosis in HCC cells addicted to aerobic glycolysis and inhibits tumor growth in mice. Oncotarget. 2015;6(15):13703–17.

30. Guzman G, Chennuri R, Chan A, Rea B, Quintana A, Patel R, Xu PZ, Xie H, Hay N. Evidence for heightened hexokinase II immunoexpression in hepatocyte dysplasia and hepatocellular carcinoma. Dig Dis Sci. 2015;60(2):420–6.

21

Evaluation of dose-efficacy of sorafenib and effect of transarterial chemoembolization in hepatocellular carcinoma patients

Wang-De Hsiao[2], Cheng-Yuan Peng[1,2], Po-Heng Chuang[2], Hsueh-Chou Lai[2], Ken-Sheng Cheng[2], Jen-Wei Chou[2], Yang-Yuan Chen[1,2], Cheng-Ju Yu[2], Chun-Lung Feng[2], Wen-Pang Su[2], Sheng-Hung Chen[2] and Jung-Ta Kao[1,2*]

Abstract

Background: Transarterial chemoembolization (TACE) and sorafenib are the therapeutic standard for intermediate and advanced stage hepatocellular carcinoma (HCC) patients respectively. High costs with adverse events (AE) of sorafenib might limit sorafenib dosage, further affecting therapeutic response. To attain greatest benefit, we evaluated the efficacy of different doses and effect of TACE during and after sorafenib discontinuation in patients representing Child-Pugh Classification Class A with venous or extra-hepatic invasion.

Methods: A total 156 patients met the criteria and were divided into Groups I ($n = 52$) accepting 800 mg/day; II ($n = 58$) accepting 800 mg/day and reduced to 400 mg/day owing to AE; and III ($n = 46$) accepting 400 mg/day. TACE was performed during and after sorafenib discontinuation and therapeutic response bimonthly to four-monthly was rated thereafter.

Results: Median duration of sorafenib treatment and patients' survival were 4.00 ± 0.45 and 7.50 ± 1.44 months in all cases; 2.50 ± 0.90 and 5.00 ± 1.10 months in Group I; 5.50 ± 1.27 and 16.50 ± 1.86 months in Group II; 4.00 ± 0.94 and 6.50 ± 2.49 months in Group III. Group II presented the best response and survival benefit ($p = 0.010$ and $p = 0.011$ respectively). Child-Pugh Classification score 5 (Hazard Ratio = 0.492, $p = 0.049$), absent AE (3.423, $p = 0.015$), tumor numbers ≤ 3 (0.313, $p = 0.009$), sorafenib duration ≤ 1 cycle (3.694, $p = 0.004$), and absent TACE (3.197, $p = 0.008$) significantly correlated with patient survival. TACE benefit appeared in separate and total cases during ($p = 0.002$, $p = 0.595$, $p = 0.074$, $p = 0.002$ respectively) and after discontinuation of sorafenib administration ($p = 0.001$, $p = 0.034$, $p = 0.647$, $p = 0.001$ respectively).

Conclusions: Low-dosage sorafenib not only appeared tolerable and lowered economic pressure but also provided satisfactory results. TACE benefited patient's survival during and after sorafenib discontinuation.

Keywords: Dose-efficacy, Sorafenib, TACE, Hepatocellular carcinoma patient

* Correspondence: garrydarkao@gmail.com
[1]School of Medicine, China Medical University, Taichung, Taiwan
[2]Division of Hepato-Gastroenterology, Department of Internal Medicine, China Medical University Hospital, No. 2, Yuh-Der Road, Taichung 404, Taiwan

Background

Worldwide, more than 711,000 new hepatocellular carcinoma (HCC) patients are diagnosed annually; 679,000 eventually die [1]. Various diagnostic and therapeutic modalities have been applied in clinical scenarios [2], with over 50 % of HCC cases showing unresectable or un-embolized condition [3]. Only palliative options are available due to limitations of vascular invasion or extra-hepatic metastases [3, 4].

Sorafenib (Nexavar, Bayer HealthCare Pharmaceuticals-Onyx Pharmaceuticals) inhibits proliferation and angiogenesis in tumors, promoting apoptosis [5, 6]. Anti-angiogenic function is via inhibition of VEGFR-2-PDGFR- and Raf-kinase properties [5–7], signaling pathways identified as a close rationale in HCC study and providing survival benefits in advanced HCC [Barcelona Clinic Liver Cancer (BCLC) stage C] [7–12]. Limitations affect patients treated with sorafenib in clinical scenarios: e.g., high cost raising economic pressure [13], while severe adverse events (AE) (26–88 %) might limit sorafenib dosage and impair therapeutic response, as well as high tumor recurrence with single agent [8, 9, 14, 15]. Therefore, combination therapy provided lesser dose of sorafenib to obtain better response for both in vitro and in vivo models [16]. In clinical settings, transarterial chemoembolization (TACE) is the current standard therapy for intermediate stage HCC (BCLC stage B) and an earlier study indicated combination of TACE with sorafenib as being more effective than TACE or sorafenib monotherapy for unresectable HCC [17]; but no data is reported on the exploration of the effect of different sorafenib dosage with subsequent TACE during or after discontinued sorafenib.

To attain the greatest benefit in clinical scenarios, we assessed two points in this study. First, investigating the relation of different therapeutic doses (initially 400 or 800 mg per day) with efficacy in unresectable HCC patients with compensated liver disease (Child-Pugh Classification Class A [18]) and venous invasion or extra-hepatic metastases. Furthermore, evaluating the effect of TACE during and after sorafenib discontinuation. We envisioned this study could afford useful references for clinical settings.

Methods

Patients

According to the standard of Taiwan's National Health Insurance Agency, sorafenib was approved for HCC patients exhibiting Child-Pugh Classification Class A (score 5 or 6) with venous invasion or extra-hepatic metastases. Excluding HCC patients not up to the standard during the period of May 2009 to June 2013, 156 cases (HCC-total group) met the criteria and accepted

sorafenib therapy at China Medical University Hospital, Taichung, Taiwan; and their response and survival results were recorded until May 2014. After reviewing their therapeutic dosage between May 2009 and June 2013, patients were divided into three groups: Group I for patients accepting 400 mg sorafenib twice daily; Group II for patients accepting initially 400 mg sorafenib twice daily with reduction to 400 mg once daily owing to intolerable AE; and Group III for patients accepting 400 mg sorafenib daily (Fig. 1). Dose reduction in Group II depended on their tolerance to sorafenib inducing AE (hand-foot skin reaction, uncontrollable hypertension, or diarrhea) rated by the National Cancer Institute (NCI) Common Terminology Criteria for Adverse Events (CTCAE) [19]. The management of AE included corticosteroid cream and painkiller pill for hand-foot skin reaction, anti-hypertension agent for hypertensive patients, as well as loperamide for diarrhea.

Evaluation of therapeutic response during sorafenib therapy

All treated patients were according to the standard of Taiwan's National Health Insurance Agency and hospital protocol. For each visit while undergoing sorafenib treatment, patients accepted detailed history and physical examination every four weeks. In addition, biochemical examination including Child-Pugh Classification score, serum AFP, renal function, and contrast-enhanced tomography (CT) were performed on those beginning sorafenib and followed up bimonthly to 4-month thereafter according to therapeutic dosage (defined as one cycle) to rate therapeutic response by Response Evaluation Criteria in Solid Tumors criteria (RECIST); only those with better response (complete response [CR], partial response [PR], or stable disease [SD]) could continue sorafenib treatment [20].

Procedure and effect comparisons of transarterial chemoembolization

In our hospital, TACE proceeds via the trans-femoral route, with arteries feeding tumors identified by angiography and then emulsion of lipiodol (10 mL) and adriamycin (20 mg) were injected, followed by embolization with absorbable particles (gelatin foam). After embolization, more angiography was used to assess extent of vascular occlusion and flow in other arteries. Effect of TACE was evaluated during and after discontinuation of sorafenib administration in separate groups, with follow-up time of either patient death or at least six months after sorafenib discontinuation due to poor therapeutic response. Patients treated with TACE were according to the standard of BCLC System and our hospital for intra-hepatic tumor.

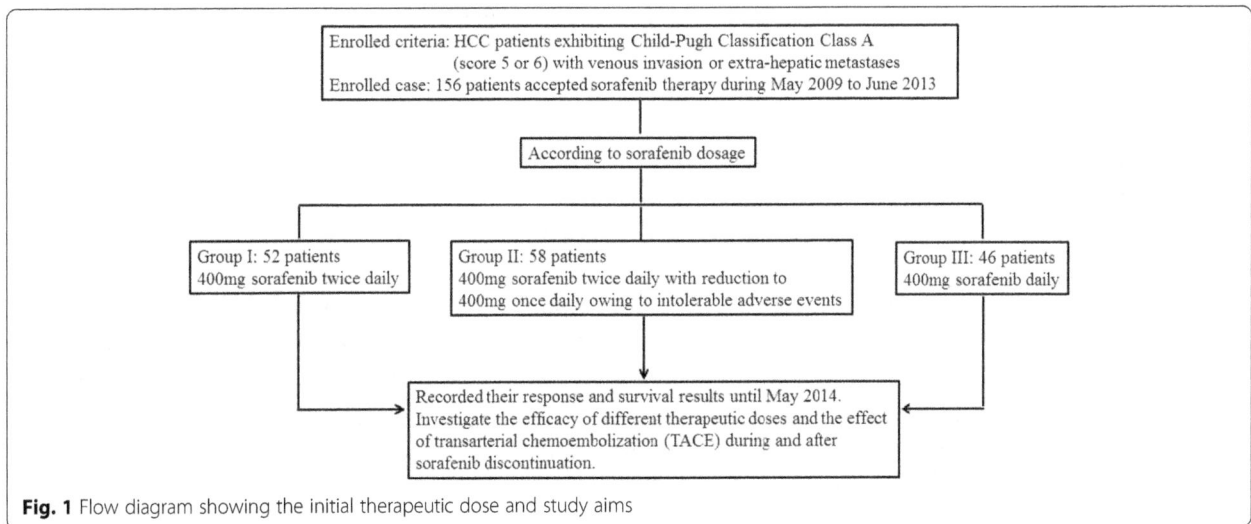

Fig. 1 Flow diagram showing the initial therapeutic dose and study aims

Serological markers and liver biochemical assay methodology

Commercial enzyme immunoassay rated HBV markers (HBsAg, HBeAg, anti-HBe) (AxSYM, Abbott, North Chicago, IL) and anti-HCV antibody (Abbott HCV EIA 2.0; Abbott Laboratories). An autoanalyzer (TBA-30FR, Toshiba, Tokyo, Japan) gauged serum albumin, bilirubin, alpha-fetoprotein (AFP), aspartate transaminase (AST), alanine Transaminase (ALT), alkaline phosphatase (Alk-p), creatinine (Cr), International Normalize Ratio (INR), and hematological count (WBC: white blood cell; Hb, hemoglobin; platelet).

Statistical analysis

All statistical analyses were performed using SPSS 17.0 (SPSS, Chicago, USA). Baseline data were expressed as mean ± standard deviation, with correlation between continuous variables assessed by Student t-test or Fisher exact test. In univariate survival analysis, the median survival times were calculated according to the Kaplan-Meier method. All variables significant in univariate analysis were entered into the multivariate model according to Cox proportional hazard regression. All statistical tests were two-tailed, P-value ≤ 0.05 defined as significant.

Results

General distribution of overall and separate hepatocellular carcinoma groups

Table 1 shows baseline characteristics of 156 HCC cases. Median durations of sorafenib treatment and patients' survival were 4.00 ± 0.45 months (95 % CI 3.13–4.87 months) and 7.50 ± 1.44 months (95 % CI 4.67–10.33 months) respectively. There were 57 patients without and 99 with AE: e.g., hand-foot skin reaction ($n = 53$ cases; 45 in grade 1 and 2; 8 in grade 3), diarrhea ($n = 24$

cases; 19 in grade 1 and 2; 5 in grade 3), hypertension ($n = 5$ cases; 4 in grade 1 and 2; 1 in grade 3), combination of hand-foot skin reaction and diarrhea ($n = 17$; 14 in grade 1 and 2; 3 in grade 3). No grade 4 or mortality case was induced from AE. According to therapeutic dosage, 52 cases belonged to Group I, 56 cases belonged to Group II, and 46 cases belonged to Group III (Fig. 1). No significant difference between the three groups besides lower albumin (3.68 ± 0.51 versus 4.05 ± 0.42 g/dL, $p < 0.001$) with advanced age (64.50 ± 12.02 versus 58.75 ± 13.33 years, $p = 0.028$) in Group III than Group I. In separate groups, median durations of sorafenib treatment and survival were 2.50 ± 0.90 months (95 % CI 0.73–4.27 months) and 5.00 ± 1.10 months (95 % CI 2.85–7.16 months) in Group I; 5.50 ± 1.27 months (95 % CI 3.01–7.99 months) and 16.50 ± 1.86 months (95 % CI 12.86–20.14 months) in Group II; 4.00 ± 0.94 months (95 % CI 2.16–5.84 months) and 6.50 ± 2.49 months (95 % CI 1.63–11.37 months) in Group III respectively.

Survival analysis in overall and separate groups

In total cases, the significant factors including Child-Pugh Classification score 5 ($p = 0.015$), absent AE ($p < 0.001$), lower ALT ($p = 0.036$), lower AFP ($p < 0.001$), tumor size ≤ 5 cm ($p = 0.046$), tumor numbers ≤ 3 ($p = 0.001$), sorafenib duration ≤ 1 cycle ($p < 0.001$), and absent TACE ($p = 0.031$) affected patient's survival. Of all significant variables, Child-Pugh Classification score 5 (Hazard Ratio = 0.492, $p = 0.049$), absent AE (Hazard Ratio = 3.423, $p = 0.015$), lower AFP (Hazard Ratio = 0.213, $p = 0.003$), tumor numbers ≤ 3 (Hazard Ratio = 0.313, $p = 0.009$), sorafenib duration ≤ 1 cycle (Hazard Ratio = 3.694, $p = 0.004$), and absent TACE (Hazard Ratio = 3.197, $p = 0.008$) significantly correlated with patient mortality (Table 2). Among separate groups, absent AE ($p = 0.008$), lower

Table 1 Baseline characteristics of total and separate hepatocellular carcinoma groups treated with sorafenib

Demographics	Total cases ($n = 156$)	Group I ($n = 52$)	Group II ($n = 58$)	Group III ($n = 46$)
Age (yrs) (range)	61.04 ± 12.76 (32.00–88.00)	58.75 ± 13.33 (32.0–84.0)	60.36 ± 12.45 (32.0–88.0)	64.50 ± 12.02 (40.0–86.0)
Sex (Male) (%)	127 (81.41)	46 (88.5)	52 (89.66)	29 (63.04)
BMI (kgs/m^2) (range)	22.69 ± 3.88(14.10–34.82)	23.05 ± 3.71 (15.24–34.82)	21.92 ± 3.48 (14.10–32.86)	23.26 ± 4.43 (15.56–33.75)
Cirrhosis (+) (%)	120 (76.92)	32 (61.5)	50 (86.21)	38 (82.61)
CPC, score 5 versus 6 (%)	81 (51.92) versus 75 (48.08)	30 (57.7) versus 22 (42.3)	31 (53.45) versus 27 (46.55)	20 (43.48) versus 26 (56.52)
Biochemical values				
Albumin (g/dL) (range)	3.88 ± 0.50 (2.80–5.10)	4.05 ± 0.42 (3.20–4.80)	3.88 ± 0.51 (2.80–5.10)	3.68 ± 0.51 (2.80–4.70)
Bilirubin (mg/dL) (range)	1.02 ± 0.46 (0.19–2.41)	0.99 ± 0.41 (0.22–1.99)	1.03 ± 0.48 (0.19–2.29)	1.05 ± 0.51 (0.38–2.41)
INR (range)	1.14 ± 0.13 (0.89–1.63)	1.13 ± 0.12 (0.90–1.63)	1.15 ± 0.13 (0.90–1.48)	1.15 ± 0.15 (0.89–1.63)
AST (IU/L) (range)	92.45 ± 105.98 (22.00–805.00)	96.20 ± 102.12 (24.00–580.00)	95.07 ± 136.90 (22.00–805.00)	84.84 ± 53.33 (23.00–237.00)
ALT (IU/L) (range)	66.54 ± 102.12 (9.00–1156.00)	65.73 ± 48.32 (15.00–251.00)	76.86 ± 157.43 (9.00–1156.00)	54.43 ± 39.91 (13.00–202.00)
ALK-P (IU/L) (range)	127.76 ± 93.34 (43.00–680.00)	124.84 ± 81.74 (50.00–421.00)	113.14 ± 93.05 (45.00–680.00)	155.0 ± 104.82 (43.00–526.00)
AFP (ng/mL) (range)	9000.31 ± 17472.65 (0.91–54001.0)	11769.7 ± 19836.59 (1.64–54001.0)	6663.7 ± 14569.6 (0.91–54001.0)	8815.86 ± 17910.81 (1.30–54001.0)
Cr (mg/dL) (range)	0.93 ± 0.35 (0.21–2.76)	0.90 ± 0.30 (0.40–2.10)	0.94 ± 0.32 (0.27–1.76)	0.95 ± 0.43 (0.21–2.76)
WBC (10^3/uL) (range)	6.90 ± 3.71 (1.70–22.62)	6.96 ± 3.33 (2.48–17.35)	6.79 ± 3.66 (1.70–19.00)	7.00 ± 4.23 (2.10–22.62)
Hb (gm/dL) (range)	12.48 ± 1.97 (7.90–17.10)	12.63 ± 1.98 (7.90–16.00)	12.64 ± 2.02 (7.90–17.10)	12.11 ± 1.89 (8.10–15.10)
Platelet (10^3/uL) (range)	171.49 ± 110.79 (16.00–796.00)	170.69 ± 82.45 (16.00–400.00)	177.19 ± 145.22 (44.00–796.0)	165.2 ± 88.18 (23.00–386.00)
Virologic values				
B or C or B + C (+) or NBNC (%)	80 (51.28) or 50 (32.05) or 5 (3.21) or 21 (13.46)	30 (57.7) or 9 (17.3) or 3 (5.8) or 10 (19.2)	33 (56.9) or 18 (31.03) or 1 (1.72) or 6 (10.34)	17 (36.96) or 23 (50.0) or 1 (2.17) or 5(10.87)
Tumor characters				
Tumor size (>5 cm) (%)	74 (47.44)	27 (51.9)	25 (43.1)	22 (47.83)
Tumor number (>3) (%)	91 (58.33)	28 (53.8)	32 (55.17)	31 (67.39)
Intra-hepatic vein (+) (%)	61 (39.10)	23 (44.2)	18 (31.03)	20 (43.48)
Extra-hepatic metastases (%)	75 (48.08)	23 (44.2)	31 (53.45)	21 (45.65)
Mixed type (vein and metastases)	20 (12.82)	6 (11.5)	9 (15.52)	5 (10.87)

Abbreviations: *CPC* child-pugh classification, *INR* international normalize ratio, *AST* aspartate transaminase, *ALT* alanine transaminase, *Alk-p* alkaline phosphatase, *GGT* gamma-glutamyltransferase, *AFP* alpha-fetoprotein, *Cr* creatinine, *WBC* white blood cell, *Hb* hemoglobin, *B* hepatitis B virus, *C* hepatitis C virus, *B + C* hepatitis B and C virus, *NBNC* non-hepatitis B or C virus

AFP ($p = 0.014$), tumor numbers ≤ 3 ($p = 0.032$), and sorafenib duration ≤ 1 cycle ($p = 0.003$) presented significant difference affecting patient's survival. Of all significant variables, lower AFP (Hazard Ratio = 0.136, $p = 0.047$) and sorafenib duration ≤ 1 cycle (Hazard Ratio = 8.112, $p = 0.040$) played independent roles to predict patient's mortality in Group I. In Group II, the factors including lower AFP ($p = 0.043$), sorafenib duration ≤ 1 cycle ($p = 0.002$), and absent TACE ($p = 0.041$) presented significant difference affecting patient's survival. Of all significant variables, sorafenib duration ≤ 1 cycle (Hazard Ratio = 7.080, $p = 0.014$) and absent TACE (Hazard Ratio = 6.742, $p = 0.022$) played independent roles to predict patient's mortality. In Group III, lower albumin ($p = 0.048$) and tumor numbers ≤ 3 ($p = 0.023$) presented significant difference affecting patient's survival. Of all significant variables, lower albumin (Hazard Ratio = 5.989, $p = 0.046$) and tumor numbers ≤ 3 (Hazard Ratio = 0.187, $p = 0.025$) played independent roles to predict patient's mortality.

Positive correlation between better sorafenib response and higher survival

There was a positive correlation between sorafenib duration and survival time ($r = 0.756$, $p < 0.001$). Group II showed the best sorafenib response and overall survival among the three groups ($p = 0.010$ and $p = 0.011$ respectively) (Fig. 2).

Table 2 Cox regression of mortality in overall hepatocellular carcinoma patients. (N = 156)

	Numbers	P-value		Hazard Ratio (95 % CI)
		Univariate	Multivariate	
Demographics				
Age (yrs), ≤65 vs. >65	100 vs. 56	0.613		
Gender, Female vs. Male	29 vs. 127	0.863		
BMI (kgs/m²), ≤22 (24) vs. >22 (24)	102 vs. 54	0.798		
Average dose (mg/kg), ≤35 vs. >35	97 vs. 59	0.848		
Cirrhosis, (-) vs. (+)	36 vs. 120	0.263		
CPC, score 5 vs. 6	81 vs. 75	0.015*	0.049*	0.492 (0.213–1.137)
AE, (-) vs. (+)	57 vs. 99	<0.001*	0.015*	3.423 (1.274–9.199)
Biochemical values				
Albumin (g/dL), ≤3.5 vs. >3.5	35 vs. 121	0.061		
Bilirubin (mg/dL), ≤1.3 vs. > 1.3	118 vs. 38	0.466		
INR, ≤1.2 vs. >1.2	116 vs. 40	0.321		
AST (IU/L), ≤34 vs. >34	25 vs. 130	0.181		
ALT (IU/L), ≤40 vs. >40	73 vs.83	0.036*		
Alk-p (IU/L), ≤126 vs. >126	87 vs.39	0.051		
AFP (ng/mL), ≤9 vs. > 9	34 vs. 122	<0.001*	0.003*	0.213 (0.078–0.583)
Creatinine (mg/dL), ≤1.3 vs. > 1.3	138 vs. 18	0.188		
WBC (10³/dL), ≤105 vs. >105	136 vs.17	0.553		
Hb (gm/dL), ≤12 vs. >12	62 vs.94	0.115		
Platelet (10³/uL), ≤130 vs. >130	61 vs. 95	0.207		
Virologic values				
HBV or HCV, (-) vs. (+)	21 vs. 135	0.873		
Tumor characters				
Tumor size, ≤5 vs. >5	82 vs. 74	0.046*		
Tumor numbers, ≤3 vs. >3	65 vs. 91	0.001*	0.009*	0.313 (0.131–0.747)
Intra-hepatic vein, (-) vs. (+)	95 vs. 61	0.661		
Extra-hepatic metastases, (-) vs. (+)	81 vs. 75	0.388		
Mixed type (vein and metastases), (-) vs. (+)	136 vs. 20	0.517		
Therapeutic response				
Sorafenib duration, cycle ≤ 1 vs. >1	75vs. 81	<0.001*	0.004*	3.694 (1.530–8.920)
TACE (-) vs. (+)	89 vs. 67	0.031*	0.008*	3.197 (1.353–7.553)

Abbreviations: *AE* adverse event, *AST* aspartate transaminase, *ALT* alanine transaminase, *Alk-p* alkaline phosphatase, *AFP* alpha-fetoprotein, *BMI* body mass index (Cut-off valve: 22 in female and 24 in male), *CPC* child-pugh classification, *Hb* hemoglobin, *B* hepatitis B virus, *C* hepatitis C virus, *INR* international normalize ratio, *NBNC* non-hepatitis B or C virus, *TACE* transarterial chemoembolization, *WBC* white blood cell
*A P-value below 0.05 is considered statistically significant

TACE increases survival during and after sorafenib discontinuation

Over the study period, presence or absence of TACE presented significant difference ($p = 0.031$) and significantly correlated with patient mortality (Hazard Ratio = 3.197, $p = 0.008$) (Table 2). During the sorafenib period, patients accepting TACE revealed lower mortality than those without TACE, particularly in total patients (39/57 versus 75/99, $p = 0.002$) and Group I (14/21 versus 28/31, $p = 0.002$) (Table 3). Patients accepting TACE had

younger age (57.54 ± 13.00 versus 63.06 ± 12.24 years, $p = 0.009$) than those without TACE among HCC total patients; lower AST (62.48 ± 37.92 versus 119.80 ± 124.85 IU/L, $p = 0.024$), higher albumin (4.20 ± 0.43 versus 3.95 ± 0.39 g/dL, $p = 0.041$), and lower BMI (21.78 ± 3.77 versus 23.91 ± 3.47 kg/m², $p = 0.041$) or higher average dose (37.85 ± 6.89 versus 34.10 ± 4.61 mg/kg, $p = 0.036$) in Group I; lower Cr (0.83 ± 0.21 versus 1.00 ± 0.36 mg/dL, $p = 0.022$) and higher rate of tumor numbers > 3 (16/21 versus 16/37, $p = 0.027$) in

(A)

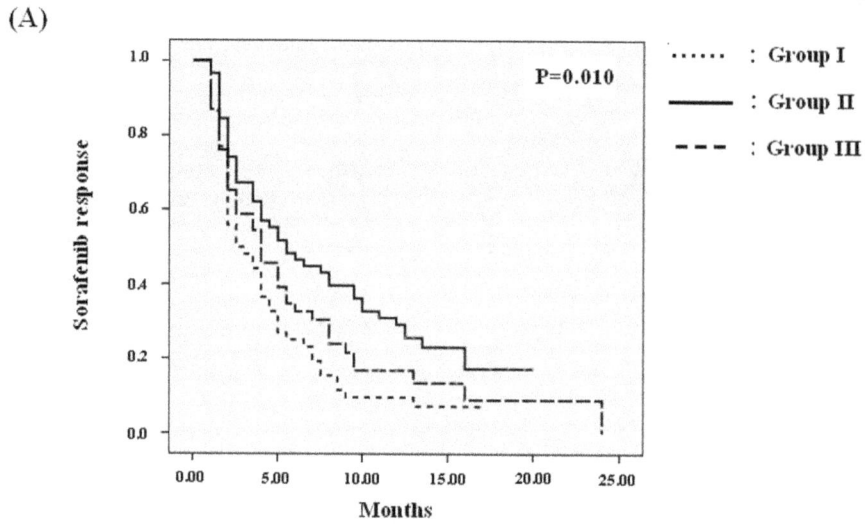

Number at risk

Group I	52	14	4	2	0	0
Group II	58	30	21	8	0	0
Group III	46	18	7	4	1	0

(B)

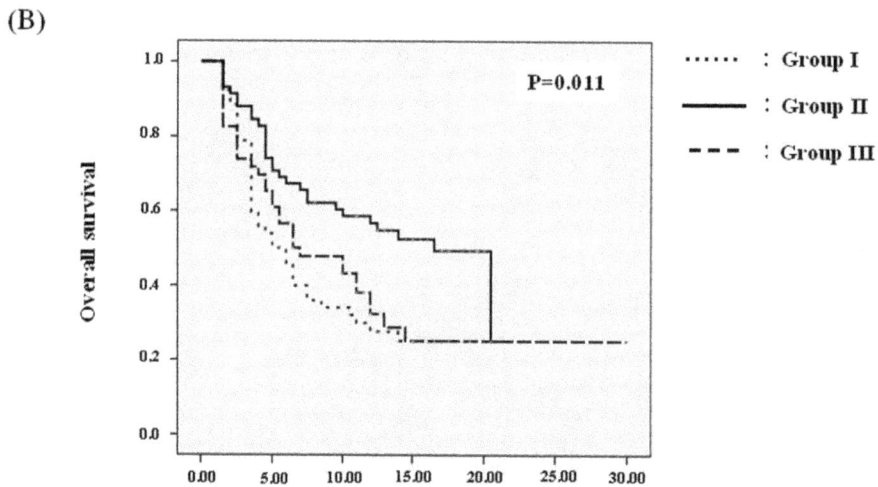

Number at risk

Group I	52	26	17	6	1	0	0
Group II	58	41	33	19	2	0	0
Group III	46	28	18	6	2	1	0

Fig. 2 Kaplan-Meier analysis of sorafenib response (**a**) and overall survival (**b**). P-value below 0.05 is considered statistically significant

Group II; higher BMI (26.35 ± 4.21 versus 22.77 ± 3.77 kg/m², $p = 0.001$), higher Hb (13.04 ± 1.98 versus 11.66 ± 1.70gm/dL, $p = 0.019$), and lower rate of tumor size < 5 cm (3/15 versus 19/31, $p = 0.012$) in Group III. After discontinued sorafenib due to poor response, patients accepting TACE also presented lower mortality than those without TACE particularly in total patients (13/26 versus 67/83, $p = 0.001$) and Groups I (6/10 versus 24/28, $p = 0.001$) with II (4/10 versus 23/30, $p = 0.034$) (Table 3). Patients accepting TACE had lower AST (56.16 ± 27.09 versus 97.35 ± 129.26 IU/L, $p = 0.008$) than those without TACE among HCC total patients; lower virology rate (6/10 versus 28/30, $p = 0.026$) in Group II; lower Alk-p (81.25 ± 18.66 versus 130.67 ± 64.17 IU/L, $p = 0.009$), lower average dose (16.04 ± 2.14 versus 20.69 ± 5.83 mg/kg, $p = 0.004$), and lower

Table 3 Comparison of mortality in presence or absence of TACE during and after discontinuation of sorafenib administration

	Sorafenib (+) TACE (+) vs. TACE (-)			Sorafenib (-) TACE (+) vs. TACE (-)
Subgroups			Subgroups	
Group I (n = 52)	14/21 vs. 28/31 p = 0.002*		Group I (n = 38)	6/10 vs. 24/28 p = 0.001*
Group II (n = 58)	13/21 vs. 23/37 p = 0.595		Group II (n = 40)	4/10 vs. 23/30 p = 0.034*
Group III (n = 46)	12/15 vs. 24/31 p = 0.074		Group III (n = 31)	3/6 vs. 20/25 p = 0.647
HCC-total Patients (N = 156)	39/57 vs. 75/99 p = 0.002*		HCC-total Patients (N = 109)	13/26 vs. 67/83 p = 0.001*

Abbreviations: Group I always accepted 800 mg/day; Group II initially accepted 800 mg/day tapering to 400 mg/day owing to adverse events; Group III always accepted 400 mg/day. *TACE* transarterial chemoembolization

*A P-value below 0.05 is considered statistically significant

cirrhotic rate (3/6 versus 23/25, $p = 0.038$) in Group III. No mortality case was induced by TACE.

Discussion

Sorafenib inhibits proliferation and angiogenesis while promoting apoptosis of tumors [5, 6], and is proven to prolong survival in advanced HCC cases [8, 9]. As in earlier studies [8, 9, 21–23], the clinical factors including superior liver preservation (score 5), lower AFP, or less aggressive tumor condition remained as the crucial roles to reflect patient results in our study (Table 2). Therefore, highly selected patients should be emphasized in initial sorafenib therapy.

Nevertheless, problems remain in clinical practice, including high sorafenib costs that raise economic pressure [13], as well as severe AE rate from 26 to 88 % that might limit sorafenib dosage and further affect therapeutic response [8, 9, 14, 15]. To attain greatest benefit, we analyzed the relationship of different sorafenib doses with efficacy. As in previous studies [8, 9], the presence of AE also played an important role predicting therapeutic response. Importantly, patients could tolerate longer duration (>1 cycles) of obtained therapeutic benefit from sorafenib (Table 2). Furthermore, we found despite Groups II and III presenting poorer baseline characteristics than I including lower albumin (3.68 ± 0.51 g/dL versus 4.05 ± 0.42 g/dL, $p < 0.001$ respectively) and older age (64.5 ± 12.02 versus 58.75 ± 13.33 years, $p = 0.028$ respectively) (Table 1), Groups II and III rather than I still showed better sorafenib response and survival benefit ($p = 0.010$ and $p = 0.011$ respectively) (Fig. 2) as our finding of poorer sorafenib response significantly correlated with higher mortality ($r = 0.756$, $p < 0.001$). This revealed sorafenib, even at lower dosages, could also provide therapeutic benefit; particularly for patients tolerating longer sorafenib duration [24]. Accordingly, this could alleviate economic pressure with tolerable dose for HCC therapy as well as wastage of medical resources.

In clinic, combination of TACE with sorafenib has proven more effective than TACE or sorafenib monotherapy for unresectable HCC [17], but no data has reported on the exploration of the effect of different sorafenib dose with subsequent TACE during or after discontinued sorafenib owing to poor response. In this study, we observed combined TACE promoted patient's survival during the period with sorafenib, which concurred with a previous finding: the sorafenib/TACE combination shows promise as an effective and tolerable treatment strategy for unresectable patients with intermediate stage/advanced HCC [17]. The benefit of TACE also appeared in patients after discontinued sorafenib, particularly in Group II where lower mortality in TACE cases existed after discontinuation than for those during sorafenib administration (Tables 2 and 3). This possibility could be attributed to AE induced by sorafenib, regarded as an indicator of better therapeutic response presenting enough anti-tumor concentrations [25, 26]. Therefore, TACE showed lower benefit during the period with sorafenib than that without sorafenib. Once tumor inhibition with sorafenib significantly decreased due to poor response and probably induced tumor re-growth, the effect of TACE became obvious. Group III rather than I or II presented insignificant benefit from TACE after discontinued sorafenib, the limited case number probably contributed to the result, and further larger studies need to be adopted in the future.

Although median overall survival in our study (7.50 ± 1.44 months) was shorter than SHARP (10.7 months) [8], better than Asian-Pacific studies (6.5 months) [9] and probably exceeded the SHARP study: 21 patients (4 in Group I, 12 in Group II, 5 in Group III) still accepted sorafenib and 42 cases (10 in Group I, 22 in Group II, 10 in Group III) had survived at end of follow-up time. Additionally, we correlated body mass index (kgs/m^2) with average sorafenib dose [$mg/(kgs/m^2)$] and patient's survival, with no significant differences in HCC total cases or separate groups (Table 2). Even after excluding TACE cases from the period with sorafenib, higher average dosage also could not promote therapeutic response [31.86 ± 9.54 versus 29.48 ± 9.78 $mg/(kgs/m^2)$, $p = 0.246$] and prolong survival [31.39 ± 9.73 versus 30.01 ± 9.32 $mg/(kgs/m^2)$, $p = 0.581$].

Conclusions

According to our interpretations, low-dosage sorafenib also provided satisfactory therapeutic result, which not only appeared tolerable but also lowered economic pressure and conserved medical resources. Beside the initial variables including the presence of AE, superior liver preservation, lower AFP, less aggressive tumor condition, and longer sorafenib duration benefited patient's survival, synergic TACE promoted patient's survival during the period of sorafenib administration and also appeared after sorafenib discontinuation. Our study provided much useful information in unresectable HCC patients with compensated liver disease and venous invasion or extra-hepatic metastases but was limited in the size of cohorts; therefore, further larger studies need to be adopted in the future.

Abbreviations

AE: adverse events; AFP: alpha-fetoprotein; Alk-p: alkaline phosphatase; ALT: alanine transaminase; AST: aspartate transaminase; CR: complete response; Cr: creatinine; CT: contrast-enhanced tomography; CTCAE: common terminology criteria for adverse events; Hb: hemoglobin; HBV: hepatitis B Virus infection platelet; HCC: hepatocellular carcinoma; HCV: hepatitis C Virus infection; INR: international normalize ratio; NCI: National Cancer Institute; PR: partial response; RECIST: response evaluation criteria in solid tumors criteria; SD: stable disease; TACE: transarterial chemoembolization; WBC: white blood cell.

Competing interests

The authors declare that they have no competing interests.

Authors' contributions

J-TK and W-DH involved in the study design, as well as in the planning, conducting, collecting and interpreting of data for this study, and in drafting/editing the manuscript. C-YP involved in the planning, collection and interpretation of data for this study, and in drafting the manuscript. P-HC and H-CL involved in data collection and drafting/editing of the manuscript. K-SC, J-WC, Y-YC, C-J, C-LF, W-PS, and S-HC involved in data collection. All the above-mentioned authors have approved the final draft submitted.

Acknowledgements

All procedures met ethical standards of the responsible committee on human experimentation (institutional and national) and with the 1975 Helsinki Declaration, as revised in 2008. The Institutional Review Board of China Medical University Hospital also approved this retrospective study (CMUH103-REC2-147). Importantly, heartfelt thanks to participants, as well as research assistants of the Liver Unit for technical assistance in data collection and case enrollment.

References

1. Garcia M, Jemal A, Ward EM, Center MM, Hao Y, Siegel RL, et al. Global Cancer Facts and Figures. 2007. https://www.cancer.org/acs/groups/content/@nho/documents/document/globalfactsandfigures2007rev2p.pdf.
2. Bruix J, Sherman M. Management of hepatocellular carcinoma: an update. Hepatology. 2011;53:1020–2.
3. Forner A, Reig ME, de Lope CR, Bruix J. Current strategy for staging and treatment: BCLC update and future prospects. Semin Liver Dis. 2010;30:61–74.
4. Imamura H, Matsuyama Y, Tanaka E, Ohkubo T, Hasegawa K, Miyagawa S, et al. Risk factors contributing to early and late phase intrahepatic recurrence of hepatocellular carcinoma after hepatectomy. J Hepatol. 2003;38:200–7.
5. Wilhelm SM, Carter C, Tang L, Wilkie D, McNabola A, Rong H, et al. BAY 43-9006 exhibits broad-spectrum oral antitumor activity and targets the RAF/MEK/ERK pathway and receptor tyrosine kinases involved in tumor progression and angiogenesis. Cancer Res. 2004;64:7099–109.
6. Chang YS, Adnane J, Trail PA, Levy J, Henderson A, Xue D, et al. Sorafenib (BAY 43-9006) inhibits tumor growth and vascularization and induces tumor apoptosis and hypoxia in RCC xenograft models. Cancer Chemother Pharmacol. 2007;59:561–74.
7. Semela D, Dufour JF. Angiogenesis and hepatocellular carcinoma. J Hepatol. 2004;41:864–80.
8. Llovet JM, Ricci S, Mazzaferro V, Hilgard P, Gane E, Blanc JF, et al. Sorafenib in advanced hepatocellular carcinoma. N Engl J Med. 2008;359:378–90.
9. Cheng AL, Kang YK, Chen Z, Tsao CJ, Qin S, Kim JS, et al. Efficacy and safety of sorafenib in patients in the Asia-Pacific region with advanced hepatocellular carcinoma: a phase III randomised, double-blind, placebo-controlled trial. Lancet Oncol. 2009;10:25–34.
10. Ito Y, Sasaki Y, Horimoto M, Wada S, Tanaka Y, Kasahara A, et al. Activation of mitogen-activated protein kinases/extracellular signal-regulated kinases in human hepatocellular carcinoma. Hepatology. 1998;27:951–8.
11. Omata M, Lesmana LA, Tateishi R, Chen PJ, Lin SM, Yoshida H, et al. Asian Pacific Association for the Study of the Liver consensus recommendations on hepatocellular carcinoma. Hepatol Int. 2010;4:439–74.
12. Calvisi DF, Ladu S, Gorden A, Farina M, Conner EA, Lee JS. Ubiquitous activation of Ras and Jak/Stat pathways in human HCC. Gastroenterology. 2006;130:1117–28.
13. Carr BI, Carroll S, Muszbek N, Gondek K. Economic evaluation of sorafenib in unresectable hepatocellular carcinoma. J Gastroenterol Hepatol. 2010;25:1739–46.
14. Ogasawara S, Kanai F, Obi S, Sato S, Yamaguchi T, Azemoto R, et al. Safety and tolerance of sorafenib in Japanese patients with advanced hepatocellular carcinoma. Hepatol Int. 2011;5:850–6.
15. Kudo M, Imanaka K, Chida N, Nakachi K, Tak WY, Takayama T, et al. Phase III study of sorafenib after transarterial chemoembolisation in Japanese and Korean patients with unresectable hepatocellular carcinoma. Eur J Cancer. 2011;47:2117–27.
16. Alsaied OA, Sangwan V, Banerjee S, Krosch TC, Chugh R, Saluja A, et al. Sorafenib and triptolide as combination therapy for hepatocellular carcinoma. Surgery. 2014;156:270–9.
17. Abdel-Rahman O, Elsayed ZA. Combination Trans Arterial Chemoembolization (TACE) Plus Sorafenib for the Management of Unresectable Hepatocellular Carcinoma: A Systematic Review of the Literature. Dig Dis Sci. 2013;58:3389–96.
18. Pugh RN, Murray-Lyon IM, Dawson JL, Pietroni MC, Williams R. Transection of the oesophagus for bleeding oesophageal varices. Br J Surg. 1973;60:646–9.
19. Trotti A, Colevas AD, Setser A, Rusch V, Jaques D, Budach V, et al. CTCAE v3.0: development of a comprehensive grading system for the adverse effects of cancer treatment. Semin Radiat Oncol. 2003;13:176–81.
20. Therasse P, Arbuck SG, Eisenhauer EA, Wanders J, Kaplan RS, Rubinstein L, et al. New guidelines to evaluate the response to treatment in solid tumors. European Organization for Research and Treatment of Cancer, National Cancer Institute of the United States, National Cancer Institute of Canada. J Natl Cancer Inst. 2000;92:205–16.
21. Changchien CS, Chen CL, Yen YH, Wang JH, Hu TH, Lee CM, et al. Analysis of 6381 hepatocellular carcinoma patients in southern Taiwan: prognostic features, treatment outcome, and survival. J Gastroenterol. 2008;43:159–70.
22. Carr BI, Pancoska P, Branch RA. Tumor and liver determinants of prognosis in unresectable hepatocellular carcinoma: a large case cohort study. Hepatol Int. 2009;4:396–405.

23. Bouattour M, Payancé A, Wassermann J. Evaluation of antiangiogenic efficacy in advanced hepatocellular carcinoma: Biomarkers and functional imaging. World J Hepatol. 2015;7:2245–63.
24. Ogasawara S, Chiba T, Ooka Y, Kanogawa N, Motoyama T, Suzuki E, et al. Is intra-patient sorafenib dose re-escalation safe and tolerable in patients with advanced hepatocellular carcinoma? Int J Clin Oncol. 2014;19:1029–36.
25. Vincenzi B, Santini D, Russo A, Addeo R, Giuliani F, Montella L, et al. Early Skin Toxicity as a Predictive Factor for Tumor Control in Hepatocellular Carcinoma Patients Treated with Sorafenib. Oncologist. 2010;15:85–92.
26. Arrondeau J, Mir O, Boudou-Rouquette P, Coriat R, Ropert S, Dumas G, et al. Sorafenib exposure decreases over time in patients with hepatocellular carcinoma. Invest New Drugs. 2012;30:2046–9.

Permissions

The contributors of this book come from diverse backgrounds, making this book a truly international effort. This book will bring forth new frontiers with its revolutionizing research information and detailed analysis of the nascent developments around the world.

We would like to thank all the contributing authors for lending their expertise to make the book truly unique. They have played a crucial role in the development of this book. Without their invaluable contributions this book wouldn't have been possible. They have made vital efforts to compile up to date information on the varied aspects of this subject to make this book a valuable addition to the collection of many professionals and students.

This book was conceptualized with the vision of imparting up-to-date information and advanced data in this field. To ensure the same, a matchless editorial board was set up. Every individual on the board went through rigorous rounds of assessment to prove their worth. After which they invested a large part of their time researching and compiling the most relevant data for our readers.

The editorial board has been involved in producing this book since its inception. They have spent rigorous hours researching and exploring the diverse topics which have resulted in the successful publishing of this book. They have passed on their knowledge of decades through this book. To expedite this challenging task, the publisher supported the team at every step. A small team of assistant editors was also appointed to further simplify the editing procedure and attain best results for the readers.

Apart from the editorial board, the designing team has also invested a significant amount of their time in understanding the subject and creating the most relevant covers. They scrutinized every image to scout for the most suitable representation of the subject and create an appropriate cover for the book.

The publishing team has been an ardent support to the editorial, designing and production team. Their endless efforts to recruit the best for this project, has resulted in the accomplishment of this book. They are a veteran in the field of academics and their pool of knowledge is as vast as their experience in printing. Their expertise and guidance has proved useful at every step. Their uncompromising quality standards have made this book an exceptional effort. Their encouragement from time to time has been an inspiration for everyone.

The publisher and the editorial board hope that this book will prove to be a valuable piece of knowledge for researchers, students, practitioners and scholars across the globe.

List of Contributors

Yachana Kataria
Department of Laboratory Medicine, Boston Children's Hospital, Boston, MA USA

Ryan J. Deaton, Erika Enk, Ming Jin, Milita Petrauskaite, Joseph R. Goldenberg and Peter H. Gann
Department of Pathology, University of Illinois at Chicago, Chicago, IL, USA

Scott J. Cotler
Department of Hepatology, Loyola University, Chicago, IL, USA

Donald M. Jensen
Center for Liver Diseases, University of Chicago, Chicago, IL, USA

Linlin Dong and Richard B. van Breemen
Department of Medicinal Chemistry & Pharmacognosy, University of Illinois at Chicago, Chicago, IL, USA

Shingo Usui, Po-Sung Chu, Nobuhiro Nakamoto and Takanori Kanai
Division of Gastroenterology and Hepatology, Department of Internal Medicine, Keio University School of Medicine, 35 Shinanomachi, Shinjuku-ku, Tokyo 160-8582, Japan

Hirotoshi Ebinuma
Division of Gastroenterology and Hepatology, Department of Internal Medicine, Keio University School of Medicine, 35 Shinanomachi, Shinjuku-ku, Tokyo 160-8582, Japan
Department of Internal Medicine, International University of Health and Welfare Mita Hospital, 1-4-3 Mita, Minato-ku, Tokyo 108-8329, Japan

Yoshiyuki Yamagishi
Division of Gastroenterology and Hepatology, Department of Internal Medicine, Keio University School of Medicine, 35 Shinanomachi, Shinjuku-ku, Tokyo 160-8582, Japan
Department of Internal Medicine, Tokyo Dental College Suidobashi Hospital, 2-9-18 Misakicho, Chiyoda-ku, Tokyo 101-0061, Japan

Hidetsugu Saito
Division of Gastroenterology and Hepatology, Department of Internal Medicine, Keio University School of Medicine, 35 Shinanomachi, Shinjuku-ku, Tokyo 160-8582, Japan
Faculty of Pharmacy, Keio University, 1-5-30 Shiba-kohen, Minato-ku, Tokyo 105-8512, Japan

Pietro Achilli
University of Milan - Fondazione IRCCS Ca' Granda Ospedale Maggiore Policlinico, Via Sforza 35, 20122 Milan, Italy

Angelo Guttadauro, Sabina Terragni and Francesco Gabrielli
Department of Surgery, University of Milan-Bicocca, Istituti Clinici Zucchi, Via Zucchi, 24, 20900 Monza, Italy

Paolo Bonfanti
Infectious Diseases Unit - A. Manzoni Hospital, Via dell'Eremo 9/ 11, 23900 Lecco, Italy

Luca Fumagalli and Marco Chiarelli
Department of Surgery, Ospedale Alessandro Manzoni, Lecco, Via dell'Eremo 9/11, 23900 Lecco, Italy

Ugo Cioffi and Matilde De Simone
Department of Surgery, University of Milan, Milan, Italy

Xiao Wei, Shan Jiang, Xiangna Zhao, Huan Li, Weishi Lin, Boxing Li, Xuesong Wang, Jing Yuan and Yansong Sun
Institute of Disease Control and Prevention, Academy of Military Medical Sciences, No. 20 Dongda Street, Fengtai District, 100071 Beijing, China

Yuye Chen
Hospital of Traditional Chinese Medicine, Liquan 713200, Shanxi, China

Ning Li
Beijing YouAn Hospital, Capital Medical University, Beijing, China

Yuan Xu
Beijing YouAn Hospital, Capital Medical University, Beijing, China
Department of Community Health Sciences, University of Calgary, Calgary, AB, Canada

Rachel J. Jolley and Hude Quan
Department of Community Health Sciences, University of Calgary, Calgary, AB, Canada

Mingshan Lu
Department of Community Health Sciences, University of Calgary, Calgary, AB, Canada
Department of Economics, University of Calgary, Calgary, AB, Canada

Elijah Dixon
Department of Community Health Sciences, University of Calgary, Calgary, AB, Canada
Division of General Surgery, Department of Medicine, University of Calgary, Calgary, AB, Canada

Robert P. Myers
Department of Community Health Sciences, University of Calgary, Calgary, AB, Canada
Liver Unit, Division of Gastroenterology and Hepatology, Department of Medicine, University of Calgary, Calgary, AB, Canada

Stian Magnus Staurung Orlien
Regional Centre for Imported and Tropical Diseases, Oslo University Hospital Ullevål, Oslo, Norway

Nejib Yusuf Ismael
Haramaya University College of Health and Medical Sciences, Harar, Ethiopia
Department of Internal Medicine, Hiwot Fana Specialized University Hospital, Harar, Ethiopia

Tekabe Abdosh Ahmed
Haramaya University College of Health and Medical Sciences, Harar, Ethiopia
Department of Internal Medicine, Jugal Hospital, Harar, Ethiopia

Nega Berhe
Regional Centre for Imported and Tropical Diseases, Oslo University Hospital Ullevål, Oslo, Norway
Aklilu Lemma Institute of Pathobiology, Addis Ababa University, Addis Ababa, Ethiopia

Trine Lauritzen
Department of Medical Biochemistry, Vestre Viken Hospital Trust, Drammen, Norway

Borghild Roald
Department of Pathology, Oslo University Hospital Ullevål, Oslo, Norway
Institute of Clinical Medicine, Faculty of Medicine, Oslo University, Oslo, Norway

Robert David Goldin
Centre for Pathology, Imperial College London, London, UK

Kathrine Stene-Johansen
Department of Molecular Biology, Norwegian Institute of Public Health, Oslo, Norway

Anne Margarita Dyrhol-Riise
Institute of Clinical Medicine, Faculty of Medicine, Oslo University, Oslo, Norway
Department of Infectious Diseases, Oslo University Hospital Ullevål, Oslo, Norway
Department of Clinical Science, University of Bergen, Bergen, Norway

Svein Gunnar Gundersen
Research Unit, Sørlandet Hospital HF, Kristiansand, Norway
Department of Global Development and Planning, University of Agder, Kristiansand, Norway

Marsha Yvonne Morgan
UCL Institute for Liver & Digestive Health, Division of Medicine, University College London, Royal Free Campus, London, UK

Asgeir Johannessen
Regional Centre for Imported and Tropical Diseases, Oslo University Hospital Ullevål, Oslo, Norway
Department of Infectious Diseases, Vestfold Hospital Trust, Tønsberg, Norway

Dana Friedrich and Frank Lammert
Department of Medicine II, Saarland University Medical Center, Saarland University, 66421 Homburg, Germany

Hanns-Ulrich Marschall
Department of Molecular and Clinical Medicine, Sahlgrenska Academy, Institute of Medicine, University of Gothenburg, Gothenburg, Sweden

Yi-Sheng Liu, Chia-Ying Lin, Ming-Tsung Chuang, Chia-Ying Lin, Yi-Shan Tsai, Chien-Kuo Wang and Ming-Ching Ou
Department of Diagnostic Radiology, National Cheng Kung University Hospital, College of Medicine, National Cheng Kung University, No. 138 Sheng Li Road, Tainan 704, Taiwan, Republic of China

Osamu Inatomi, Takayuki Imai, Takehide Fujimoto, Kenichiro Takahashi, Yoshihiro Yokota, Noriaki Yamashita, Hiroshi Hasegawa, Atsushi Nishida and Akira Andoh
Division of Gastroenterology, Department of Medicine, Shiga University of Medical Science, Seta Tsukinowa-cho, Otsu, Shiga 520-2192, Japan

Shigeki Bamba
Division of Clinical Nutrition, Department of Medicine, Shiga University of Medical Science, Otsu, Japan

Mitsushige Sugimoto
Division of Digestive Endoscopy, Shiga University of Medical Science Hospital, Otsu, Japan

Wolfgang Huber and Roland Schmid
II. Medizinische Klinik und Poliklinik, Klinikum rechts der Isar, Technische Universität München, Ismaninger Straße 22, D-81675 Munich, Germany

Benedikt Henschel
Klinik für Anaesthesiologie der Universität München, Campus Großhadern, Marchioninistraße, 15 81377 Munich, Germany

Ahmed Al-Chalabi
Jamaica Hospital Medical Center, 8900 Van Wyck Expy, Jamaica, NY 11418, USA

Naglaa F. A. Youssef and Amany Farag
Faculty of Nursing, Cairo University, Cairo 11562, Egypt

Mohamed El Kassas
Faculty of Medicine, Helwan University, Cairo, Egypt

Ashley Shepherd
Faculty of Health Sciences and Sport, University of Stirling, Stirling FK9 4LA, Scotland, UK

Raffaella Lissandrin, Giovanna Ferraioli, Laura Maiocchi and Carlo Filice
Ultrasound Unit, Department of Infectious Diseases, Fondazione IRCCS Policlinico San Matteo, University of Pavia, Viale Camillo Golgi 19, Pavia 27100, Italy

Corrado Regalbuto, Daniela Larizza and Valeria Calcaterra
Pediatric Unit, Department of the Mother and Child Health, Fondazione IRCCS Policlinico San Matteo, University of Pavia, Pavia, Italy

Marinella Guazzotti and Gloria Pelizzo
Pediatric Surgery Unit, Department of the Mother and Child Health, Fondazione IRCCS Policlinico San Matteo, University of Pavia, Pavia, Italy

Carmine Tinelli and Annalisa De Silvestri
Clinical Epidemiology and Biometric Unit, Fondazione IRCCS Policlinico San Matteo, Pavia, Italy

Sónia Bernardo, Sofia Carvalhana, Teresa Antunes, Paula Ferreira, Helena Cortez-Pinto and José Velosa
Departament of Gastroenterology and Hepatology, Hospital de Santa Maria, CHLN.Av. Prof. Egas Moniz, 1649-028 Lisbon, Portugal

Jie-wen Lei, Yan Chen and Jia Guo
Department of Ultrasound, Eastern Hepatobiliary Surgery Hospital (EHBH), Second Military Medical University, Shanghai, China

Xiao-yu Ji
People's Liberation Army Military Academy, Second Military Medical University, Shanghai, China

Jun-feng Hong
Department of Ultrasound, Eastern Hepatobiliary Surgery Hospital (EHBH), Second Military Medical University, Shanghai, China
Department of Ultrasound, FuZhou General Hospital (Dongfang Hospital), Xiamen University, Fuzhou, Fujian, China

Wan-bin Li
Department of Ultrasound, Shanghai First People's Hospital, Shanghai, China

Yan Pan
Department of Ultrasound, Yuhuangding Hospital, Yantai, Shandong, China

Norio Akuta, Yusuke Kawamura, Yasuji Arase, Satoshi Saitoh, Shunichiro Fujiyama, Hitomi Sezaki, Tetsuya Hosaka, Masahiro Kobayashi, Yoshiyuki Suzuki, Fumitaka Suzuki, Kenji Ikeda and Hiromitsu Kumada
Department of Hepatology, Toranomon Hospital and Okinaka Memorial Institute for Medical Research, 2-2-2 Toranomon, Minato-ku, Tokyo 105-0001, Japan

Mariko Kobayashi
Liver Research Laboratory, Toranomon Hospital, Tokyo, Japan

Anna Chiara Dall'Aglio, Francesca Dazzani, Arianna Lanzi, Sara Savini, Gaia Saini, Francesco Giuseppe Foschi and Giuseppe Francesco Stefanini
Department of Internal Medicine, Ospedale di Faenza, AUSL Romagna Faenza, Italy

Claudio Tiribelli and Giorgio Bedogni
Liver Research Center, Italian Liver Foundation, Basovizza, Trieste, Italy

Marco Domenicali and Mauro Bernardi
Department of Medical and Surgical Sciences, University of Bologna, Via Massarenti 9, 40138 Bologna, Italy

Fabio Conti
Department of Medical and Surgical Sciences, University of Bologna, Via Massarenti 9, 40138 Bologna, Italy
Research Center for the Study of Hepatitis, Department of Medical and Surgical Sciences, University of Bologna, Bologna, Italy

Pierluigi Giacomoni
Department of Internal Medicine, Ospedale di Lugo, AUSL Romagna, Locarno, Italy

Pietro Andreone
Research Center for the Study of Hepatitis, Department of Medical and Surgical Sciences, University of Bologna, Bologna, Italy

Amalia Gastaldelli
Institute of Clinical Physiology, National Research Council, Pisa, Italy

Andrea Casadei Gardini
Department of Medical Oncology, Istituto Scientifico Romagnolo per lo studio e la cura dei tumori (IRST) IRCCS, Meldola, Italy

Stefano Bellentani
Gastroenterology and Hepatology Service, Clinica Santa Chiara, Locarno, Switzerland

Xiaoqin Wang, Jian Hu and Nianyue Wang
Department of Clinical Laboratory, The First Affiliated Hospital of Xi'an Jiaotong University, 277 West Yanta Road, Xi'an 710061, People's Republic of China

Yongfeng Yang and Li Ma
Department of Clinical Laboratory and Liver Diseases, The Second Hospital of Nanjing, Affiliated to Medical School of Southeast University, Nanjing 210000, China

Ruilin Han and Cunling Yan
Department of Clinical Laboratory, Peking University First Hospital, Beijing 100000, China

Wei Zhang
Department of Mathematics & Statistics, University of Arkansas at Little Rock, Little Rock, AR 72204, USA

Yijie Zheng
Medical Scientific Affairs, Abbott Diagnostics Division, Abbott Laboratories, Shanghai 200032, China

Kelly L. Hayward
School of Medicine, The University of Queensland, Translational Research Institute, Brisbane, Australia
Pharmacy Department, Princess Alexandra Hospital, Brisbane, Australia

Patricia C. Valery
QIMR Berghofer Medical Research Institute, Brisbane, Australia

W. Neil Cottrell
School of Pharmacy, The University of Queensland, Brisbane, Australia

Katharine M. Irvine, Leigh U. Horsfall and Brittany J Ruffin
Centre for Liver Disease Research, The University of Queensland, Brisbane, Australia

Elizabeth E. Powell
Centre for Liver Disease Research, The University of Queensland, Brisbane, Australia
Department of Gastroenterology and Hepatology, Princess Alexandra Hospital, Woolloongabba 4102, Brisbane, Queensland, Australia

Caroline J. Tallis
Department of Gastroenterology and Hepatology, Princess Alexandra Hospital, Woolloongabba 4102, Brisbane, Queensland, Australia

Veronique S. Chachay
School of Human Movement and Nutrition Sciences, The University of Queensland, Brisbane, Australia

Jennifer H. Martin
School of Medicine and Public Health, The University of Newcastle, Newcastle, Australia

Chang Seok Bang, Hyo Sun Kim, Ki Tae Suk, Sung Eun Kim, Ji Won Park, Hyoung Su Kim, Myoung Kuk Jang, Sang Hoon Park, Myung Seok Lee, Choong Kee Park and Dong Joon Kim
Department of Internal Medicine, Hallym University College of Medicine, Chuncheon, Gangwon-do 24253, South Korea

Seung Ha Park
Department of Internal Medicine, Inje University Haeundae-Paik Hospital, Busan, South Korea

Zhi-Feng Zhang, Xiao-Sha Feng, He Chen, Zhi-Jun Duan, Li-Xia Wang and Dong Yang
Department of Gastroenterology, The First Affiliated Hospital of Dalian Medical University, 116000 Dalian, Liaoning Province, China

Pi-Xu Liu and Han Liu
Institute of Cancer Stem Cell, Dalian Medical University, 116000 Dalian, Liaoning Province, China

Qiu-Ping Zhang, Yan-Ling Jin and Zhi-Gang Sun
Department of Pathology, The First Affiliated Hospital of Dalian Medical University, 116000 Dalian, Liaoning Province, China

Cheng-Yuan Peng, Yang-Yuan Chen and Jung-Ta Kao
School of Medicine, China Medical University, Taichung, Taiwan
Division of Hepato-Gastroenterology, Department of Internal Medicine, China Medical University Hospital, No. 2, Yuh-Der Road, Taichung 404, Taiwan

Wang-De Hsiao, Po-Heng Chuang, Hsueh-Chou Lai, Ken-Sheng Cheng, Sheng-Hung Chen, Jen-Wei Chou, Cheng-Ju Yu, Chun-Lung Feng and Wen-Pang Su
Division of Hepato-Gastroenterology, Department of Internal Medicine, China Medical University Hospital, No. 2, Yuh-Der Road, Taichung 404, Taiwan

Index

www.ingramcontent.com/pod-product-compliance
Lightning Source LLC
Chambersburg PA
CBHW082025190326
41458CB00010B/3272